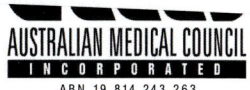

AUSTRALIAN MEDICAL COUNCIL
INCORPORATED
ABN 19 814 243 263

Anthology of Medical Conditions

- Integrated multidisciplinary index of clinical conditions and presentations
- Guidelines for clinical problem-solving
- Legal, ethical and organisational aspects of clinical medicine

EDITORIAL COMMITTEE

Vernon C Marshall

Kerry J Breen   Barry P McGrath
Peter G Devitt   Neil S Paget
Reuben D Glass   Roger J Pepperell
Frank P Hume   Alan T Rose
Michael R Kidd   Bryan W Yeo

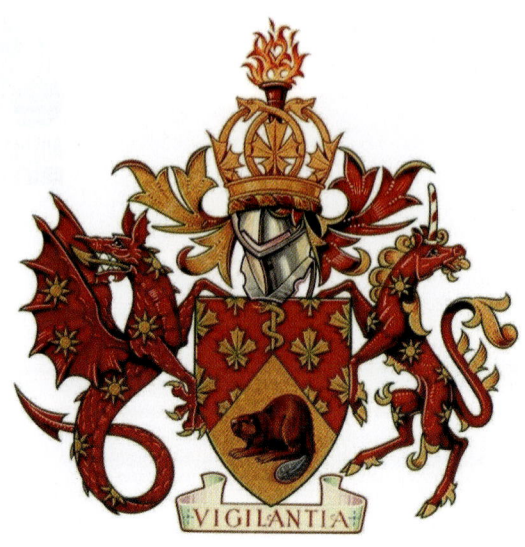

Published and distributed by the Australian Medical Council Limited
PO Box 4810
KINGSTON ACT 2604
AUSTRALIA
Phone: (02) 6270 9777
Facsimile: (02) 6270 9799
website: www.amc.org.au (order form available)

National Library of Australia Cataloguing-in-Publication entry.
Anthology of medical conditions.

Includes index.
ISBN 978-1-875440-28-3

1. Diseases - Textbooks. 2. Medicine - Textbooks. I.
Australian Medical Council.

616

Designed by Art Attack Pty Ltd, Brisbane
Printed by BPA Print Group, Melbourne

Table of Contents

Foreword

In 1997 the Australian Medical Council (AMC) published the book, *Annotated Multiple Choice Questions,* to assist overseas-trained doctors preparing for the AMC examinations. This current book represents the second in what the AMC intends to be a series of publications to familiarise overseas-trained doctors with the standards and principles of medical practice in Australia.

The *Anthology of Medical Conditions* publication aims to assist clinical problem-solving based on presenting clinical conditions. The AMC believes that this book will be a valuable clinical reference tool for medical students, AMC candidates and medical practitioners.

This book has been derived from the Canadian publication *Objectives for the Qualifying Examination* and has been adapted to reflect clinical conditions in the Australian community. The AMC wishes to acknowledge the generous support of the Medical Council of Canada (MCC) in the development of this project.

Lloyd A Toft

President of the Australian Medical Council
March 2003

Preface

This book has been prepared by a group of clinicians and educators who examine in both university undergraduate examinations for Australian medical students, and in the assessments, held by the Australian Medical Council, which assess the adequacy of knowledge and ability of overseas-trained doctors who wish to practise medicine in Australia.

The Australian Medical Council hopes that in providing this *Anthology of Medical Conditions*, overseas and local candidates will be helped in their preparation for assessment for registration within this country, whether it be for work in the metropolitan area, in large country towns or even in the 'outback' where medical facilities may be less than ideal and certain medical conditions more common. Clearly such preparation must be complemented by the use of recommended texts and medical journals; but the *Anthology of Medical Conditions*, Council believes, overviews appropriately the spectrum of medical knowledge and skills required of the graduating clinician in Australia.

Roger J Pepperell

Chairman of the Board of Examiners
Australian Medical Council
March 2003

Contributors

Editorial Committee

Vernon C Marshall
MBBS,FRACS,FACS
> Editor-in-Chief – Australian Medical Council
> Emeritus Professor of Surgery, Monash University
> Consultant Surgeon, Monash Medical Centre
> Senior Examiner in Surgery for the Australian Medical Council
> Former Chairman of the Board of Examiners, MCQ Panel of Examiners and
> Clinical Panel of Examiners of the Australian Medical Council

Kerry J Breen
MBBS,MD,FRACP
> Associate Professor of Medicine, University of Melbourne
> Gastroenterologist, St Vincent's Hospital Melbourne
> Past President, Medical Practitioners Board of Victoria
> Past President, Australian Medical Council
> Chairman, Australian Health Ethics Committee (NHMRC)

Peter G Devitt
MBBS,MS,FRACS
> Associate Professor of Surgery, University of Adelaide
> Senior Visiting Surgeon, Royal Adelaide Hospital
> Senior Examiner in Surgery for the Australian Medical Council
> Member – Board of Examiners, MCQ Panel of Examiners and Clinical Panel
> of Examiners of the Australian Medical Council

Reuben D Glass
MBBS,FRACP,DipEd
> Formerly Senior Lecturer in Paediatrics, Monash University
> Consultant Paediatrician, Monash Medical Centre
> Senior Examiner in Paediatrics for the Australian Medical Council
> Member – Board of Examiners, MCQ Panel of Examiners and Clinical Panel
> of Examiners of the Australian Medical Council

Frank P Hume
MBBS,FRACP,MRC Psych
> Clinical Lecturer, School of Psychiatry, University of New South Wales
> Senior Examiner in Psychiatry for the Australian Medical Council
> Member – Board of Examiners, MCQ Panel of Examiners and Clinical Panel
> of Examiners of the Australian Medical Council

Michael R Kidd
MBBS,MD,FRACGP,DipRACOG,DCCH
> President, Royal Australian College of General Practitioners
> Professor of General Practice, The University of Sydney
> Senior Examiner in General Practice for the Australian Medical Council
> Member – Board of Examiners, MCQ Panel of Examiners and Clinical Panel
> of Examiners of the Australian Medical Council

Additional Contributors

Heather Alexander
BSc,DipNutrDiet,MAppSc(Research),PhD
>Manager, Research and Policy Branch, Queensland Studies Authority
>Technical Advisor on Assessment for the Australian Medical Council
>Member – Clinical Panel of Examiners of the Australian Medical Council

Anthony J Buzzard
MBBS,FRCS,FRACS,FACS
>Senior Lecturer – Monash University Department of Surgery, Alfred Hospital, Melbourne
>Honorary Senior Fellow, Department of Anatomy & Cell Biology – Faculty of Medicine, Dentistry & Health Sciences, The University of Melbourne
>Senior Examiner in Surgery for the Australian Medical Council
>Member – MCQ Panel of Examiners and Clinical Panel of Examiners of the Australian Medical Council
>Chairman of Staff, The Avenue Hospital, Melbourne

Charles Bryan Campbell AM
MBBS,MD,FRACP,FRACMA
>Chief Health Officer, Queensland Health
>Professor of Medicine, University of Queensland
>Member, Medical Board of Queensland
>Member, National Health and Medical Research Council
>Former Head of the Graduate School of Medicine, University of Queensland

Chris W Cooper
MBBS,MRCGP,MPH,DTPH
>Lecturer, Department of General Practice, University of Sydney
>Visiting Medical Officer, Royal North Shore Hospital
>Visiting Medical Officer, Liverpool Hospital (Sexual Assault Unit)
>Senior Examiner in General Practice for the Australian Medical Council

Alan E Davis
MBBS,MD,MA(Oxon),BSc(Oxon),FRCP,FRACP
>Formerly Associate Professor in Medicine, University of New South Wales
>Formerly Consultant Physician and Head, Gastroenterology Department, Prince of Wales Hospital
>Senior Examiner in Medicine for the Australian Medical Council
>Member – MCQ Panel of Examiners and Clinical Panel of Examiners of the Australian Medical Council

Richard R Doherty
MBBS,DObstRCOG,FRACP
>Professor of Paediatrics, Monash University
>Consultant Paediatrician and Head, Paediatric Infectious Diseases, Monash Medical Centre
>Senior Examiner in Paediatrics for the Australian Medical Council
>Member – Board of Examiners, MCQ Panel of Examiners and Clinical Panel of Examiners of the Australian Medical Council

David Gillies
MBBS,MD,FRACP
Formerly Senior Lecturer in Medicine, University of New South Wales
Consultant Neurologist, Institute of Neurological Sciences, Prince of Wales
Hospital
Senior Examiner in Medicine for the Australian Medical Council
Member – MCQ Panel of Examiners of the Australian Medical Council

Phillipa J Hay
MBBS,MD,DPhil,FRANZCP
Senior Lecturer in Psychiatry, University of Adelaide
Senior Consultant Psychiatrist and Clinical Director, Community Mental
Health Services at the Royal Adelaide Hospital
Senior Examiner in Psychiatry for the Australian Medical Council
Member – MCQ Panel of Examiners of the Australian Medical Council

Reginald S A Lord
MBBS,MD,FRCS,FRACS
Professor of Surgery, University of New South Wales
Chair, Surgical Professorial Unit, St Vincent's Hospital, Sydney
Senior Examiner in Surgery for the Australian Medical Council
Member – Clinical Panel of Examiners of the Australian Medical Council

John E Murtagh AM
MBBS,MD,FRACGP,DipObsRCOG,BSc,BEd
Adjunct Professor of General Practice, Monash University
Professorial Fellow, Department of General Practice, The University of
Melbourne
Adjunct Professor, Graduate School Integrative Medicine, Swinburne
University
General Practitioner, East Bentleigh Murrumbeena Medical Group
Senior Examiner in General Practice for the Australian Medical Council
Member – Clinical Panel of Examiners of the Australian Medical Council

Diane B Neill
MBBS,FFPsych(SA),FRANZCP
Monash University Clinical Assistant (Teaching & Research), The Alfred
Hospital, Melbourne
Consultant Psychiatrist, Millswyn Clinic
Member – Committee for Examinations, Royal Australian and New Zealand
College of Psychiatrists
Senior Examiner in Psychiatry for the Australian Medical Council
Member – Clinical Panel of Examiners of the Australian Medical Council

Michael Oldmeadow
MBBS,FRACP
Senior Lecturer, Monash University Department of Medicine
Consultant Physician, Professorial General Medical Unit, The Alfred Hospital,
Melbourne
Senior Examiner in Medicine for the Australian Medical Council
Member – MCQ Panel of Examiners of the Australian Medical Council

Leon Piterman

MBBS,MMed,MEdSt,MRCP,FRACGP

Professor of General Practice, Monash University

Head of School of Primary Health Care and Deputy Dean, Faculty of Medicine, Nursing and Health Services, Monash University

Member of Panel of Examiners, Royal Australian College of General Practitioners

Senior Examiner in General Practice for the Australian Medical Council

Member – MCQ Panel of Examiners of the Australian Medical Council

Alexander (Sandy) L A Reid

MBBS,FRACGP

Emeritus Professor of General Practice, University of Newcastle, New South Wales

Professor and Director, University of New South Wales School of Rural Health

Censor, Royal Australian College of General Practitioners

Examiner Royal Australian College of General Practitioners

Senior Examiner in General Practice for the Australian Medical Council

Member – Clinical Panel of Examiners of the Australian Medical Council

Ross Sweet

MBBS,FRCOG,FRANZCOG,FACLM

Senior Clinical Lecturer in Obstetrics and Gynaecology, University of Adelaide

Medical Chief, Women's and Babies' Division, Women's and Children's Hospital, Adelaide, South Australia

Senior Examiner in Obstetrics and Gynaecology for the Australian Medical Council

Member – MCQ Panel of Examiners of the Australian Medical Council

Jane Vernon-Roberts

MBBS,MPH,GradDipPsychotherapy,FACPsychMed

Head of Clinical Studies, The University of Adelaide

Clinical Studies Advisor, The Royal Adelaide Hospital

Senior Visiting Medical Practitioner, Department of Endocrinology, The Royal Adelaide Hospital

Senior Examiner in General Practice for the Australian Medical Council

Member – Clinical Panel of Examiners of the Australian Medical Council

Poroor Vikraman

MBBS,FRACP

Tutor – Final Year Medical Students, Royal Melbourne Hospital

Tutor – Foreign Practitioners, Victorian Medical Postgraduate Foundation

Formerly Tutor – Final Year Medical Students, Western Hospital

Formerly Tutor – Final Year Medical Students, Monash University

Consultant Nephrologist and General Physician, Royal Melbourne Hospital

Senior Examiner in Medicine for the Australian Medical Council

Member – Clinical Panel of Examiners of the Australian Medical Council

Peter J Vine

MBBS,FRACP

Senior Lecturer and Campus Coordinator, University of New South Wales School of Rural Health

Senior Examiner in Paediatrics for the Australian Medical Council

Member – MCQ Panel of Examiners and Clinical Panel of Examiners of the Australian Medical Council

AMC Secretariat

Susan Buick
> Examinations Officer, Multiple Choice Questions (MCQ)
> Administrator of the Editorial Committee, Australian Medical Council

Ian Frank
> Executive Officer, Australian Medical Council

Acknowledgements

The editorial panel wishes to acknowledge the support of the additional contributing authors of the Board of Examiners and Multiple Choice Question (MCQ) and Clinical panels of examiners, and to the other academic and clinical staff of Australian medical schools who provided assistance, advice and contributions to this book. We are unaware of any of the additional material having prior copyright and apologise for any omission in this regard.

The help of the Medical Council of Canada in allowing use of their publications on assessment objectives is again acknowledged.

We are very grateful to Ian Frank for his contributions within the editorial panel, and to the staff of the Australian Medical Council (AMC) secretariat.

Cherie Hart deserves our special thanks for her painstaking and meticulous co-ordinating efforts in preparation and in transcribing this material through multiple revisions. Damien Krikowa was active in the initiating stages of the project.

We are grateful to Michael Oakey, Head, Medical Illustration Unit, University of New South Wales and to Bryan Yeo and the clinicians of the Prince of Wales Hospital for making available to us the MIDAS clinical illustration image bank; and to Peter Devitt and the clinicians of the Royal Adelaide Hospital for granting similar access to the MEDICI imaging bank.

Peter Jamison of Art Attack Pty Ltd, who has a long experience of collaboration with the Australian Medical Council in preparation of publications, has expertly formatted the text and visual material.

Finally, a very special note of thanks is due to Susan Buick, who has inspired, guided and co-ordinated the project with care and flair through all phases since its inception. Her tireless efforts in the roles of production co-ordinator and editorial panel member have ensured successful completion of the project.

Introduction

This *Anthology of Medical Conditions* lists common and important medical conditions encountered in clinical practice. Conditions are defined and classified to assist a problem-solving approach.

The Australian Medical Council, through accreditation of Australian university clinical programmes and assessments of overseas-trained doctors, monitors and evaluates the testing of cognitive abilities, clinical reasoning, communication and management skills and professional attitudes required of all clinicians entering medical practice in Australia, to maintain equivalent standards of registration for practice nationwide.

The medical conditions discussed have been developed from the Medical Council of Canada's publication, *Medical Council of Canada – Objectives for the Qualifying Examination*. They have been adapted and modified for Australian conditions by a multidisciplinary editorial review committee of the Board of Examiners of the Australian Medical Council. The educational foundations and procedures used by the Medical Council of Canada are described in detail as seven guiding principles in the 'Mandin, Dauphinée' article published in Academic Medicine 2000[1].

The Australian Medical Council wishes to express its gratitude to the Medical Council of Canada for allowing use of the assessment objectives publication for Canadian final year graduates, from which this present book derives. The Australian Medical Council and the Medical Council of Canada have initiated previous interchanges of examination material, beginning with multiple choice questions (MCQs). This present interchange of clinical assessment guidelines continues this cooperation, which has aided monitoring and validation of Australian Medical Council examination content at the appropriate level for Australian final year medical students and for their international equivalents.

Australia is a land similarly extensive in area to Canada, and ranges from temperate Southern Tasmania to tropical Northern Queensland; from large littoral capital cities (40% of the population live in Sydney and Melbourne, the two largest cities) to a central sparsely populated desert hinterland. Our population mix is a multicultural mosaic of different ethnicities and religions and includes indigenous native aboriginal Australians and migrants from a diverse spread of countries. More than one in five (23%) of the population were born overseas. The multiculturalism of the current Australian environment is reflected in the many overseas-trained doctors who, after passing their assessments, enter our community as medical practitioners, enriching the provision of healthcare in Australia. Modifications made to the original Canadian publication have taken account of the differences noted above and the differences in organisation of health services between the two countries.

Nonetheless, similarities of consensus best practice far outweigh any differences; and these illustrate strikingly the basic universality and internationality of competent clinical practice, facilitation of which is the major thrust of this book. The sets of objectives for basic medical education stated by the Australian Medical Council and the Medical Council of Canada confirm these similarities, and both are presented in full.

---

1 Mandin H, Dauphinée WD. Conceptual guidelines for developing and maintaining curriculum and examination objectives: the experience of the Medical Council of Canada. Acad Med 2000;75(10):1031-37.

Medical conditions do not define a medical curriculum; but patients present with conditions, clinical scenarios and related problems, rather than with identified diseases. The conditions discussed in this publication cover most domains of knowledge and clinical reasoning and management skills and professional attitudes evaluated by the Australian Medical Council assessments.

Each condition has been reviewed by a multidisciplinary editorial panel of experienced clinicians and educators and by additional contributing authors. The *Anthology of Medical Conditions* is designed to help students at final year undergraduate level in recognising, evaluating, and managing clinical problems.

Definition of the patient's principal presenting clinical condition and problem is a fundamental first step in diagnosis[2]. The **condition** may present as: a symptom presented by a patient (back pain, dysphagia, dyspnoea, dysmenorrhoea, pruritus, tinnitus), a physical sign (abdominal distension, goitre, hepatomegaly, jaundice, a swollen leg), a grouping of symptoms and signs to form a definable syndrome (shock, anaemia, child abuse, pregnancy, hyperthyroidism, renal failure), or as the result of a diagnostic test examination (screening mammogram, hypercalcaemia, abnormal liver function test). The condition may seem obviously focal (a lump or ulcer, nipple discharge) but the alert clinician must be aware of possible focal manifestations of a systemic problem.

Once the main clinical presenting condition or problem has been defined, its rationale should be considered by a critical overview focusing on the most likely key issues raised by the identified complaint. Experienced clinicians tend to do such screening automatically and semi-intuitively. This mature clinical approach is different from the all-embracing 'questionnaire' used by junior doctors and students. The mature approach seeks as rapidly as possible to gather appropriately focused data leading to a definitive diagnosis, and to discard unhelpful clinical 'noise', while maintaining sympathetic communication with the patient.

Identifying the most helpful and most valuable nuggets of diagnostic information can be difficult and is helped by accurate knowledge of the probable significance of the presenting condition: which aspects are important, and which are not. Thus, dysphagia is always likely to be a significant and major problem whereas backache is much less commonly so. Backache and headache are so common that infrequent but serious causes may be overlooked. A discrete breast lump is of far greater significance than nipple discharge or breast pain. Scrotal lumps are commonly of minor significance, particularly in the elderly, while acute scrotal pain in a child or youth is very likely to be a surgical emergency. Hypercalcaemia, even when of minor degree, will usually require investigation whereas hyponatraemia is a common, often transient finding in hospitalised patients and rarely of major import unless severe and persistent.

Graduating doctors need to develop an appreciation of the natural history and prognosis of individual clinical conditions and their causative diseases and an ability to come expeditiously to the pith of the problem in order to formulate appropriate diagnostic and management plans. This book aims to help the imminent graduate to develop and hone these clinical reasoning skills. The book provides guidelines to a problem-solving focused approach to individual conditions, which is both comprehensive but geared in its perspective to the most common and important causes.

---

2   Hunt P, Marshall VC. Clinical problems in general surgery. Sydney: Butterworth-Heinemann Medical; 1991.

The *clinical conditions* presented in this book are grouped alphabetically and for each, four problem-solving steps are outlined as follows.

1. Overview

This briefly sets the scene, providing an appropriate rationale and perspective for approaching the problem. Critical clinical cues may be highlighted and will suggest which facets of the problem are most important for the competent clinician to consider.

2. Causes

Whilst being comprehensive, this section aims to provide a *manageable* list of diseases which are the most likely diagnostic probabilities for the problem. Where these are numerous, the presenting problem appears in systematised, logical sub-categories. This approach is utilised where the complete list of important causes is such that it would be cumbersome and unhelpful if the list was to be considered in isolation.

For example, the problem of *abdominal pain* is sub-classified into acute versus chronic and further into right upper quadrant, left upper quadrant, epigastric pain and so on. Similarly, *bleeding from the gastrointestinal tract* will appear as different clinical syndromes such as acute upper gastrointestinal bleeding (haematemesis and/or melaena), acute lower gastrointestinal bleeding (acute colonic haemorrhage), intermittent fresh blood loss with defaecation (bleeding of anorectal origin – 'bleeding PR') and occult blood loss (presenting as iron deficiency anaemia). The common causes will then be listed under each subcategory, such as peptic ulcer, colonic diverticula, haemorrhoids and caecal cancer, in this last example.

3. Key Objectives

This section highlights the key issues to be addressed in solving the particular problem and presents one or two of the most important determinants of a successful outcome being achieved.

4. General and Specific Objectives

General objectives mostly relate to data collection through *history*, *examination* and *relevant investigation*. These are followed by objectives which relate more to the *specific* presentation and encompass the formulation of appropriate *diagnostic* and *management* plans. These objectives will include self-learning exercises directed, in particular, to formulating pathways in diagnosis and management using sequential or stepwise decision trees and algorithms.

General objectives enable gathering of subjective and objective information relating to the presenting problem in an expeditious, focused, efficient and empathetic manner. Choosing investigations with careful discrimination is an important part of this process.

5. Illustrations

Captioned illustrations have been added to complement and highlight the text; and to provide a background of clinical and investigative visual examples over a broad range of clinical conditions. The illustrations aim to exemplify the diversity of clinical medicine; they are not designed to comprise a comprehensive medical atlas, or to indicate priorities of diagnosis or investigation.

In practice, it is important to remain aware that algorithmic protocols and pathways are primarily to facilitate optimum and efficient individual diagnostic and management plans and are not a substitute for the broader requirements of holistic patient management and care. Furthermore, at each branch in the pathway, consideration must be given to whether available diagnostic tests in relation to a particular patient's problems, will significantly alter the management plan. The tendency for those lacking clinical judgement and for ultracautious junior doctors is to accumulate unnecessary clinical data through prolonged questioning and excessive investigation. Best use of available protocols will help avoid such an approach, which is of necessity, wasteful of time and of other valuable resources. For example, a previously fit patient with clinically apparent *acute appendicitis* needs early appendicectomy, **not** additional (but unnecessary) tests of full blood examination (FBE) and differential leucocyte count, abdominal X-rays, ultrasound or computed tomography (CT) scanning.

Readers are encouraged in using this book to consider individual problems and to attempt first to categorise their approach to the condition (under the headings listed above) prior to consulting the text.

Decision trees and algorithms are particularly useful in formalising clinical practice among groups of doctors working together in clinical departments and have the potential to provide fail-safe protocols for short segments of management. An example of this is shown in the Life Support Protocol (Figure 1) which provides a flowchart for use in hospital emergency departments.

Candidates preparing for assessments are thus encouraged to use the book to facilitate individual self-education, as a guide and *vade mecum* in formulating general management plans for each condition listed and as a base for more detailed study of history-taking and physical examination techniques as well as individual diseases, found in other texts such as those cited in the List of References for Further Study.

Legal, Ethical and Organisational Aspects of Medical Practice (LEO)

Legal, ethical and organisational aspects of medical practice were considered in a supplementary booklet by the Medical Council of Canada (*CLEO – Consideration of the Legal, Ethical and Organisational Aspects of Medical Practice*). These topics have been incorporated also in the current Australian Medical Council *Anthology of Medical Conditions*. Legal, ethical and organisational aspects have been presented as an individual block, rather than being interleaved alphabetically with the clinical presenting conditions.

Medicine is an ethical profession. The ethics of medicine range across all aspects of practice and involve ideals and traditions, morals, and social and cultural mores. They link the humanitarian and holistic aspects of practice (the 'art' of medicine) with its scientific basis. Ethical issues and attitudes evolve over time, as does medical science. Ethics are influenced by the cultural traditions of the society in which medicine is practised. By their nature, ethics tend to involve broad and controversial topics concerning problems of life, death and the intervening period; and to engender intense public debate and discussion while being codified into guidelines for practice or codes of consensus best practice. Thus, aspects of methods of diminishing or increasing fertility, abortion, euthanasia, consent to treatment and withdrawal of treatment, protection of the rights of minors, and doctor-patient relationships have been the subject of discussion and debate since the beginnings of medicine.

It behoves all doctors to be familiar with the laws of the society in which they practise medicine. The law, with its emphasis on due process and precedent, often lags behind evolving ethical issues, particularly when new treatments are being introduced. LEO summarises the legal aspects of local and Federal laws relevant to medicine in Australia.

Organisational aspects of Australian medicine at national, state and territory level are also summarised; these outline the details of university clinical schools, the functions and administration of the Australian Medical Council, and details of state and territory medical boards responsible for registration of medical practitioners, and of the specialist colleges.

These three components of LEO, as with the other *Anthology of Medical Conditions* sections, have been modified from the Canadian booklet to conform with Australian practice. We are again grateful to the Medical Council of Canada for allowing us to build upon their framework and experience.

Cautionary statement: As with other Australian Medical Council publications, these guidelines are a work in progress based on the best currently available evidence and clinical advice and will regularly be reviewed and modified.

Vernon C Marshall

Editor-in-Chief of the Australian Medical Council
March 2003

Life Support Protocol Flow Chart

On finding a collapsed patient

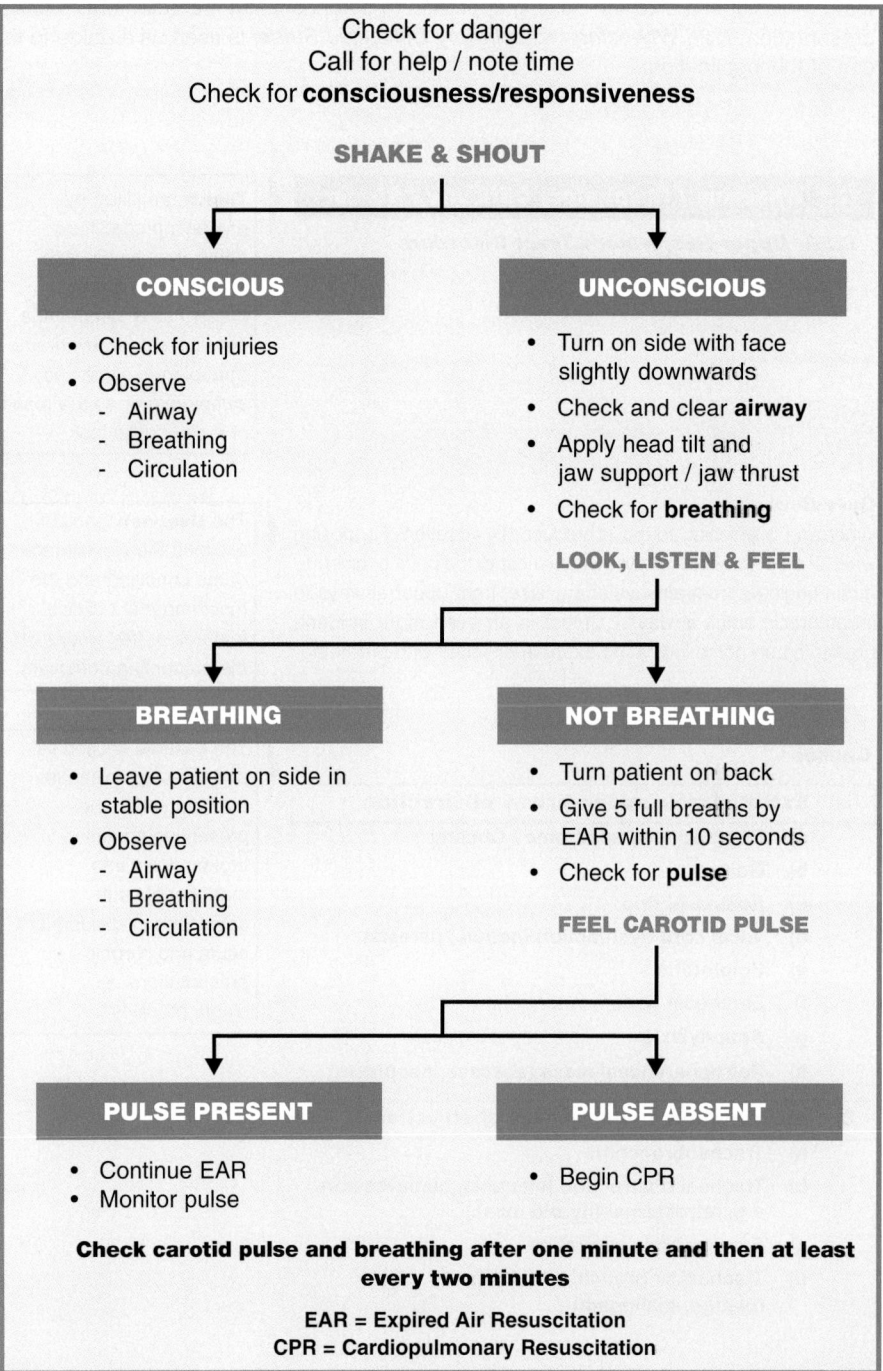

Check for danger
Call for help / note time
Check for **consciousness/responsiveness**

SHAKE & SHOUT

CONSCIOUS

- Check for injuries
- Observe
  - Airway
  - Breathing
  - Circulation

UNCONSCIOUS

- Turn on side with face slightly downwards
- Check and clear **airway**
- Apply head tilt and jaw support / jaw thrust
- Check for **breathing**

LOOK, LISTEN & FEEL

BREATHING

- Leave patient on side in stable position
- Observe
  - Airway
  - Breathing
  - Circulation

NOT BREATHING

- Turn patient on back
- Give 5 full breaths by EAR within 10 seconds
- Check for **pulse**

FEEL CAROTID PULSE

PULSE PRESENT

- Continue EAR
- Monitor pulse

PULSE ABSENT

- Begin CPR

Check carotid pulse and breathing after one minute and then at least every two minutes

EAR = Expired Air Resuscitation
CPR = Cardiopulmonary Resuscitation

Figure 1

How To Use the *Anthology of Medical Conditions*

The *Anthology of Medical Conditions* lists presenting clinical conditions and classifies them to assist in a problem-solving approach to diagnosis and management. Clinical presentation *#126 Wheezing / Respiratory Difficulty / Stridor* is used as a guide to the use of this publication.

126 Wheezing / Respiratory Difficulty / Stridor

126A Upper Respiratory Tract Disorders

> **Topics** are listed by presenting conditions rather than by disease. The conditions may present as a symptom, a physical sign, a syndrome (grouping of signs and symptoms) or as the result of a diagnostic test.

Overview

Wheezing, a whistling sound, is produced by vibration of opposing walls of an airway that is narrowed almost to the point of closure. It can originate from airways of any size, from upper airways to intrathoracic small airways. Stridor is an even more strident, urgent, harsh noise indicating extreme difficulty with breathing.

> The **Overview** section explains the significance of the condition and the most important clinical features or key issues of the presenting complaint.

Causes

1) Extrathoracic upper airway obstruction

a) Sleep-apnoea syndrome / Obesity

b) Goitre

c) Postnasal drip

d) Vocal cord dysfunction (nodule, paresis)

e) Epiglottitis

f) Laryngeal oedema/stenosis

g) Anaphylaxis

h) Retropharyngeal mass (abscess, neoplasm)

2) Intrathoracic upper airway obstruction

a) Tracheobronchitis

b) Tracheal obstruction (stenosis, compression e.g. retrosternal thyroid mass)

c) Foreign body aspiration

d) Tracheal or bronchial tumours (benign, malignant)

> The **Causes** section lists and classifies diseases that can cause the presenting condition broken down into manageable sub-categories or divided into acute and chronic presentations as diagnostic aids.

Key Objectives

- Determine whether the wheezing is associated with chronic dyspnoea and cough, because this triad is highly suggestive of asthma.

- Appreciate that asthma is **not** the sole or most common cause of wheezing; identify extrathoracic/intrathoracic upper airway obstruction (e.g. from thyroid).

The **Key Objectives** section explains the *key issues* to be addressed in solving the problem or managing the condition.

General/Specific Objectives

- Through efficient, focused, data gathering:

  - Determine whether the wheezing is polyphonic, since if so it is more likely to originate from more central airways.

  - Determine if wheezing is maximum in inspiration or expiration, and whether accompanied by stridor.

  - Determine the most likely site of obstruction, whether large or small intrathoracic airway or extrathoracic airway.

  - From history and clinical examination, determine the most likely cause and the urgency of management.

- Interpret critical clinical and laboratory findings which are key in the processes of exclusion, differentiation, and diagnosis:

  - List indications for diagnostic imaging.

  - Select pulmonary function studies as one means to differentiate between causes once diagnostic possibilities have been narrowed by clinical means.

- Conduct an effective plan of management for a patient with upper respiratory tract disorders:

  - Outline the use of bronchodilator therapy for diagnostic purposes.

  - Select patients in need of specialised care.

The **General/Specific Objectives** section summarises the steps in the effective diagnosis and management of the condition and suggests self-learning exercises.

Retrosternal goitre extension causing stridor

Captioned illustrations complement the text.

List of References for Further Study

Textbooks

There are many medical textbooks available and most of them are of high standard. They range from quite short texts, which cover essential knowledge, to long and comprehensive treatises which most people use as reference books. The Australian Medical Council has drawn up the following list, as a guide to some useful texts. The list includes larger reference works as well as shorter books written as undergraduate texts in disciplines of general practice, internal medicine, obstetrics and gynaecology, paediatrics, psychiatry and surgery, plus some integrated texts. **They are intended for guidance only and not as prescribed reading.**

American Psychiatric Association. Diagnostic and statistical manual of mental disorders: DSM-IV-TR. 4th edn, text revision. Washington, DC: American Psychiatric Association; 2000. ISBN 0890420246 (hardcover); ISBN 0890420254 (softcover).
http://www.psych.org

Beischer NA, Mackay EV. Obstetrics and the newborn: an illustrated text. 3rd edn. Sydney: WB Saunders; 1998. ISBN 0702021237.
http://www.us.elsevierhealth.com

Bloch S, Singh BS, editors. Foundations of clinical psychiatry. 2nd edn. Carlton South, Vic: Melbourne University Press; 2001. ISBN 0522849245.
http://www.mup.com.au

Braunwald E, Fauci A, Kasper D, Hauser S, Longo D, Jameson J. Harrison's principles of internal medicine. 15th edn. New York: McGraw-Hill; 2001. ISBN 0070072744 (hardcover); ISBN 0071374795 (CD-ROM)
http://www.bookstore.mcgraw-hill.com

Breen KJ, Pleuckhan VD, Cordner SM. Ethics, law and medical practice. Sydney: Allen & Unwin; 1997. ISBN 1864484071.
http://www.allen-unwin.com.au

Burkitt HG, Quick CRG. Essential surgery: problems, diagnosis and management. 3rd edn. London: Churchill Livingstone Inc; 2001. ISBN 0443063753.
http://www.us.elsevierhealth.com

Devitt PG, Barker JN, Mitchell J, Hamilton-Craig C. Clinical problems in general medicine and surgery. 2nd edn. Edinburgh: Churchill Livingstone; 2003.
http://www.elsevierhealth.com

Gelder MG, Lopez-Ibor JJ, Andreasen N. New Oxford textbook of psychiatry. New York: Oxford University Press; 2000. ISBN 0192629700
http://mnemosyne.oup-usa.org/medical

Haslett C, Chilvers ER, Boon NA, Colledge N, Hunter JA, editors. Davidson's principles and practice of medicine. 19th edn. Edinburgh: Churchill Livingstone; 2003. ISBN 0443070350.
http://www.us.elsevierhealth.com

Healey PM, Jacobson EJ. Common medical diagnoses: an algorithmic approach. 3rd edn. WB Saunders; 2000. ISBN 0721677320.
http://www.us.elsevierhealth.com

Hull D, Johnston D. Essential paediatrics. 4th edn. Edinburgh: Churchill Livingstone; 1999. ISBN 0443059586.
http://www.us.elsevierhealth.com

Lau L. Imaging guidelines. 4th edn. Melbourne: The Royal Australian and New Zealand College of Radiologists; 2001. ISBN 0959285415.
http://www.ranzcr.edu.au

Llewellyn-Jones D. Fundamentals of obstetrics and gynaecology. 7th edn. London: Mosby; 1999. ISBN 0723431507.
http://www.mosby.com

Mackay EV, Beischer NA, Pepperell R, Wood C. Illustrated textbook of gynaecology. 2nd edn. Sydney: WB Saunders; 1992. ISBN 0729512118.
http://www.us.elsevierhealth.com

Morris PJ, Wood WE. Oxford textbook of surgery. 2nd edn. New York: Oxford University Press; 2001. ISBN 0192628844 (three volume set).
http://mnemosyne.oup-usa.org/medical

Murtagh J. General practice. 2nd edn. Sydney: McGraw Hill Australia; 1999. ISBN 0074707191 (softcover); ISBN 0074704362 (hardcover 1998).
http://www.bookstore.mcgraw-hill.com

Robinson MJ, Roberton DM. Practical paediatrics. 5th edn. Melbourne: Churchill Livingstone; 2002. ISBN 044307139X.
http://www.us.elsevierhealth.com

Royal Children's Hospital (Melbourne, Vic.). Paediatric handbook. 6th edn. Carlton South, Vic: Blackwell Science Asia; 2000. ISBN 086793011X.
http://www.blacksci.co.uk/australi/books.htm

Talley NJ, O'Connor S. Clinical examination: a systematic guide to physical diagnosis. 4th edn. Sydney: MacLennan & Petty; 2001. ISBN 0864331444.
http://www.maclennanpetty.com.au

Tjandra JJ, Clunie GJA, Thomas RSJ, editors. Textbook of surgery. 2nd edn. Melbourne: Blackwell Science Asia; 2001. ISBN 0867930233.
http://www.blacksci.co.uk/australi/books.htm

Weatherall DJ, Ledingham JGG, Warrell DA, editors. Oxford textbook of medicine. 3rd edn. Oxford: Oxford University Press; 1996. ISBN 0192621408 (set of 3); ISBN 0192684299 (Version 1.0 on CD-ROM).
http://mnemosyne.oup-usa.org/medical

Williamson R, Waxman BP. Scott: an aid to clinical surgery. 6th edn. Edinburgh: Churchill Livingstone; 1998. ISBN 044305603X.
http://www.us.elsevierhealth.com

Miscellaneous
Therapeutic Guidelines from Therapeutic Guidelines Limited, North Melbourne, Vic.
http://www.tg.com.au

Therapeutic Guidelines: Analgesic Version 4, 2002

Therapeutic Guidelines: Antibiotic Version 12, 2003

Therapeutic Guidelines: Cardiovascular Version 3, 1999

Therapeutic Guidelines: Dermatology Version 1, 1999

Therapeutic Guidelines: Endocrinology Version 2, 2001

Therapeutic Guidelines: Gastrointestinal Version 3, 2002

Therapeutic Guidelines: Neurology Version 2, 2002

Therapeutic Guidelines: Palliative Care Version 1, 2001

Therapeutic Guidelines: Psychotropic Version 4, 2000

Therapeutic Guidelines: Respiratory Version 2, 2000

Note: Available in print individually or as a complete set in the form of an electronic subscription ('eTG complete').

Manual of use and interpretation of pathology tests. 3rd edn. Sydney: The Royal College of Pathologists of Australasia; 2002. ISBN 0646409646. This edition is available on CD-ROM or online only.
http://www.rcpa.edu.au

MIMS Australia. St Leonards, NSW: MediMedia Australia Pty Limited. Subscriptions: ISSN 10355723 (MIMS Bi-monthly), ISSN 0725-4709 MIMS Annual, ABNRID 000012656851 (eMIMS – CD-ROM or MIMS on PDA (Personal digital assistant)).
http://www.mims.com.au

Australian medicines handbook. 4th edn. Adelaide: Australian Medicines Handbook Pty Ltd; 2003. ISBN 0957852126. Online version via Health Communication Network.
http://www.hcn.com/au/products/kro_druginfo.html

National Health and Medical Research Council (NHMRC). The Australian immunisation handbook. 7th edn. Canberra: Australian Government Publishing Service; 2000. ISBN 0644475781.
http://www.health.gov.au/pubhlth/immunise/publications.htm

Journals
In addition to the major texts, journals should be read selectively, using editorials, annotations and review articles. The following journals are suggested as source material: *Australian Family Physician* (http://www.racgp.org.au/publications), *Australian Prescriber* (http://www.australianprescriber.com), *British Medical Journal* (http://www.bmj.com), *Hospital Medicine* (http://www.hospitalmedicine.co.uk), *Current Therapeutics* (http://www.ctonline.com.au), *Lancet* (http://www.thelancet.com), *Medical Journal of Australia* (http://www.mja.com.au), *New England Journal of Medicine* (http://content.nejm.org).

AMC *Annotated Multiple Choice Questions*
The Australian Medical Council (AMC) has prepared a selection of over 600 multiple choice questions (MCQs) from its MCQ Question Bank with commentaries and explanations on each question. These questions have been used in previous AMC examinations and will provide candidates with a comprehensive guide to the scope and standard of the AMC MCQ examination. This book is essential reading for those intending to sit the AMC examination. The book *Annotated Multiple Choice Questions* may be purchased from: Blackwell Science Asia Pty Ltd, 550 Swanston Street, CARLTON VIC 3053, AUSTRALIA, (http://www.blackwell-science.com).

OBJECTIVES OF THE AUSTRALIAN MEDICAL COUNCIL

The Australian Medical Council (AMC) established a set of objectives for basic medical education to guide and assist students in the learning and assessment of appropriate competencies. These are grouped in three areas for convenience, although it is recognised that the management of patients always requires combinations of attributes from each of these three domains. The three areas are: Knowledge and Understanding; Skills; and Attitudes as they affect Professional Behaviour.

Attributes of Medical Graduates

The goal of medical education is to develop junior doctors who possess attributes that will ensure they are initially competent to practise safely and effectively as interns in Australia or New Zealand, and that they have an appropriate foundation for further training in any branch of medicine and for lifelong learning. Attributes should be developed to an appropriate level for the graduates' stage of training.

Included below is the list of knowledge and understanding, skills and attitudes required of graduates completing basic medical education that is included in the AMC's *Assessment and Accreditation of Medical Schools: Standards and Procedures*.

Knowledge and Understanding

Graduates completing basic medical education should have knowledge and understanding of:

1   Scientific method relevant to biological, behavioural and social sciences at a level adequate to provide a rational basis for present medical practice, and to acquire and incorporate the advances in knowledge that will occur over their working life.

2   The normal structure, function and development of the human body and mind at all stages of life, the factors that may disturb these, and the interactions between body and mind.

3   The aetiology, pathology, symptoms and signs, natural history, and prognosis of common mental and physical ailments in children, adolescents, adults and the aged. A more detailed knowledge is required of those conditions that require urgent assessment and treatment.

4   Common diagnostic procedures, their uses and limitations.

5   Management of common conditions including pharmacological, physical, nutritional and psychological therapies.

6   Normal pregnancy and childbirth, the more common obstetrical emergencies, the principles of antenatal and postnatal care, and medical aspects of family planning.

7   The principles of health education, disease prevention and screening.

8   The principles of amelioration of suffering and disability, rehabilitation, and the care of the dying.

9   Factors affecting human relationships, the psychological well-being of patients and their families, and the interactions between humans and their social and physical environment.

10 Systems of provision of health care including their advantages and limitations, the principles of efficient and equitable allocation and use of finite resources.

11 The principles of ethics related to health care and the legal responsibilities of the medical profession.

Skills
Graduates completing basic medical education should have developed the following skills:

12 The ability to take a tactful, accurate, organised and problem-focused medical history.

13 The ability to perform an accurate physical and mental state examination.

14 The ability to choose from the repertoire of clinical skills, those that are appropriate and practical to apply in a given situation.

15 The ability to interpret and integrate the history and physical examination findings to arrive at an appropriate diagnosis or differential diagnosis.

16 The ability to select the most appropriate and cost-effective diagnostic procedures.

17 The ability to interpret common diagnostic procedures.

18 The ability to formulate a management plan, and to plan management in concert with the patient.

19 The ability to communicate clearly, considerately and sensitively with patients and their families, doctors, nurses, other health professionals and the general public.

20 The ability to counsel patients sensitively and effectively, and to provide information in a manner that ensures patients and families can be fully informed when consenting to any procedure.

21 The ability to recognise serious illness and to perform common emergency and life-saving procedures such as caring for the unconscious patient and cardiopulmonary resuscitation.

22 The ability to interpret medical evidence in a critical and scientific manner, and to use libraries and other information resources to pursue independent inquiry relating to medical problems.

23 The ability to use information technology appropriately as an essential resource for modern medical practice.

Attitudes as they affect professional behaviour
At the end of basic medical education, students should demonstrate the following professional attitudes that are fundamental to medical practice:

24 Recognition that the doctor's primary professional responsibilities are the health interests of the patient and the community.

25 Recognition that the doctor should have the necessary professional support, including a primary care physician, to ensure his or her own well-being.

26 Respect for every human being, including respect of sexual boundaries.

27 Respect for community values, including an appreciation of the diversity of human background and cultural values.

28 A commitment to ease pain and suffering.

29 A realisation that it is not always in the interests of patients or their families to do everything that is technically possible to make a precise diagnosis or to attempt to modify the course of an illness.

30 An appreciation of the complexity of ethical issues related to human life and death, including the allocation of scarce resources.

31 An appreciation of the need to recognise when a clinical problem exceeds their capacity to deal with it safely and efficiently and of the need to refer the patient for help from others when this occurs.

32 An appreciation of the responsibility to maintain standards of medical practice at the highest possible level throughout a professional career.

33 An appreciation of the responsibility to contribute towards the generation of knowledge and the professional education of junior colleagues.

34 An appreciation of the systems approach to health care safety, and the need to adopt and practise health care that maximises patient safety.

35 An awareness of the need to communicate with patients and their families, and to involve them fully in planning management.

36 A desire to achieve the optimal patient care for the least cost, with an awareness of the need for cost-effectiveness to allow maximum benefit from the available resources.

37 A willingness to work effectively in a team with other health care professionals.

OBJECTIVES OF THE MEDICAL COUNCIL OF CANADA

The definition and grouping of objectives by the Medical Council of Canada has been guided by the seven principles underpinning the development of their *Objectives for the Qualifying Examination* (1999) as outlined in the article by 'Mandin and Dauphinée' (2000). It was also informed by the definition of roles identified through the CANMeds 2000 project of the Royal College of Physicians and Surgeons of Canada. These roles were employed to characterise the future needs for training medical specialists: as medical expert; as communicator; as collaborator; as learner; as gatekeeper; as advocate; and professional. The Canadian objectives are grouped under these areas: Rationale; Objectives; Communication Skills; History; Physical Examination; Investigations; Clinical Judgement and Decision-making, Management Skills; Health Promotion and Maintenance; Critical Appraisal/Medical Economics; Law and Ethics.

Rationale

An appropriate history-taking and physical examination are essential for the candidate's identification of the clinical presentation, derivation of possible diagnoses, and rational plans for investigation and management. Frequently however, the unique social, cultural and behavioural characteristics of the patient may make it difficult to obtain the clinical data. Despite these potential obstacles, the candidate must be able to implement timely and appropriate plans for investigation and management based on the information obtained.

Objectives

Faced by a patient with a clinical problem, candidates will:

- Obtain pertinent information about the patient.

- Perform an appropriate physical examination.

- Order relevant investigations.

- Arrive at a reasonable diagnosis(es).

- Formulate management plans for short and long term care.

Communication Skills

Competent candidates will communicate effectively with patients, families, and other relevant persons by:

- Demonstrating a compassionate interest, respect, and understanding of the patient as an individual, while maintaining a professional relationship.

- Listening and interpreting information.

- Eliciting the concerns of the patient using non-directive (open-ended) and directive (closed-ended) questions, paraphrasing and summarising when appropriate.

- Evaluating information gained from nonverbal communication.

- Describing the effect of their own affective response on the doctor/patient relationship.

- Demonstrating nonjudgemental behaviour.

- Outlining the socio-cultural and individual influences that affect the doctor/patient relationship, such as:

    - sex role and gender identity of both the physician and patient

    - socio-cultural and religious differences

    - lifestyle

- Demonstrating ways of dealing effectively with difficult situations (e.g. excessively talkative and rambling, reticent, excessively quiet, crying, hostile and/or angry patients).

- Demonstrating ways of dealing effectively with the mentally and physically disabled patient.

- Eliciting and interpreting the anxieties related to embarrassment, fear of disease and confidentiality.

- Discussing sensitive issues such as sexual dysfunction, family dysfunction (including marital dysfunction), homicidal and suicidal risks.

- Discussing the emotional effects of physiological events.

- Demonstrating emotional and social support to gain confidence and cooperation.

- Evaluating the interaction between members of a family where appropriate.

- Discussing information at the appropriate intellectual level for all ages and conditions.

History
Competent candidates will:

- Elicit and interpret pertinent events from the patient, family or other sources.

- Demonstrate the ability to modify their history according to the severity and urgency of the problem at hand.

- Demonstrate the ability to record and/or summarise information in a timely manner.

- Provide a clear definition of the patient's problems upon which to base further investigation, diagnosis and ongoing management.

Physical examination
Competent candidates will:

- Perform a physical examination appropriate to the age of the patient and nature of the clinical problem(s) presented.

- Elicit and interpret information through continuous observation.

- Demonstrate the ability to record and/or summarise information in a timely manner.

- Provide a clear definition of the patient's problems upon which to base further investigation, diagnosis and ongoing management.

Investigations
Competent candidates will:

- Select and interpret appropriate laboratory and other diagnostic procedures that confirm the diagnosis; exclude other important diagnoses or determine the degree of dysfunction.

- Discuss the limitations and contraindications of common investigations.

- Determine the reliability and predictive value of common investigations.

- State the effect of demographic considerations on the sensitivity and specificity of diagnostic tests.

- Demonstrate ways to deal effectively with unexpected findings, ill-defined results or normal variance not indicative of disease.

- Outline the physiological, biochemical and pathological principles of common investigations.

- Perform common procedures using the appropriate instruments and materials.

- Describe any discomfort, harm or inconvenience to the patient associated with the investigations they have selected.

Clinical judgement and decision-making

Competent candidates will:

- Differentiate between important and spurious information.

- Interpret pertinent data in order to:

    - list and prioritise a differential diagnosis for common clinical problems

    - diagnose specific common diseases

    - diagnose more rare, but life-threatening diseases

- Differentiate among acute emergency situations, acute exacerbations of chronic illnesses and serious but nonemergency situations.

- List the indications for specialised care and/or consultation.

- Discuss pertinent information with other members of the healthcare team including consultants.

- Evaluate critically, their own professional competencies and determine their personal learning needs.

Management skills

Competent candidates will:

- Outline the initial management for both common and more rare but life-threatening conditions.

- Determine the importance of time and place in determining appropriate management.

- Evaluate the response to therapy and other management.

- State the pharmacologic effects, the clinical application including indications, contraindications, major side-effects and interactions of commonly used drugs.

- Discuss the diagnosis, treatment plan and prognosis with the patient, family and other concerned individuals, where appropriate.

- Outline the contribution and expertise of other healthcare professionals and community agencies.

- Select the appropriate multidisciplinary teams for the optimal care of patients.

- Select psychological methods of treatment where appropriate.

Health promotion and maintenance

Competent candidates will:

- Formulate preventive measures into their management strategies.

- Communicate with the patient, the patient's family and concerned others with regard to risk factors and their modification where appropriate.

- Describe programmes for the promotion of health including screening for, and the prevention of, illness.

- Describe the concept of illness behaviour and its influence on healthcare.

Critical appraisal / Medical economics
Competent candidates will:

- Evaluate medical evidence in both clinical and academic situations.

- Evaluate scientific literature in order to critically assess the benefits and risks of current and proposed methods of investigation, treatment and prevention of illness.

- Demonstrate the use of the computer for appropriate data retrieval and function.

- Define the socio-economic rationales, implications and consequences of medical care.

- Outline the principles of cost containment, cost-benefit analysis and cost-effectiveness.

Law and ethics
Competent candidates will:

- Discuss the principles of law, biomedical ethics and other social aspects related to common practice situations.

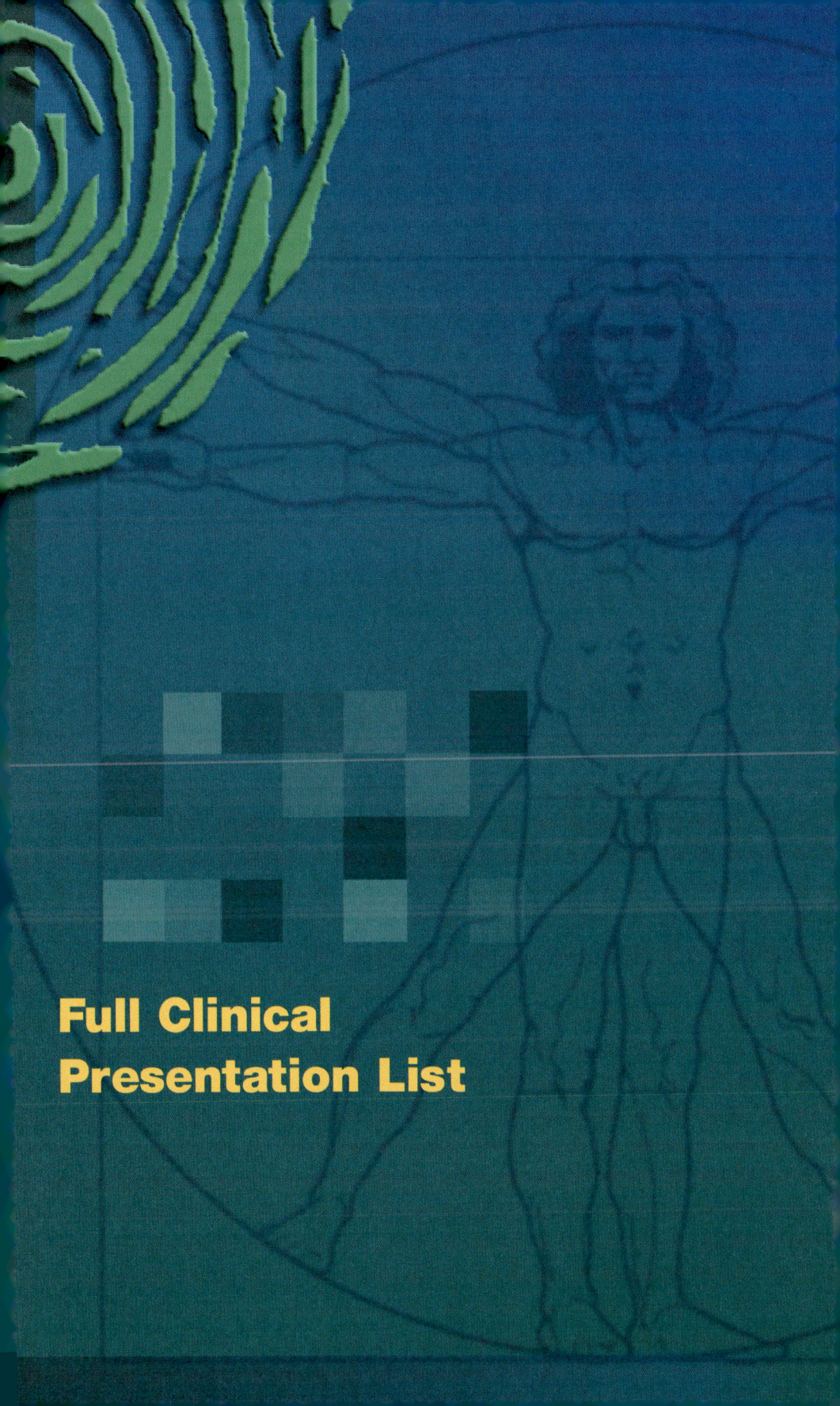

Full Clinical
Presentation List

Definition

A clinical condition, presentation or problem represents a common or important way in which a patient, group of patients, community or population presents to a medical practitioner. Graduating medical students and trainees would be expected to show appropriate clinical competence in dealing with each of the conditions listed, over a further period of clinical practice and supervised training in hospitals and at other sites, prior to full medical registration.

The clinical conditions have been listed numerically, in alphabetical sequence, in colour emboldened main headings. Conditions covering a wide field have additional emboldened subdivisions. Synonyms for entries included under other headings through the text are also ordered alphabetically, but are not assigned a number nor emboldened, and are in lower case.

001 Abdominal Distension/Ileus (Ascites, Bowel Obstruction) *{Med/Surg/Primary}*

Abdominal hernia – see #002G Abdominal Hernia under Abdominal Mass

Abdominal injuries – see #113A Abdominal Injuries under Trauma/Accidents/Prevention

002 Abdominal Mass *{Med/Surg/Primary/Paed}*

002A Epigastric Mass
002B Right Hypochondrial Mass
002C Left Hypochondrial Mass
002D Right Iliac Fossa Mass
002E Suprapubic/Pelvic Mass
002F Left Iliac Fossa Mass
002G Abdominal Hernia
002H Adrenal Mass

003 Abdominal Pain *{Med/Surg/Primary/Paed}*

003A Abdominal Pain in Adults
003B Non-acute/Recurrent Abdominal Pain in Infancy and Early Childhood
003C Chronic Recurrent Abdominal Pain
003D Heartburn/Dyspepsia
003E Anal Pain
003F Acute Abdominal Pain in Children

Abnormal ECG / Arrhythmia – see #072 Palpitations (Abnormal Electrocardiogram (ECG) / Arrhythmia)

004 Abnormal Serum Calcium/Phosphate
{Med/Surg/Paed}

004A **Hypercalcaemia**
004B **Hypocalcaemia**
004C **Hypophosphataemia / Fanconi Syndrome**

005 Abnormal Serum Hydrogen Ion Concentration
{Med/Surg}

005A **Metabolic Acidosis**
005B **Metabolic Alkalosis**
005C **Respiratory (Gaseous) Acidosis**
005D **Respiratory Alkalosis**
005E **Mixed Acid-base Disturbances**

006 Abnormal Serum Lipids {Med}

Abnormal stature – see #110 Tall Stature / Short Stature / Abnormal Stature

007 Abnormal Liver Function Tests {Med/Surg}

008 Abnormal Serum Potassium Concentration / Magnesium {Med/Surg}

008A **Hypokalaemia**
008B **Hyperkalaemia**
008C **Hypomagnesaemia**

009 Abnormal Serum Sodium Concentration
{Med/Surg/Paed}

009A **Hyponatraemia**
009B **Hypernatraemia**

010 Abnormalities of White Blood Cells {Med/Paed}

011 Acutely Ill Infant/Child {Paed}

011A **Paediatric Emergencies**
011B **Crying/Fussing Child**
011C **Hypotonia / Floppy Infant**

Accidents – see #113 Trauma/Accidents/Prevention

Acute abdominal pain in children – see #003F Acute Abdominal Pain in Children under Abdominal Pain

Acute brain syndrome – see #022 Confusion/Delirium / Acute Brain Syndrome

Acute, children – see #003F Acute Abdominal Pain in Children under Abdominal Pain

Acute diarrhoea – see #027A Acute Diarrhoea under Diarrhoea/Constipation

Acute life-threatening event (ALTE) – see #099 Sudden Infant Death Syndrome (SIDS) (Acute Life-Threatening Event (ALTE))

Acute lower gastrointestinal bleeding – see #016 Bleeding with Defaecation / Acute Lower Gastrointestinal Bleeding / Melaena / Occult Blood in Stool / Prevention of Cancer

Acute renal failure (ARF) – see #090 Renal Failure, Acute (Anuria/Oliguria / Acute Renal Failure (ARF))

Addiction – see #107 Substance Abuse/Addiction

Adrenal mass – see #002H Adrenal Mass under Abdominal Mass

Adult constipation – see #027E Adult Constipation under Diarrhoea/ Constipation

Aggression and mental illness – see #119 Violence/Aggression and Mental Illness

Allergic Reactions (see #127 Allergic Reactions) *{Med/Paed}*

Allergic rhinitis – see #092 Rhinorrhoea / Sore Throat and #127 Allergic Reactions

Amblyopia – see #106 Strabismus and/or Amblyopia

Amenorrhoea – see #063A Amenorrhoea under Menstrual Cycle Abnormal and #064 Menopause

Anal pain – see #003E Anal Pain under Abdominal Pain

Anaphylaxis – see #098A Anaphylaxis under Shock / Hypotension

Anasarca – see #034 Oedema

012   Anaemia and Pallor *{Med}*

Angina – see #092 Rhinorrhoea / Sore Throat and #102B Childhood Communicable Diseases with or without Skin Rash under Skin Rash / Dermatitis

Angina pectoris – see #020 Chest Discomfort

Angio-oedema – see #102B Childhood Communicable Diseases with or without Skin Rash under Skin Rash / Dermatitis

Anorexia – see #125 Weight Loss / Eating Disorders / Anorexia / Nutritional Disorders and #014 under Behaviour Disorder

Antepartum care – see #081A Antepartum Care under Pregnancy

Anuria/Oliguria / Acute renal failure (ARF) – see #090 Renal Failure, Acute (Anuria/Oliguria / Acute Renal Failure (ARF))

Anxiety – see #073 Panic and Anxiety and #013 Attention Deficit / Learning Disability

Apnoea – see #023A Cyanosis / Hypoxia / Apnoea in Children under Cyanosis/ Hypoxaemia / Hypoxia, #056 Insomnia / Sleep and Circadian Rhythm Disorders / Sleep-Apnoea Syndrome and #099 Sudden Infant Death Syndrome (SIDS) (Acute Life-Threatening Event (ALTE))

Aphasia – see #050 Hemiplegia / Hemisensory Loss / Stroke with or without Aphasia / Prevention of Stroke and #103 Speech and Language Abnormalities / Dysphonia / Hoarseness

Arrhythmias – see #072 Palpitations (Abnormal Electrocardiogram (ECG) / Arrhythmia)

Arthritis – see #059 Joint Pain, Mono-Articular (Acute, Chronic) and #060 Joint Pain, Poly-Articular (Acute, Chronic)

Ascites – see #001 Abdominal Distension/Ileus (Ascites, Bowel Obstruction) and see #034 Oedema

Asthma – see #126 Wheezing / Respiratory Difficulty / Stridor

Ataxia – see #042 Gait Disturbances – Ataxia and #057 Involuntary Movement Disorders / Tic Disorders

Atopy – see #127 Allergic Reactions

013 Attention Deficit / Learning Disability
{Med/Paed/Psych}

Back pain – see #089B Low Back Pain and 089C Neck Pain under Regional Pain

014 Behaviour Disorder (see also #026 Development Disorder / Developmental Delay) {Med/Paed/Psych}

Bipolar disorders – see #065 Mood Disorders

Bites, Stings and Envenomations (see #128 Bites, Stings and Envenomations) {Med/Surg/Primary}

015 Bleeding Tendency / Bruising {Med/Surg/Paed}

Blindness – see #120A Visual Disturbance/Loss and #106 Strabismus and/or Amblyopia

016 Bleeding with Defaecation / Acute Lower Gastrointestinal Bleeding / Melaena / Occult Blood in Stool / Prevention of Cancer (see #027 Diarrhoea/Constipation) {Med/Surg/Paed/Surg}

Boils – see #101 Skin Blisters – Boils – Comedones – Ulcers

Bone/Joint injury – see #041 under Fractures / Dislocations

Bowel obstruction – see #001 Abdominal Distension/Ileus (Ascites, Bowel Obstruction)

Brain death – see #045 Head Injuries / Brain Death / Transplant Donation

017 Breast Disorders {Med/Surg/Surg/Obs-Gyn}

017A **Male (Gynaecomastia)**
017B **Female (Breast Lump / Prevention of Cancer / Screening)**
017C **Nipple Discharge / Galactorrhoea**
017D **Breast Pain (Mastalgia)**
017E **Breast – Skin Changes**

Breathing difficulty – see #032 under Dyspnoea and/or Cough / Prevention of Cancers and Chronic Respiratory Diseases

Bruising – see #015 Bleeding Tendency / Bruising

Bruit – see #111 Tinnitus/Bruit

018 Burns *{Paed/Primary/Surg}*

Cancer pain – see #089K Cancer Pain under Regional Pain

019 Cardiac Arrest / Respiratory Arrest
{Med/Surg/Primary/Paed/Obs-Gyn}

Cervicitis – see #118 Vaginal Discharge / Urinary Symptoms, Vulvar Lesions, Sexually Transmitted Diseases (STDs)

020 Chest Discomfort *{Med/Primary}*

Chest injuries – see #113D Chest Injuries under Trauma/Accidents/Prevention

Child abuse – see #119A Child Abuse under Violence/Aggression and Mental Illness

Childhood communicable diseases – see #102B Childhood Communicable Diseases with or without Skin Rash under Skin Rash / Dermatitis

Chills – see #040 under Fever and Chills (Adult and Paediatric)

Chronic diarrhoea – see #027B Chronic Diarrhoea under Diarrhoea/Constipation

Chronic leg ulcer – see #101A Chronic Leg Ulcer under Skin Blisters – Boils – Comedones – Ulcers

Chronic musculo fascial pain – see #089A Chronic Musculo Fascial Pain under Regional Pain

Chronic recurrent abdominal pain – see #003C Chronic Recurrent Abdominal Pain under Abdominal Pain

Chronic respiratory diseases – see #032 Dyspnoea and/or Cough / Prevention of Cancers and Chronic Respiratory Diseases

Circadian rhythm disorders – see #056 Insomnia / Sleep and Circadian Rhythm Disorders / Sleep-Apnoea Syndrome

Cold injuries – see #040D Hypothermia under Fever and Chills (Adult and Paediatric)

Colic (infantile) – see #003F Acute Abdominal Pain in Children under Abdominal Pain

021 Coma / Impaired Consciousness *{Med/Surg/Psych}*

Comedones – see #101 Skin Blisters – Boils – Comedones – Ulcers

Communicable diseases (childhood) – see #102B Childhood Communicable Diseases with or without Skin Rash under Skin Rash / Dermatitis

Congenital malformations – see 129A Congenital Malformations under Deformities/Malformations

Congestive heart failure – see #032 under Dyspnoea and/or Cough / Prevention of Cancers and Chronic Respiratory Diseases

022 Confusion/Delirium / Acute Brain Syndrome
{Med/Surg/Psych}

Constipation – see #027 Diarrhoea/Constipation, #027C Constipation/ Encopresis, Paediatric and #027E Adult Constipation under Diarrhoea/ Constipation

Contraception – see #082 Contraception / Pregnancy Prevention/Termination

Convulsions – see #095 Seizures (Epilepsy)

Cough – see #032F Cough under Dyspnoea and/or Cough / Prevention of Cancers and Chronic Respiratory Diseases

Crying/Fussing child – see #011B Crying/Fussing Child under Acutely Ill Infant/ Child

023 Cyanosis/Hypoxaemia / Hypoxia *{Med/Paed}*

023A Cyanosis / Hypoxia / Apnoea in Children
Deafness – see #047 Hearing Loss / Deafness

Deformities – see #060 Joint Pain, Poly-Articular (Acute, Chronic)

Deformities, hand – see #129B Hand Deformities under Deformities/ Malformations

Deformities/Malformations (See #129 Deformities/Malformations) *{Paed/ Med/Surg/Primary}*

Delirium – see #022 Confusion/Delirium / Acute Brain Syndrome

Dehydration – see #027D Diarrhoea, Paediatric under Diarrhoea/Constipation and #009B Hypernatraemia under Abnormal Serum Sodium Concentration

024 Dementia / Memory Disturbances *{Med/Psych}*

025 Newborn in Poor Condition / Depressed Breathing
{Paed/Obs-Gyn}

Depressed mood / Depression – see #065 Mood Disorders

Dermatitis and/or fever – see #102 Skin Rash / Dermatitis

026 Development Disorder / Developmental Delay
(see also #014 Behaviour Disorder) *{Paed/Psych}*

Diabetes mellitus – see #053 Hyperglycaemia / Diabetes Mellitus and #114B Urinary Frequency: Associated with 'Polyuria/Polydipsia' under Urinary Frequency

027 Diarrhoea/Constipation *{Med/Primary/Paed/Psych/Surg}*

027A Acute Diarrhoea
027B Chronic Diarrhoea

027C **Constipation/Encopresis, Paediatric**
027D **Diarrhoea, Paediatric**
027E **Adult Constipation**

Diastolic murmur – see #067B Diastolic Murmur under Murmur / Extra Heart Sounds

Difficulty swallowing – see #031 Dysphagia

028 Diplopia (Double Vision) *{Med/Surg/Primary}*

Dislocations – see #041 Fractures / Dislocations

Disordered thought – see #087 Psychosis / Disordered Thought

029 Dizziness/Vertigo *{Med/Surg/Primary}*

Double vision – see #028 Diplopia (Double Vision)

Drug addiction – see #107A Substance Abuse / Drug Addiction/Withdrawal under Substance Abuse/Addiction

030 Dying Patient *{Med/Surg/Primary/Paed/Psych/Obs-Gyn}*

Dysmenorrhoea – see #117 Vaginal Bleeding, Excessive in Amount or Irregular in Timing and #063B Pre-Menstrual Syndrome / Dysmenorrhoea under Menstrual Cycle Abnormal

Dysmorphic features – see #043 Genetic Concerns, Dysmorphic Features and #110 Tall Stature / Short Stature / Abnormal Stature

Dyspepsia – see #003D Heartburn/Dyspepsia under Abdominal Pain and see #032 under Dyspnoea and/or Cough / Prevention of Cancers and Chronic Respiratory Diseases

031 Dysphagia *{Med/Surg/Primary}*

Dysphonia – see #103 under Speech and Language Abnormalities / Dysphonia / Hoarseness

032 Dyspnoea and/or Cough / Prevention of Cancers and Chronic Respiratory Diseases
{Med/Primary/Paed/Surg}

032A **With Diffuse Chest X-Ray Abnormality**
032B **With Pleural Chest X-Ray Abnormality**
032C **With Fever**
032D **With Local Chest X-Ray Abnormality**
032E **With Normal Chest X-Ray**
032F **Cough**
032G **Dyspnoea / Respiratory Distress, Paediatric**

Dysuria – see #114A Urinary Frequency: Associated with 'Dysuria and/or Pyuria / Urethral Discharge under Urinary Frequency'

033 Ear Pain *{Primary/Paed/Med/Surg}*

Eating disorders – see #125 Weight Loss / Eating Disorders / Anorexia / Nutritional Disorders, #124 Weight Gain / Obesity and #077 Periodic Health Examination / Growth and Development

034 Oedema *{Med}*

034A Generalised Oedema
034B Unilateral Limb Oedema (Swollen Limb)

Elderly abuse – see #119B Elder Abuse under Violence/Aggression and Mental Illness

Elevated haemoglobin – see #080 Polycythaemia / Elevated Haemoglobin

Elevated mood – see #065 under Mood Disorders

Emergencies, life-threatening – see #131A Life-Threatening Emergencies under Medical Emergencies

Emergencies, medical – see #131 Medical Emergencies

Emotional abuse – see #119A Child Abuse, #119B Elder Abuse and #119C Violence: Domestic/Family under Violence/Aggression and Mental Illness and #070A Somatic Complaints / Somatoform Disorders under Pain

Encopresis – see #027C Constipation/Encopresis, Paediatric under Diarrhoea/Constipation

Enuresis – see #115A Urinary Incontinence, Paediatric Enuresis under Urinary Incontinence / Enuresis

Envenomations – see #128 Bites, Stings and Envenomations

Environment – see #077H Environment under Periodic Health Examination / Growth and Development

Epigastric mass – see #002A Epigastric Mass under Abdominal Mass

Epigastric pain – see #003 Abdominal Pain and #003D Heartburn/Dyspepsia under Abdominal Pain and #054B Pregnancy-Associated Hypertension under Hypertension

Epilepsy – see #095 Seizures

Extra heart sounds – see #067 Murmur / Extra Heart Sounds

Eye injuries – see #035 Eye Redness, #120 Visual Disturbance/Loss and #113F Eye Injuries

035 Eye Redness *{Primary/Med/Surg}*

Facial injuries – see #045 Head Injuries / Brain Death / Transplant Donation, #104 under Spinal injuries and #113G Facial Injuries

Facial pain – see #089D Facial Pain under Regional Pain

043 Genetic Concerns, Dysmorphic Features
{Med/Surg/Obs-Gyn/Paed/ Psych}

043A   Genetic Concerns, Screening

Glomerular haematuria – see #049 Haematuria

Goitre – see #068 Neck or Facial Mass / Goitre / Thyroid Disease

Growth and development – see #077 Periodic Health Examination / Growth and Development and #036A Infant/Child under Failure to Thrive

Gynaecomastia – see #017A Male (Gynaecomastia) under Breast Disorders

Haemorrhage – see #117 Vaginal Bleeding, Excessive in Amount or Irregular in Timing and #098 Shock / Hypotension

044 Hair and Nail Disorders {Med/Surg/Paed}

044A Hair Disorders
044B Nail Disorders

Hand deformities – see #129B Hand Deformities under Deformities/ Malformations

Hand/Wrist injuries – see #113H Hand/Wrist Injuries under Trauma/Accidents/ Prevention

Hand/Wrist/Elbow pain – see #089F Hand/Wrist/Elbow Pain under Regional Pain

045 Head Injuries / Brain Death / Transplant Donation
{Surg/Med/Paed}

046 Headache {Med/Primary}

Health examination – see #077 Periodic Health Examination / Growth and Development

Health of special populations – see #077F Health of Special Populations under Periodic Health Examination / Growth and Development

047 Hearing Loss / Deafness {Med/Surg}

Heartburn/Dyspepsia – see #003D Heartburn/Dyspepsia under Abdominal Pain

Heart failure – see #032 under Dyspnoea and/or Cough / Prevention of Cancers and Chronic Respiratory Diseases

Heart sounds, pathological – see #067C Heart Sounds, Pathological under Murmur / Extra Heart Sounds

048 Haematemesis/Melaena {Med/Surg}

049 Haematuria {Med/Surg}

050 Hemiplegia / Hemisensory Loss / Stroke with or without Aphasia / Prevention of Stroke {Med}

050A Paraplegia/Paraparesis

051 Haemoptysis {Med/Surg}

Hepatomegaly – see #002 Abdominal Mass

Hesitancy – see #116 Urinary Obstruction / Hesitancy / Prostatic Cancer / Screening

Hip pain – see #089G Hip Pain under Regional Pain

052 Hirsutism and Virilisation {Med}

History – see under General Objectives

Hoarseness – see #103 Speech and Language Abnormalities / Dysphonia / Hoarseness and #092 Rhinorrhoea / Sore Throat

Hypercalcaemia – see #004A Hypercalcaemia under Abnormal Serum Calcium/Phosphate

053 Hyperglycaemia / Diabetes Mellitus {Med/Primary/Paed}

053A Hypoglycaemia
Hyperkalaemia – see #008B Hyperkalaemia under Abnormal Serum Potassium Concentration / Magnesium

Hypernatraemia – see #009B Hypernatraemia under Abnormal Serum Sodium Concentration

Hyperthermia – see #040E Hyperthermia under Fever and Chills (Adult and Paediatric)

Hyperthyroidism – see #068 Neck or Facial Mass / Goitre / Thyroid Disease

054 Hypertension {Med/Primary/Obs-Gyn/Paed}

054A Hypertension in Childhood
054B Pregnancy-associated Hypertension
054C Hypertension in the Elderly
054D Malignant Hypertension
Hypocalcaemia – see #004B Hypocalcaemia under Abnormal Serum Calcium/Phosphate

Hypochondrial mass, left – see #002C Left Hypochondrial Mass under Abdominal Mass

Hypochondrial mass, right – see #002B Right Hypochondrial Mass under Abdominal Mass

Hypoglycaemia – see #053A Hypoglycaemia under Hypoglycaemia / Diabetes Mellitus

Hypokalaemia – see #008A Hypokalaemia under Abnormal Serum Potassium Concentration / Magnesium

Hypomagnesaemia – see #008C Hypomagnesaemia under Abnormal Serum Potassium Concentration / Magnesium

Hyponatraemia – see #009A Hyponatraemia under Abnormal Serum Sodium Concentration

Hypophosphataemia – see #004C Hypophosphataemia / Fanconi Syndrome under Abnormal Serum Calcium/Phosphate

Hypotension – see #098 Shock / Hypotension

Hypothermia / Cold intolerance – see #040D Hypothermia under Fever and Chills (Adult and Paediatric)

Hypothyroidism – see #068 Neck or Facial Mass / Goitre / Thyroid Disease

Hypotonia – see #011C Hypotonia / Floppy Infant under Acutely Ill Infant/Child

Hypoxaemia / Hypoxia – see #023 Cyanosis/Hypoxaemia / Hypoxia

Ileus – see #001 Abdominal Distension/Ileus (Ascites, Bowel Obstruction)

Iliac fossa mass, left – see #002F Left Iliac Fossa Mass under Abdominal Mass

Iliac fossa mass, right – see #002D Right Iliac Fossa Mass under Abdominal Mass

Infections, tropical – see #130 Travel Medicine and Tropical Infections

Intra-uterine growth aberration – see #123 Weight (Low) at Birth / Intra-uterine Growth Aberration

Impaired consciousness – see #021 Coma / Impaired Consciousness

Impotence – see #055 Infertility / Impotence / Sexual Dysfunction

Immunisation – see #077B Infant and Child Immunisation under Periodic Health Examination / Growth and Development

Incontinence – see #115 Urinary Incontinence / Enuresis

055 Infertility / Impotence / Sexual Dysfunction
{Med/Obs-Gyn/Surg}

056 Insomnia / Sleep and Circadian Rhythm Disorders / Sleep-apnoea Syndrome {Med/Psych/Primary}

Intra-uterine growth aberration – see #123 Weight (Low) at Birth / Intra-uterine Growth Aberration

Intrapartum/Postpartum care – see #081B Intrapartum/Postpartum Care under Pregnancy

057 Involuntary Movement Disorders / Tic Disorders
{Med/Psych}

Itching – see #086 Pruritus

058   Jaundice *{Med/Paed/Surg}*

058A   Neonatal Jaundice

Joint injuries – see #041 Fractures / Dislocations

059   Joint Pain, Mono-articular (Acute, Chronic) *{Med/Surg/Primary/Paed/Surg}*

060   Joint Pain, Poly-articular (Acute, Chronic) *{Med/Surg/Primary/Paed}*

Knee pain – see #089H Knee Pain under Regional Pain

Labour (normal, abnormal) – see #081B Intrapartum/Postpartum Care under Pregnancy

Language abnormalities – see #103 Speech and Language Abnormalities / Dysphonia / Hoarseness

Learning disorder, disability – see #013 Attention Deficit / Learning Disability

Leukaemia, leucocytosis – see #010 Abnormalities of White Blood Cells

Life-threatening emergencies – see #131A Life-Threatening Emergencies under Medical Emergencies

Limp – see #061 Limp / Pain in Lower Extremity in Children

Loss of consciousness – see #109 Syncope / Pre-Syncope / Loss of Consciousness

Low back pain – see #089B Low Back Pain under Regional Pain

Lower extremities – see #071B Pain in the Lower Extremities under Painful Limb

Lower respiratory tract disorders – see #126B Lower Respiratory Tract Disorders under Wheezing / Respiratory Difficulty / Stridor

061   Limp / Pain in Lower Extremity in Children *{Paed/Med/Surg}*

062   Lymphadenopathy *{Med/Surg/Paed}*

Magnesium – see #008 Abnormal Serum Potassium Concentration / Magnesium

Malformations, congenital – see #129A Congenital Malformations under Deformities/Malformations

Malformations/Deformities – see #129 Deformities/Malformations

Malignant hypertension – see #054D Malignant Hypertension

Medical Emergencies (See #131 Medical Emergencies) *{Paed/Med/Surg/Primary/Obs-Gyn/LEO/Psych}*

Medicine, travel – see #130 Travel Medicine and Tropical Infections

Melaena – see #016 Bleeding with Defaecation / Acute Lower Gastrointestinal Bleeding / Melaena / Occult Blood in Stool / Prevention of Cancer

Memory disturbances – see #024 Dementia / Memory Disturbances

063   Menstrual Cycle Abnormal {Obs-Gyn}

063A   Amenorrhoea (also Oligomenorrhoea)
063B   Pre-menstrual Syndrome / Dysmenorrhoea

064   Menopause {Obs-Gyn}

Metabolic acidosis/alkalosis – see #005A Metabolic Acidosis and #005B Metabolic Alkalosis under Abnormal Serum Hydrogen Ion Concentration

Mixed acid-base disturbances – see #005E Mixed Acid-Base Disturbances under Abnormal Serum Hydrogen Ion Concentration

065   Mood Disorders {Primary/Psych}

066   Mouth Problems {Med/Surg/Paed}

Movement disorders – see #057 Involuntary Movement Disorders / Tic Disorders

067   Murmur / Extra Heart Sounds {Med}

067A   Systolic Murmur
067B   Diastolic Murmur
067C   Heart Sounds, Pathological

Nail and hair complaints – see #044 Hair and Nail Disorders

Nausea – see #121 Vomiting, Nausea

068   Neck or Facial Mass / Goitre / Thyroid Disease {Med/Surg}

Neck pain – see #089C Neck Pain under Regional Pain

Neglect – see #119A Child Abuse under Violence/Aggression and Mental Illness

Neonatal jaundice – see #058A Neonatal Jaundice under Jaundice

Nerve injuries – see #113J Nerve Injuries under Trauma/Accidents/Prevention

Neuropathy – see #069 Numbness and Tingling

Newborn assessment/nutrition – see #077A Newborn Assessment/Nutrition under Periodic Health Examination / Growth and Development

Nipple discharge – see #017C Nipple Discharge / Galactorrhoea under Breast Disorders

Non-acute abdominal pain in infancy and early childhood – see #003B Non-Acute/Recurrent Abdominal Pain in Infancy and Early Childhood under Abdominal Pain

Non-reassuring fetal status – see #039 Fetal Distress / Non-Reassuring Fetal Status

069   Numbness and Tingling *{Med/Surg}*

Nutrition / Newborn assessment – see #077A Newborn Assessment/Nutrition under Periodic Health Examination / Growth and Development

Nutritional disorders and deficiencies – see #125B Nutritional Disorders and Deficiencies

Obesity – see #124 Weight Gain / Obesity

Obstetrical complications – see #081D Obstetrical Complications under Pregnancy

Occult blood in stool – see #016 Bleeding with Defaecation / Acute Lower Gastrointestinal Bleeding / Melaena / Occult Blood in Stool / Prevention of Cancer

Oedema – see #034 Oedema, #034A Generalised Oedema and #034B Unilateral Limb Oedema (Swollen Limb)

Oligomenorrhoea – see #063A Amenorrhoea (also Oligomenorrhoea) under Menstrual Cycle Abnormal

Oliguria – see #090 Renal Failure, Acute (Anuria/Oliguria / Acute Renal Failure (ARF))

Osteoporosis – see #077 Periodic Health Examination / Growth and Development and #089B Low Back Pain and #089C Neck Pain under Regional Pain

Paediatric emergencies – see #011A Paediatric Emergencies under Acutely Ill Infant/Child

070   Pain *{Med/Surg/Paed/Psych}*

070A   Somatic Complaints / Somatoform Disorders

071   Painful Limb *{Med/Surg/Primary}*

071A   Pain In The Upper Extremities
071B   Pain In The Lower Extremities – see also #061 Limp /
Pain   in Lower extremity in Children

071C   Painful Lower Limb – Varicose Veins

Pallor – see #012 Anaemia and Pallor

072   Palpitations (Abnormal Electrocardiogram (ECG) / Arrhythmia) *{Med}*

073   Panic and Anxiety *{Primary/Psych}*

074   Papanicolaou (Pap) Smear / Screening / Prevention *{Obs-Gyn}*

Paresis/Paralysis – see #122 Weakness/Paralysis/Paresis

Pathological/Problem gambling – #107B Pathological/Problem Gambling under Substance Abuse/Addiction

Pelvic inflammatory disease – see #076 Pelvic Pain, #118 Vaginal Discharge / Urinary Symptoms, Vulvar Lesions, Sexually Transmitted Diseases (STDs), #003 Abdominal Pain, and #040 Fever and Chills (Adult and Paediatric)

Pelvic/Suprapubic mass – see #002E Suprapubic/Pelvic Mass under Abdominal Mass

075 Pelvic Mass *{Obs-Gyn}*

076 Pelvic Pain *{Obs-Gyn/Paed}*

Pelvic relaxation – see #084 Prolapse / Pelvic Relaxation

Performance drugs – see #107A Substance Abuse / Drug Addition/Withdrawal under Substance Abuse/Addiction

077 Periodic Health Examination / Growth and Development *{Med/Primary/Paed/Surg}*

077A Newborn Assessment/Nutrition
077B Infant and Child Immunisation
077C Preoperative Assessment
077D Postoperative Patient Evaluation and Care
077E Work-related Health Issues
077F Health of Special Populations
077G Population
077H Environment

078 Personality Disorders *{Psych}*

Phosphate – see #004 Abnormal Serum Calcium/Phosphate

Physical abuse – see #119A Child Abuse under Violence/Aggression and Mental Illness and #070A Somatic Complaints / Somatoform Disorders under Pain

Physical examination – see #077 Periodic Health Examination / Growth and Development and see under General Objectives

Pleuritis – see #020 Chest Discomfort and #032B With Pleural Chest X-Ray Abnormality under Dyspnoea and/or Cough / Prevention of Cancers and Chronic Respiratory Diseases

079 Poisoning *{Med/Paed}*

080 Polycythaemia / Elevated Haemoglobin *{Med}*

Polyuria/Polydipsia – see #114B Urinary Frequency: Associated with 'Polyuria/ Polydipsia' under Urinary Frequency and see #053 Hyperglycaemia / Diabetes Mellitus

Population – see #077G Population under Periodic Health Examination / Growth and Development

Postoperative assessment – see #077D Postoperative Assessment under Periodic Health Examination / Growth and Development

Postpartum haemorrhage – see #081B Intrapartum/Postpartum Care under Pregnancy

Pre-menstrual syndrome – see #063B Pre-Menstrual Syndrome / Dysmenorrhoea under Menstrual Cycle Abnormal

Pre-syncope – see #109 Syncope / Pre-Syncope / Loss of Consciousness

081   Pregnancy *{Primary/Obs-Gyn}*

081A   Antepartum Care
081B   Intrapartum/Postpartum Care
081C   Haemorrhage (see #117 Vaginal Bleeding, Excessive in Amount or Irregular in Timing)
081D   Obstetrical Complications

082   Contraception / Pregnancy Prevention/Termination *{Primary/Obs-Gyn/Paed}*

Pregnancy-associated hypertension – see #054B Pregnancy-Associated Hypertension under Hypertension

083   Prematurity *{Paed}*

Prenatal – see #081A Antepartum Care under Pregnancy

Preoperative assessment – see #077C Preoperative Assessment under Periodic Health Examination / Growth and Development

Prevention of cancer – see #016 Bleeding with Defaecation / Acute Lower Gastrointestinal Bleeding / Melaena / Occult Blood in Stool / Prevention of Cancer

Prevention of cancer / screening – see #017B Female (Breast Lump / Prevention of Cancer / Screening)

084   Prolapse / Pelvic Relaxation (see also #115B Urinary Incontinence, Elderly under Urinary Incontinence / Enuresis) *{Obs-Gyn}*

Prostatic cancer – see #116 Urinary Obstruction / Hesitancy / Prostatic Cancer / Screening

085   Proteinuria *{Med}*

086   Pruritus *{Med}*

086A   Pruritus Ani

087   Psychosis / Disordered Thought *{Psych}*

Psychological abuse – see #119A Child Abuse under Violence/Aggression and Mental Illness

Pulmonary oedema – see #032A With Diffuse Chest X-Ray Abnormality under Dyspnoea and/or Cough / Prevention of Cancers and Chronic Respiratory Diseases

088   Pupil Abnormalities *{Med/Surg}*

Pyuria – see #114A Urinary Frequency: Associated with 'Dysuria and/or Pyuria / Urethral Discharge under Urinary Frequency'

Rape – see #119A Child Abuse, #119B Elder Abuse, #119C Violence: Domestic/Family and #119D Rape / Violence Against Women under Violence/ Aggression and Mental Illness

Rash – see #102 Skin Rash / Dermatitis

Recurrent fever – see #040B Fever in the Immune-Compromised Host / Recurrent Fever under Fever and Chills (Adult and Paediatric)

089   Regional Pain *{Surg/Med/Primary}*

089A   Chronic Musculo Fascial Pain
089B   Low Back Pain
089C   Neck Pain
089D   Facial Pain
089E   Shoulder Pain
089F   Hand/Wrist/Elbow Pain
089G   Hip Pain
089H   Knee Pain
089I   Foot and Ankle Pain
089J   Spinal Compression / Osteoporosis
089K   Cancer Pain

090   Renal Failure, Acute (Anuria/Oliguria / Acute Renal Failure (ARF)) *{Med/Surg/Paed}*

091   Renal Failure, Chronic *{Med/Surg/Paed}*

Respiratory acidosis/alkalosis – see #005C Respiratory Acidosis and #005D Respiratory Alkalosis under Abnormal Serum Hydrogen Ion Concentration

Respiratory arrest – see #019 Cardiac Arrest / Respiratory Arrest

Respiratory difficulty – see #126 Wheezing / Respiratory Difficulty / Stridor

092   Rhinorrhoea / Sore Throat *{Primary/Paed/Med/Surg}*

Screening – see #043A Genetic Concerns, Screening under Genetic Concerns, Dysmorphic Features and see under the Index for further presentations

School failure – see #013 Attention Deficit / Learning Disability

093   Scrotal Mass *{Primary/Surg/Paed}*

094   Scrotal Pain (Acute) *{Primary/Surg/Paed}*

095   Seizures (Epilepsy) *{Med/Paed}*

Self-inflicted – see #022 Confusion/Delirium / Acute Brain Syndrome

Sensory disturbance – see #069 Numbness and Tingling

Serum sickness – see #062 Lymphadenopathy

Sexual abuse – see #119A Child Abuse under Violence/Aggression and Mental Illness and see under the Index for further presentations

Sexual dysfunction – see #055 Infertility / Impotence / Sexual Dysfunction and #097 Sexual Concerns and Gender Identity Disorders

096 Sexual Maturation {Paed}
096A Sexual Maturation, Normal
096B Sexual Maturation, Abnormal

097 Sexual Concerns and Gender Identity Disorders {Psych/Paed}

Sexually transmitted diseases (STDs) – see #118 Vaginal Discharge / Urinary Symptoms, Vulvar Lesions, Sexually Transmitted Diseases (STDs)

098 Shock / Hypotension {Med/Paed/Surg/Obs-Gyn}
098A Anaphylaxis
Short stature – see #110 Tall Stature / Short Stature / Abnormal Stature

Shortness of Breath – see #032A With Diffuse Chest X-ray Abnormality under Dyspnoea and/or Cough / Prevention of Cancers and Chronic Respiratory Diseases

Shoulder pain – #089E Shoulder Pain under Regional Pain

Skin injuries – see #113K Skin Injuries under Trauma/Accidents/Prevention

Sleep and circadian rhythm disorders – see #056 Insomnia / Sleep and Circadian Rhythm Disorders / Sleep-Apnoea Syndrome

Sleep-apnoea syndrome – see #056 Insomnia / Sleep and Circadian Rhythm Disorders / Sleep-Apnoea Syndrome

Spinal compression / osteoporosis – see #089J Spinal Compression / Osteoporosis under Regional Pain

Stings – see #128 Bites, Stings and Envenomations

Stridor – see #126 Wheezing / Respiratory Difficult / Stridor

099 Sudden Infant Death Syndrome (SIDS) (Acute Life-Threatening Event (ALTE)) {Paed}

100 Skin and Subcutaneous Lesions {Surg/Primary/Med}
100A Focal Skin Lesions – Benign Lesions
100B Focal Skin Lesions – 'Suspicious Lesions'
100C Focal Subcutaneous Lumps
100D Red, Hot, Tender, Swollen Skin and Subcutaneous Layers

101   Skin Blisters – Boils – Comedones – Ulcers
{Paed/Primary}

101A   Chronic Leg Ulcer

102   Skin Rash / Dermatitis *{Med/Primary/Paed}*

102A   Skin Rash / Dermatitis and/or Fever, Urticaria/Angio-oedema

102B   Childhood Communicable Diseases with or without Skin Rash

Somatic complaints – see #070A Somatic Complains / Somatoform Disorders under Pain

Sore mouth – see #066 Mouth Problems and #036B Failure to Thrive in the Elderly under Failure to Thrive

Sore throat – see #092 Rhinorrhoea / Sore Throat and #102B Childhood Communicable Diseases with or without Skin Rash under Skin Rash / Dermatitis

103   Speech and Language Abnormalities / Dysphonia / Hoarseness *{Med/Paed/Psych/Surg/Primary}*

104   Spinal Injuries *{Surg/Med}*

105   Splenomegaly *{Med/Surg/Paed}*

Spouse abuse – see #119C Violence: Domestic/Family under Violence/ Aggression and Mental Illness

Steatorrhoea – see #004C Hypophosphataemia / Fanconi Syndrome under Abnormal Serum Calcium/Phosphate and #008C Hypomagnesaemia under Abnormal Serum Potassium Concentration / Magnesium

106   Strabismus and/or Amblyopia *{Paed/Med/Surg}*

Stroke – see #042 Gait Disturbances – Ataxia and see under the Index for further presentations

107   Substance Abuse/Addiction *{Psych/Med/Paed}*

107A   Substance Abuse / Drug Addiction/Withdrawal
107B   Pathological/Problem Gambling

108   Suicidal Behaviour/Prevention *{Psych/Paed}*

Suprapubic/Pelvic mass – see #002E Suprapubic/Pelvic Mass under Abdominal Mass

109   Syncope / Pre-syncope / Loss of Consciousness *{Med}*

Systolic murmur – see #067A Systolic Murmur under Murmur / Extra Heart Sounds

Tall stature – see #110 Tall Stature / Short Stature / Abnormal Stature

110   Tall Stature / Short Stature / Abnormal Stature
{Med/Paed}

Tendon injuries – see #113H Hand/Wrist Injuries under Trauma/Accidents/Prevention

Termination – see #082 Contraception / Pregnancy Prevention/Termination

Thyroid disease – see #068 Neck or Facial Mass / Goitre / Thyroid Disease and under associated signs and symptoms of hypo- and hyperfunction

Tic disorders – see #057 Involuntary Movement Disorders / Tic Disorders

Tingling and numbness – see #069 Numbness and Tingling and #042 Gait Disturbances – Ataxia

111   Tinnitus/Bruit *{Med}*

112   Torticollis (see also #057 Involuntary Movement Disorders / Tic Disorders) *{Paed}*

Transplant donation – see #045 Head Injuries / Brain Death / Transplant Donation

Travel Medicine and Tropical Infections (See #130 Travel Medicine and Tropical Infections) *{Primary/Med}*

113   Trauma/Accidents/Prevention *{Paed/Surg}*

113A	**Abdominal Injuries**
113B	**Bone and Joint Injuries** – see also #041 Fractures / Dislocations
113C	**Burn Injuries** – see #018 Burns
113D	**Chest Injuries**
113E	**Cold Injuries** – see #040D Hypothermia under Fever and Chills (Adult and Paediatric)
113F	**Eye Injuries** – see #035 Eye Redness and #120 Visual Disturbance/Loss
113G	**Facial Injuries** – see #045 Head Injuries / Brain Death / Transplant Donation and #104 Spinal Injuries
113H	**Hand/Wrist Injuries**
113I	**Head Injuries** – see #045 Head Injuries / Brain Death / Transplant Donation
113J	**Nerve Injuries**
113K	**Skin Injuries**
113L	**Spinal Injuries** – see #104 Spinal Injuries
113M	**Urinary Tract Injuries** – see #049 Haematuria
113N	**Vascular Injuries**

Tropical infections – see #130 Travel Medicine and Tropical Infections

Ulcers – see #101 Skin Blisters – Boils – Comedones – Ulcers

Unilateral limb oedema – see #034B Unilateral Limb Oedema (Swollen Limb) under Oedema

119 Violence/Aggression and Mental Illness
{Primary/Obs-Gyn/Paed/Psych}

119A Child Abuse
119B Elder Abuse
119C Violence: Domestic/Family
119D Rape / Violence Against Women (see #119C)
Virilisation – see #052 Hirsutism and Virilisation and #055 Infertility / Impotence / Sexual Dysfunction

120 Visual Disturbance/Loss *{Med/Surg}*

Volume loss/depletion – see #090 Renal Failure, Acute (Anuria/Oliguria / Acute Renal Failure (ARF))

121 Vomiting, Nausea *{Med/Paed/Surg/Obs-gyn}*

Vulvar lesions – see #118 under Vaginal Discharge / Urinary Symptoms, Vulvar Lesions, Sexually Transmitted Diseases (STDs)

122 Weakness/Paralysis/Paresis *{Med/Surg/Paed}*

123 Weight (Low) at Birth / Intra-uterine Growth Aberration *{Paed}*

124 Weight Gain / Obesity
{Med/Surg/Primary/Psych/Paed}

125 Weight Loss / Eating Disorders / Anorexia / Nutritional Disorders *{Med/Surg/Paed/Psych}*

125A Weight Loss / Eating Disorders / Anorexia
125B Nutritional Disorders and Deficiences

126 Wheezing / Respiratory Difficulty / Stridor
{Med/Paed}

126A Upper Respiratory Tract Disorders
126B Lower Respiratory Tract Disorders
Withdrawal – see #107 Substance Abuse/Addiction and see under the Index for further presentations

Work-related health issues – see #077E Work-Related Health Issues under Periodic Health Examination / Growth and Development

127 Allergic Reactions

128 Bites, Stings and Envenomations *{Med/Surg/Primary}*

129 Deformities/Malformations *{Paed/Med/Surg/Primary}*

129A Congenital Malformations
129B Hand Deformities

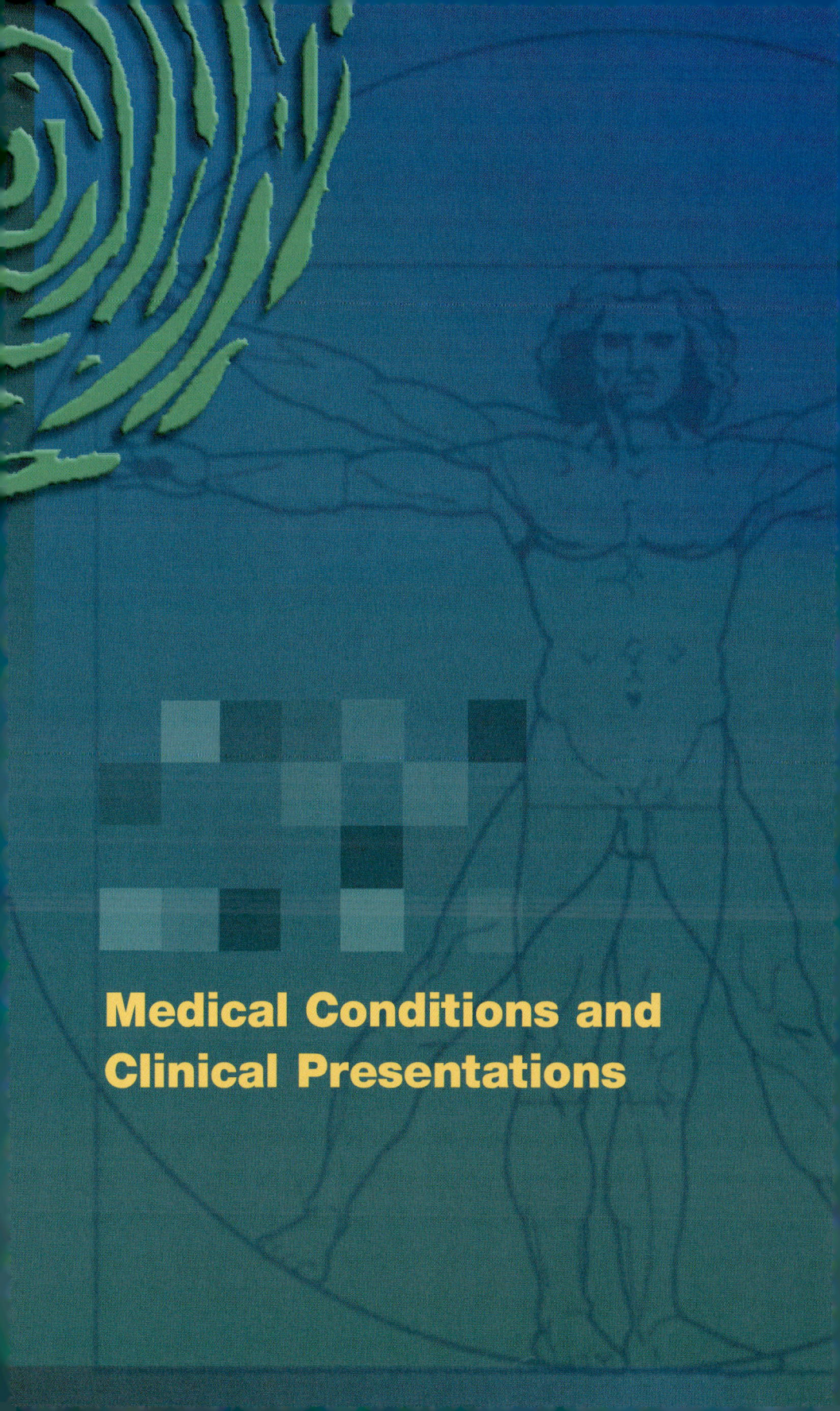

Medical Conditions and Clinical Presentations

Overview

Abdominal distension is common and may indicate the presence of serious intra-abdominal or systemic disease. Clinically, distension is separable into two main types of presentation: **Acute** distension (usually painful and predominantly surgical), or **Chronic/Subacute** distension (usually painless and associated with obstetrical/gynaecological and medical causes). Remember all the 'F's, which cover many of the causes over both groups: **Fluid, Flatus, Faeces, Fat, Fetus**, large **Focal** masses, and the **False** impressions of pseudopregnancy.

Causes

1) Acute abdominal distension

a) Mechanical intestinal obstruction (luminal, wall, extrinsic – usually painful)

The most common causes are **adhesions, tumours, hernias, volvulus**

- ❏ Gastric outlet obstruction – 'pyloric' stenosis
- ❏ Small intestine – adhesions, hernias, tumours etc.
- ❏ Large intestine – tumours, diverticular disease, volvulus

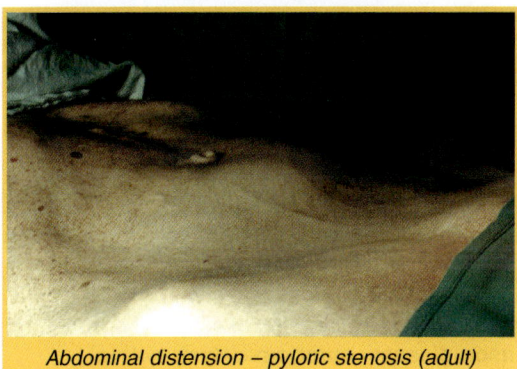

Abdominal distension – pyloric stenosis (adult)

b) Non-mechanical intestinal obstruction (acute intestinal pseudo-obstruction – sometimes painless)

- ❏ Acute gastric dilatation
- ❏ Small and large intestine – 'paralytic' or 'spastic' ileus
  - • Transient postoperative physiological ileus
  - • Secondary to peritonitis from any cause
  - • Secondary to ischaemia (mesenteric infarction, ischaemic enteritis)
  - • Toxic inflammatory bowel disease (IBD) (toxic megacolon)
  - • Secondary to severe systemic illness or retroperitoneal pathology (haemorrhage, tumours, etc.)

2) Chronic abdominal distension (usually painless)

a) **Ascites**

b) **Faecal impaction**

c) **Large abdominal or pelvic mass**
- ❏ Hepatosplenomegaly
- ❏ Neoplasms
- ❏ Abdominal aneurysms
- ❏ Ovarian cysts
- ❏ Gross bladder distension

d) **Pregnancy (exclude first in females)**

e) **Subjective (false pregnancy, irritable bowel syndrome, obesity)**

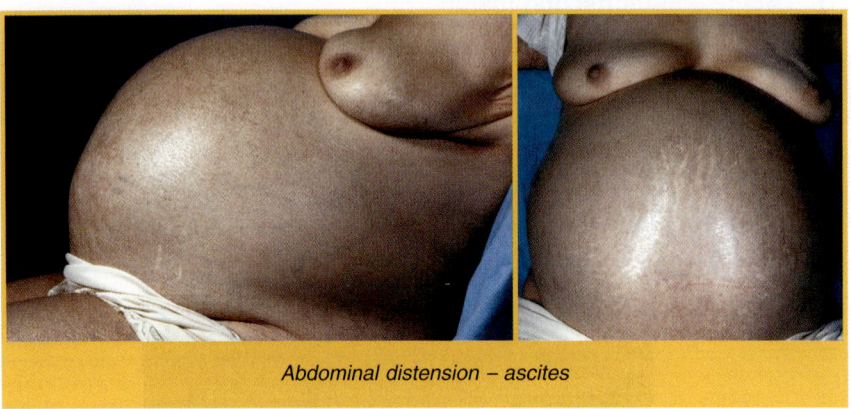

Abdominal distension – ascites

3) Chronic nonmechanical intestinal pseudo-obstruction

a) **Enteric nervous system (amyloidosis, diabetes, paraneoplastic)**

b) **Extrinsic nervous system (stroke, spinal cord injury, multiple sclerosis, Parkinson disease, autonomic dysfunction)**

c) **Smooth muscle (scleroderma)**

Key Objectives

- Differentiate between causes of abdominal distension based on history and physical findings.

- Identify causes of acute abdominal distension requiring urgent early care.

General/Specific Objectives

- Through efficient, focused data gathering:

  - Differentiate clinically the aetiology of abdominal distension.

  - Elicit information on risk factors which would predispose to the various causes for abdominal distension.

- Interpret the critical clinical and laboratory findings which were key in the processes of exclusion, differentiation and diagnosis:

  - Select and interpret abdominal X-rays and other appropriate investigations used in cases of abdominal distension.

  - Recommend paracentesis when indicated and interpret the results.

- Conduct an effective plan of management for a patient with abdominal distension/ileus:

  - Outline the short term medical and surgical management of patients with gaseous distension.

  - Contrast the immediate and long term management of a patient with cirrhotic ascites versus malignant ascites.

  - Select patients in need of specialised care.

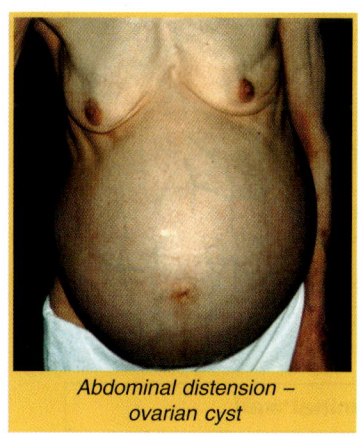

*Abdominal distension –
ovarian cyst*

Overview

Most abdominal masses represent significant underlying disease requiring complete investigation. Intra-abdominal masses must be differentiated from abdominal wall masses. The large number of possible causes can be made more manageable by focusing on the site and physical characteristics of the mass. (See #002A Epigastric Mass – #002F Left Iliac Fossa Mass.)

Causes

1) Organomegaly

    a) Hepatomegaly

    b) Splenomegaly

    c) Enlarged kidneys

    d) Retroperitoneal masses

2) Gastrointestinal system masses

    a) Gastric, colonic, appendiceal

    b) Stool

    c) Pancreatic (pseudocyst)

    d) Gallbladder mass

3) Vascular (abdominal aortic aneurysm)

4) Gynaecologic / Pelvic

    a) Pregnant uterus

    b) Ovarian mass

    c) Enlarged bladder

5) Lymphadenopathy

    a) Lymphomas

    b) Metastases

    c) Infectious causes

6) Masses in abdominal wall

    (see #002G Abdominal Hernia)

    a) Rectus sheath haematoma

    b) Desmoid tumour

    c) Umbilical lump/discharge

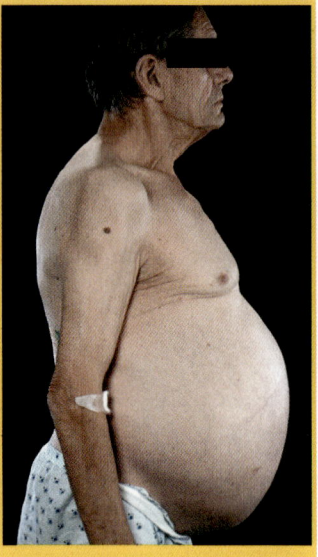

Retroperitoneal liposarcoma

- ❏ Intertrigo, concretions, granulomas
- ❏ Malignant nodule (Sister Mary Joseph nodule)
- ❏ Pilonidal sinus
- ❏ Endometriosis
- ❏ Embryological remnants (vitelline duct, urachus)

Key Objectives

- Distinguish the cause of an abdominal mass based on history and physical findings.

- Distinguish intra-abdominal from abdominal wall masses.

General/Specific Objectives

- Through efficient, focused data gathering:

  - Exclude pregnancy as cause of the abdominal mass.

  - Determine which patients are likely to have a neoplasm causing the abdominal mass.

  - Determine the physical characteristics enabling diagnosis of masses arising in specific organs.

  - Describe the risk factors which would predispose to the various causes for abdominal mass.

- Interpret critical clinical and laboratory findings which were key in the processes of exclusion, differentiation and diagnosis:

  - Select and interpret abdominal imaging (radiography, computed tomography (CT) scan, ultrasound, etc.) in patients with an abdominal mass.

  - Interpret and discuss the role of serum tumour marker testing.

- Conduct an effective plan of management for a patient with an abdominal mass:

  - Discuss the medical and surgical management of patients with an abdominal mass.

  - Select patients in need of specialised care.

002A Epigastric Mass

Overview

Epigastric masses are most commonly due to pathology in stomach or liver; or may indicate retroperitoneal pathology (aneurysm, pancreatic or lymph node mass).

Causes

1)	Abdominal aortic aneurysm

2)	Gastric mass (neoplasm, gastric dilatation)

3)	Liver mass (left lobe)

4)	Pancreatic mass (pseudocyst, tumour)

5)	Lymph node mass (para-aortic nodes)

Key Objective

• Distinguish the cause of an epigastric mass based on history and physical findings.

General/Specific Objectives

• Through efficient, focused data gathering:

- Identify site of origin and likely cause of an epigastric mass based on clinical findings.

• Interpret the critical clinical and laboratory findings in diagnosis.

• Outline an effective management plan for a patient with an epigastric mass.

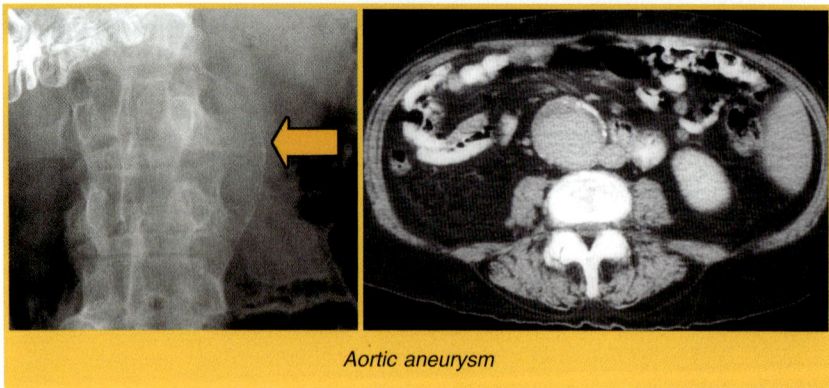

Aortic aneurysm

002B Right Hypochondrial Mass

Overview
Masses in the right hypochondrium arise most commonly from the liver or gallbladder. The normal liver is impalpable, except in children. The liver becomes palpable when abnormally firm and enlarged or when it contains a mass.

Causes

1) Hepatomegaly

    a) **General enlargement**

        ❏ Cirrhosis

        ❏ Heart failure

    b) **Focal masses**

        ❏ Neoplasms, parasitic cysts, etc.

2) Enlarged gallbladder

    a) **Acute cholecystitis**

    b) **Mucocele / Empyema**

    c) **Courvoisier sign and law (underlying pancreatic neoplasm)**

3) Hepatic flexure colonic mass

4) Right renal mass

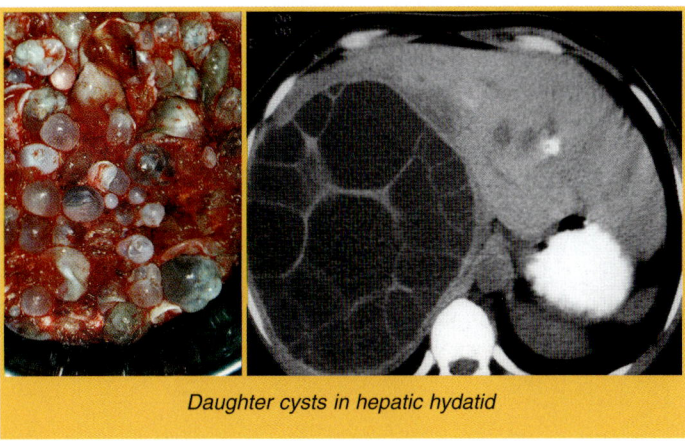

Daughter cysts in hepatic hydatid

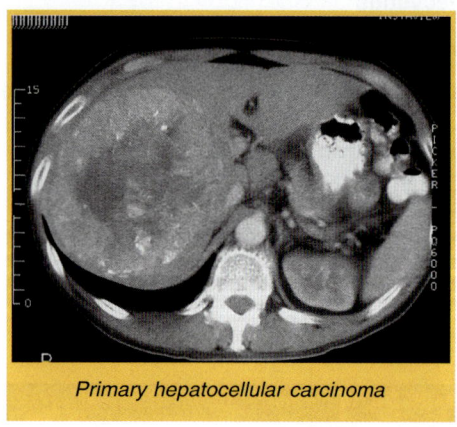

Primary hepatocellular carcinoma

002C Left Hypochondrial Mass

Overview

Masses in the left hypochondrium are most commonly caused by splenic enlargement, which must be differentiated from renal, colonic or pancreatic tail lesions.

Causes

1)	**Splenomegaly**

2)	**Left renal mass**

3)	**Colonic mass (splenic flexure)**

4)	**Pancreatic tail mass**

Key Objective
- Distinguish the cause of a left hypochondrial mass based on history and physical findings.

General/Specific Objectives
- Through efficient, focused data gathering:

  - Differentiate splenic from other masses.

- Outline an effective management plan in a patient with a left hypochondrial mass due to splenomegaly.

- Outline effective diagnostic and management plans in patients with a left renal mass.

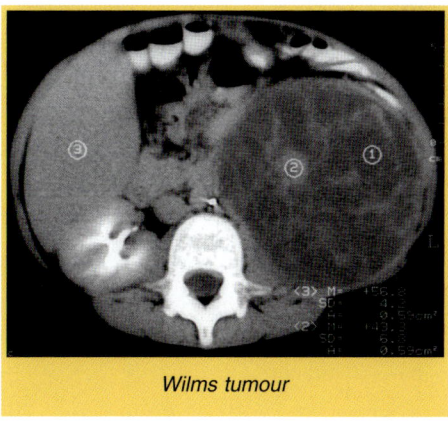

Wilms tumour

002D Right Iliac Fossa Mass

Overview

Painful right iliac fossa masses commonly are associated with appendiceal or colonic pathology and require prompt surgical assessment.

Causes

1) Appendiceal mass (phlegmon or abscess)

2) Caecal mass (carcinoma)

3) Other infectious/inflammatory causes

   a) Crohn disease

   b) Actinomycosis

   c) Ileocaecal tuberculosis (TB)

   d) Psoas abscess

4) Iliac lymph node swellings

   a) Lymphoma

   b) Metastatic

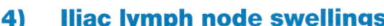

Crohn ileitis

Key Objective

- Distinguish the cause of a right iliac fossa mass based on history and physical findings.

General/Specific Objectives

- Outline a management plan for a patient presenting with a right iliac fossa mass.

- Select and interpret imaging investigations (radiography, computed tomography (CT) scans, ultrasound, etc.) in patients presenting with a right iliac fossa mass.

002E Suprapubic/Pelvic Mass

Overview

In women a pregnant uterus must first be excluded. Other gynaecologic causes include large ovarian or uterine abdominopelvic masses. In both sexes, a distended bladder is an important cause.

Causes

1)	**Pregnant uterus**

2)	**Urinary bladder**

3)	**Ovarian mass**

Key Objective
- Distinguish the cause of a suprapubic mass on the basis of history and physical findings.

General/Specific Objective
- Outline effective diagnostic/management plans for a patient with a suprapubic mass.

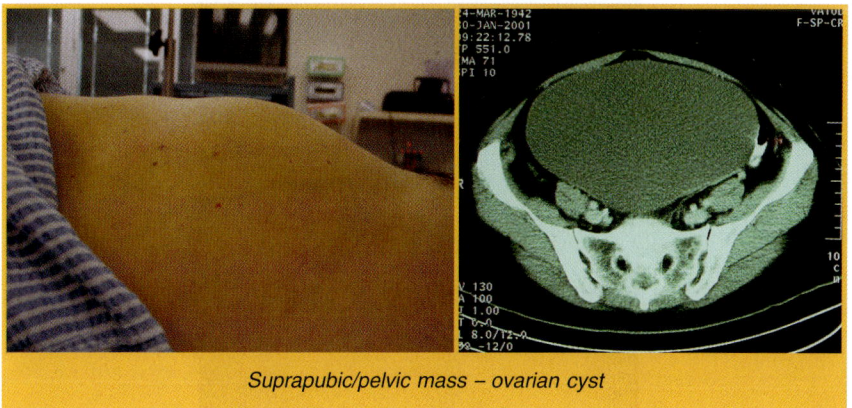

Suprapubic/pelvic mass – ovarian cyst

002F Left Iliac Fossa Mass

Overview

Left iliac fossa masses are most commonly due to significant colonic pathology.

Causes

> **1) Colonic mass**

      a) Carcinoma sigmoid colon

      b) Colonic diverticular disease

      c) Faeces

> **2) Lymph node mass**

Key Objective

- Distinguish the cause of a left iliac fossa mass based on history and physical findings.

General/Specific Objectives

- Outline effective diagnostic/management plans for a patient with a left iliac fossa mass.

- Outline the diagnostic plans for a patient presenting with left iliac fossa mass due to iliac lymph node enlargement.

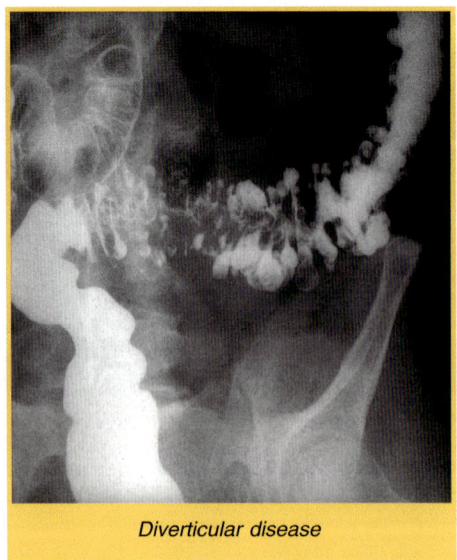

Diverticular disease

002G Abdominal Hernia

Overview

Herniorrhaphy is the commonest surgical procedure performed by general surgeons. Twenty-five per cent of males will develop an inguinal hernia in their lifetime. Interference with the blood supply of the hernial contents (strangulation) is a surgical emergency.

Causes

1)   Groin hernias

    a) Inguinal hernia (direct, indirect)
- ❏ Commoner in males

    b) Femoral hernia
- ❏ Commoner in females

2)   Umbilical hernias

    a) Congenital umbilical hernia of infancy
- ❏ Most settle spontaneously

    b) Adult umbilical/para-umbilical hernia
- ❏ Multiparity in females major causal factor

3)   Incisional (wound) hernia

    a) Commoner with vertical incisions

    b) Wound infection commonest cause

4)   Less common abdominal wall hernias

    a) Epigastric hernia (fatty hernia of linea alba)

    b) Spigelian (linea semilunaris) hernia
- ❏ Characteristically interstitial

    c) Lumbar hernia

    d) Perineal hernia (usually after abdomino-perineal excision of rectum)

Indirect inguinoscrotal inguinal hernia

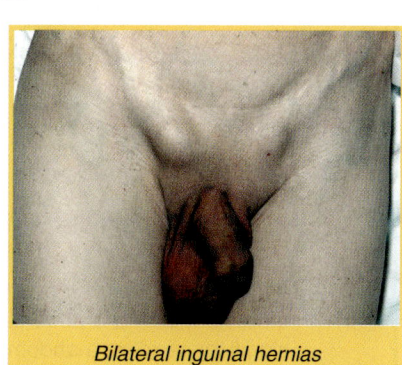

Bilateral inguinal hernias

5) Divarication of recti

a) Diffuse epigastric bulge between recti in epigastrium due to obesity and spreading of linea alba – not a true hernia

6) Internal abdominal hernias

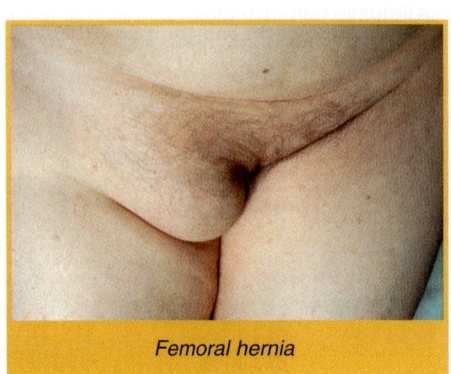

Femoral hernia

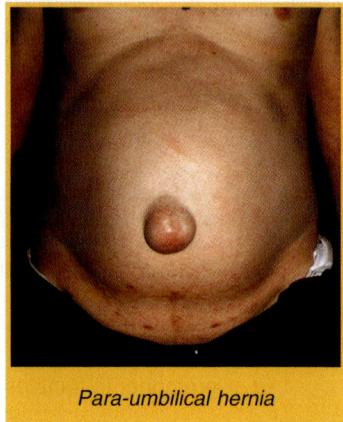

Para-umbilical hernia

Key Objectives

- Identify abdominal wall hernias requiring immediate rather than elective repair.

- Recognise factors predictive of hernia recurrence postoperatively (such as wound sepsis, obesity, ascites and malnutrition).

General/Specific Objectives

- Through efficient, focused data gathering:

  - Recognise symptoms and signs of strangulated hernia, as opposed to irreducibility.

  - Differentiate inguinal and femoral hernias from other causes of a groin (or inguinoscrotal) mass such as lymphadenopathy, varicocele, hydrocele, saphena varix or femoral aneurysm.

  - Differentiate inguinal from femoral hernia on the basis of physical signs including visual inspection, palpation and special manoeuvres.

- Conduct an effective diagnostic and management plan for a patient with an abdominal wall hernia:

  - Identify patients in need of surgical repair (emergency and elective).

  - Identify factors predisposing to abdominal wall hernia.

  - Counsel and educate patients on the risks associated with uncorrected hernias and identify hernias at special risk of strangulation.

  - Identify possible sites of intra-abdominal herniation by considering embryology of intra-abdominal structures; and outline the potential clinical significance of intra-abdominal hernias.

002H Adrenal Mass

Overview

Adrenal masses are at times found incidentally after computed tomography (CT) scan, magnetic resonance imaging (MRI), or ultrasound examination done for unrelated reasons. The incidence is about 3% (almost 10% of autopsies). Larger masses are likely to require investigation. Functioning adrenal masses comprise a group causing important treatable causes of hypertension.

Causes

1) **Non-functioning adenoma**

2) **Functioning adenoma**

   a) **Cushing syndrome (glucocorticoid excess)**

   b) **Conn syndrome (aldosterone excess)**

   c) **Androgen excess**

   d) **Phaeochromocytoma**

3) **Adrenal carcinoma**

4) **Metastasis**

5) **Neuroblastoma (in children)**

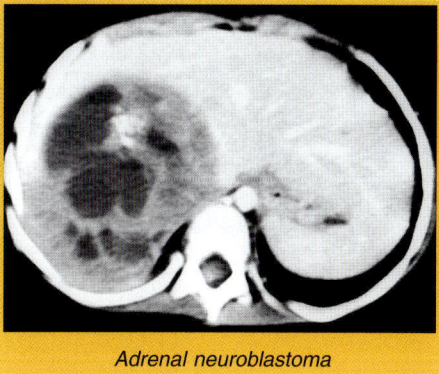

Adrenal neuroblastoma

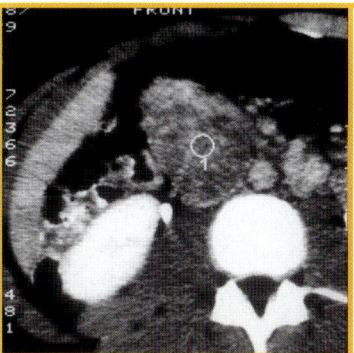

Serum / Plasma	
Sodium	139 mmol/L
Potassium	⇩ 2.4 mmol/L
Chloride	96 mmol/L
Bicarbonate	⇧ 34 mmol/L
Urea	3.8 mmol/L
Creatinine	71 μmol/L
Ionised calcium	⇩ 1.11 mmol/L
Aldosterone	⇧ 2029 pmol/L
Renin	<7.0 mU/L

Adrenal mass on CT, with serum chemistry – Conn syndrome

Key Objectives
- Determine whether the mass is malignant or not.

- Determine whether the mass is functional or not.

General/Specific Objectives
- Through efficient, focused data gathering:

  - Differentiate benign functioning adenomas from those that are non-functioning.

  - Differentiate benign from malignant masses by inquiring and examining for primary tumours which metastasise to the adrenal glands.

- Interpret critical clinical and laboratory findings which were key in the processes of exclusion, differentiation, and diagnosis:

  - Select and interpret investigations for the exclusion of functioning adrenal masses.

  - List features noted on diagnostic imaging techniques suggestive of malignancy.

  - Select patients and list indications for fine needle aspiration cytological (FNAC) biopsy.

- Conduct an effective plan of management for a patient with an adrenal mass:

  - Outline initial plan of management for patients with adrenal masses which are functioning.

- Select patients in need of specialised care; list those requiring referral to endocrinology / internal medicine, and those requiring surgical referral.

003A Abdominal Pain in Adults

Overview
Abdominal pain may result from intra-abdominal inflammation or disorders of the abdominal wall. Pain may also be referred from sources outside the abdomen such as retro-peritoneal processes as well as intrathoracic processes. Thorough clinical evaluation is the most important 'test' in the diagnosis of acute abdominal pain. Localisation of the pain site, and awareness of characteristic symptom sequences, can reduce the list of possible causes to manageable size.

Causes

1) Right upper quadrant pain

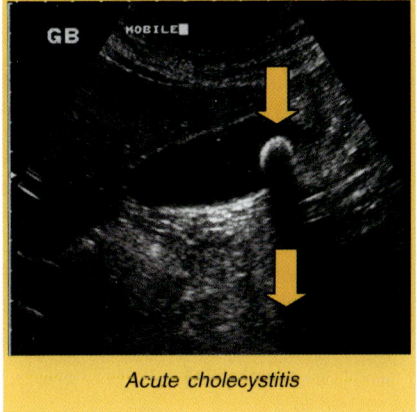

Acute cholecystitis

   a) **Biliary tract**
- ❏ Biliary 'colic'
- ❏ Acute cholecystitis
- ❏ Cholangitis

   b) **Liver (hepatitis, hepatic abscess, neoplasms)**

   c) **Pancreatitis**

   d) **Renal pain (pyelonephritis, tumours, infarction and polycystic kidney)**

   e) **Extra-abdominal (myocardial infarction (MI), pulmonary embolus, pneumonia)**

2) Epigastric pain

   a) **Peptic ulcer disease**

   b) **Pancreatitis**

   c) **Cholangitis**

   d) **Functional dyspepsia**

   e) **Neoplasms (hepatic, gastric, pancreatic)**

   f) **Abdominal aortic aneurysm**

   g) **Epigastric hernia**

3) Left upper quadrant pain

   a) **Peptic ulcer disease**

   b) **Pancreatitis**

   c) **Gastric and pancreatic neoplasms**

   d) **Renal pain**

4) Right/Left lower quadrant pain

a) Bowel (appendicitis, colitis, diverticulitis: large and small bowel)

b) Mesenteric lymphadenitis

c) Gynaecologic causes (complicated ovarian cyst, ectopic pregnancy, pelvic inflammatory disease)

d) Ureteric/Renal 'colic'

e) Urinary retention

f) Pyelonephritis and cystitis

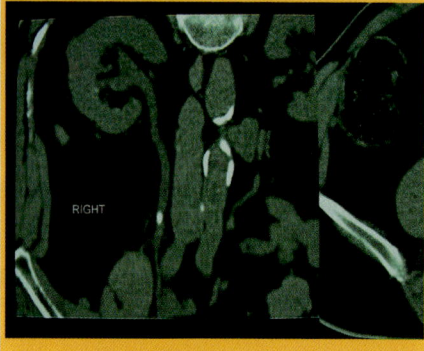

Ureteric calculus – renal 'colic'

5) Generalised

a) Functional gut disorders (functional dyspepsia, irritable bowel syndrome)

b) Peritoneal inflammation (ruptured viscus, bacterial peritonitis)

c) Bowel obstruction

d) Vascular (ischaemic bowel, ruptured abdominal aortic aneurysm)

e) Metabolic (diabetic ketoacidosis, porphyria)

f) Neurogenic (herpes zoster)

g) Other (Mediterranean/Malta fever (brucellosis), sickle cell crisis, etc.)

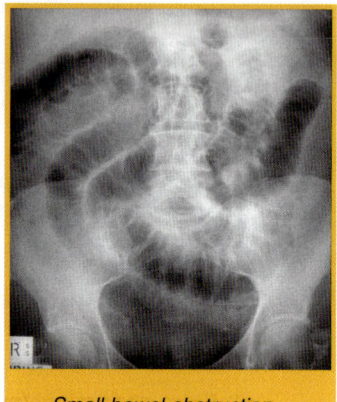

Small bowel obstruction – adhesions

6) Special group 'acute abdomen – acute abdominal surgical emergency'

a) Perforated viscus (peptic ulcer, appendix, gallbladder, colon)

- ❏ Perforated peptic ulcer
- ❏ Perforated appendicitis / cholecystis
- ❏ Perforated colonic diverticulitis with faecal peritonitis

b) Strangulated intestinal obstruction

c) Ruptured aortic aneurysm

d) Acute haemorrhagic pancreatitis (pancreatic necrosis)

e) Ruptured ectopic pregnancy

f) Acute massive mesenteric vascular infarction

g) Blunt or penetrating trauma with peritonitis

h) Primary bacterial peritonitis

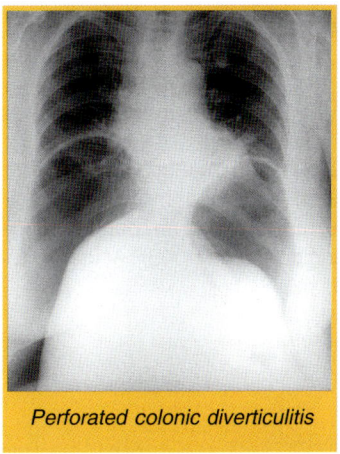

Perforated colonic diverticulitis

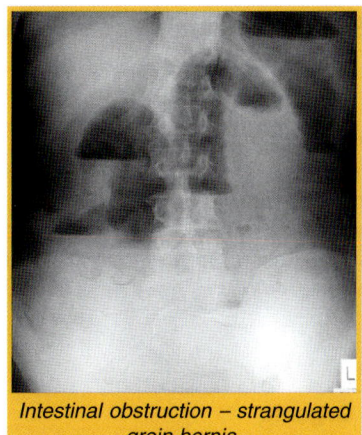

Intestinal obstruction – strangulated groin hernia

Key Objectives
- Recognise patients with abdominal pain who require emergency treatment, medical or surgical.
- Recognise the special group of 'acute abdomen – acute abdominal surgical emergency' where early surgical referral and exploration is likely to be required.
- Determine whether extra-abdominal causes listed above (MI, etc.) may be causing the pain.

General/Specific Objectives
- Through efficient, focused data gathering:
  - Elicit clinical findings and their sequence which are key to establishing the most likely source of the pain.
  - Differentiate intra-abdominal from extra-abdominal or metabolic causes of acute abdominal pain.
- Interpret the critical clinical and laboratory findings which were key in the processes of exclusion, differentiation and diagnosis:
  - Interpret abdominal X-rays and other imaging modalities diagnostic of various causes.
- Conduct an effective plan of management for a patient with acute abdominal pain:
  - Select patients who require emergency surgery and who require emergency medical care.
  - Outline a plan of management for common causes of abdominal pain.
  - Select patients in need of specialised care and/or further investigation.
  - Understand the common and life-threatening causes of acute abdominal pain.

003B   Non-Acute/Recurrent Abdominal Pain in Infancy and Early Childhood

Overview

Abdominal pain is a common and disconcerting problem in infants and children. In an infant or child presenting with *chronic* but persistent intermittent abdominal pain, the probable causes should be rapidly identified so that directed management can be initiated. Causes of *acute* abdominal pain are considered in #003F Acute Abdominal Pain in Children.

Causes

1)   Organic

a) **Abdominal**

❏   Infantile colic

❏   Infectious (*Giardia lamblia*)

❏   Obstructive (chronic constipation)

❏   Trauma

❏   Vasculitic

❏   Miscellaneous

b) **Extra-abdominal**

❏   Miscellaneous (peptic ulceration, intermittent porphyria)

2)   Functional

a) **Psychogenic (family disruption, school failure)**

Key Objective

•   It is important to differentiate between functional and organic causes and to recognise how causes of abdominal pain in infants and children differ from those in adulthood.

General/Specific Objectives

•   Through efficient, focused data gathering:

-    In an infant, identify the acute organic causes and differentiate from infantile colic.

-    Differentiate acute from chronic and functional abdominal pain.

•   Interpret critical clinical and laboratory findings which were key in the processes of exclusion, differentiation and diagnosis:

-    Select appropriate laboratory investigations to differentiate those conditions requiring acute management.

- Investigate colic and functional pain with the minimum investigations to establish the diagnosis.

- Identify from investigations, the key essentials differentiating acute from chronic pain.

• Conduct an effective plan of management for a patient with abdominal pain:

- In infants, outline the initial stages for management of acute intestinal obstruction.

- Manage infantile colic with the infant's interests as the focus.

- Manage functional abdominal pain with the child's interests as the focus.

- Outline the treatment programme for a child with chronic abdominal pain utilising the support of the parents, family and community services.

003C Chronic Recurrent Abdominal Pain

Overview

Chronic and recurrent abdominal pain is a common symptom with an extensive differential diagnosis and heterogeneous pathophysiology. The history and physical examination frequently differentiate between functional and more serious underlying diseases.

Causes

1) Intestinal tract

    a) Oesophageal (oesophagitis)

    b) Gastric (peptic ulcer disease, neoplasm)

    c) Duodenal (peptic ulcer disease)

    d) Small bowel (inflammatory bowel disease (IBD), neoplasm)

    e) Colon (IBD, irritable bowel syndrome, neoplasm, diverticulosis)

2) Related organs

    a) Gallbladder / Biliary tract (cholelithiasis / biliary 'colic')

    b) Pancreas (chronic pancreatitis, neoplasm)

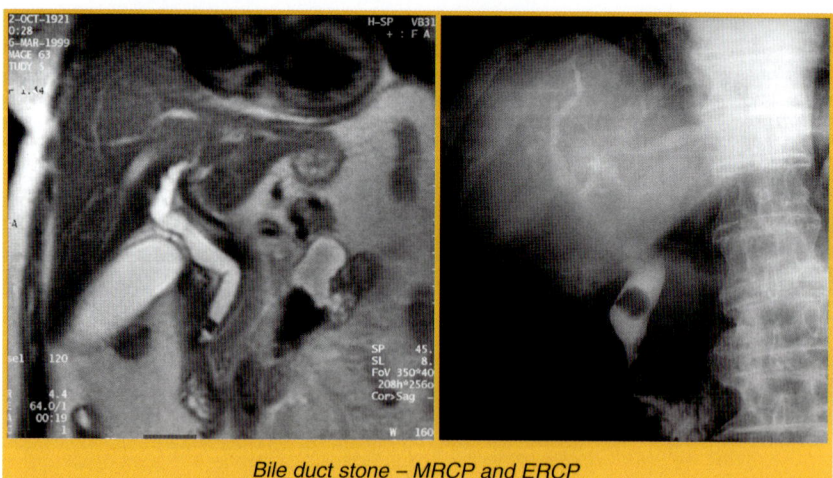

Bile duct stone – MRCP and ERCP

Other

   a) **Psychogenic factors (malingering, functional dyspepsia)**

   b) **Abdominal wall**

   c) **Gynaecologic causes**

   d) **Visceral neoplasms/lymphomas**

   e) **Collagen / Vascular**

   f) **Lactose intolerance**

Key Objective
- Recognising that visceral pain is typically poorly localised and often referred to distal sites, differentiate between various causes of chronic abdominal pain.

General/Specific Objectives
- Through efficient, focused data gathering:

  - Differentiate between organic and non-organic causes of chronic abdominal pain.

  - Select patients in need of further laboratory and radiological investigation.

- Interpret the critical clinical and laboratory findings which were key in the processes of exclusion, differentiation and diagnosis:

  - Outline the significance of common findings on ultrasound or computed tomography (CT) imaging of the abdomen as well as barium contrast studies.

- Conduct an effective plan of management for a patient with chronic abdominal pain:

  - Contrast the medical, surgical, nutritional and psychological management of chronic abdominal pain.

  - Select narcotics appropriately for patients and manage complications arising from the use of these drugs.

  - Select patients in need of referral to other healthcare professionals.

  - Counsel and provide appropriate education for patients with chronic abdominal pain syndromes.

003D Heartburn/Dyspepsia

Overview

'Heartburn' and 'dyspepsia' are common gastrointestinal complaints, since studies from various countries report an incidence of the symptoms in 20–40% of adults. Although serious complications can arise with few premonitory symptoms, appropriate management can generally avert such sequelae.

Causes

1)	**Functional dyspepsia / Somatoform disorders**

2)	**Gastro-oesophageal reflux disease with/without oesophagitis**

3)	**Motility disorders of the oesophagus**

   a) Achalasia

   b) Scleroderma

4)	**Peptic ulcer disease (including drugs)**

5)	**Miscellaneous (biliary disease, irritable bowel, chronic pancreatitis, diabetic gastroparesis, ischaemic heart disease, etc.)**

Key Objectives
- Diagnose somatoform disorders by inclusion rather than exclusion; always exclude the possibility of ischaemic heart disease.
- Outline conservative management measures including dietary counselling.

General/Specific Objectives
- Through efficient, focused data gathering:
  - Differentiate between dyspepsia and chest pain or referred pain resulting from ischaemic heart disease.
- Interpret the critical clinical and laboratory findings which were key in the processes of exclusion, differentiation and diagnosis:
  - List or outline indications for radiological or endoscopic investigation of patients with symptoms suggestive of gastro-oesophageal reflux or peptic ulcer.
- Conduct an effective plan of management for a patient with 'heartburn':
  - Discuss the current concepts of pathophysiology in the management of gastro-oesophageal reflux and peptic ulcer disease.

- Counsel patients regarding lifestyle modification which can ameliorate symptoms of gastro-oesophageal reflux and peptic ulcer disease.
- Select patients in need of specialised care.

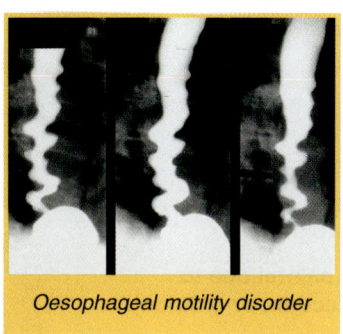

Oesophageal motility disorder

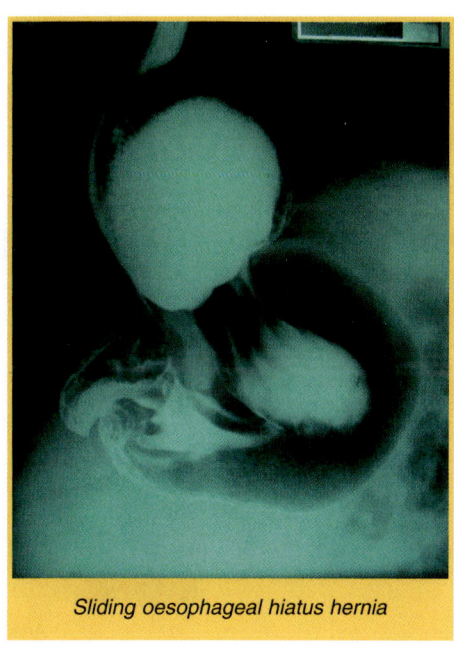

Sliding oesophageal hiatus hernia

003E Anal Pain

Overview
While almost all causes of anal pain are treatable, some can be destructive locally if left untreated. Anal pain is *not* a feature of uncomplicated haemorrhoids.

Causes

1) Identifiable

    a) Perianal haematoma

    b) Haemorrhoids (painful due to thrombosis, infection, or erosion)

    c) Anal fissure

    d) Anal ulcer / Anal cancer

    e) Perianal fistula (due to Crohn disease)

    f) Perirectal abscess

2) Other

    a) Proctalgia fugax, neuropathic pain syndrome

    b) Coccygeal pain, other pelvic floor muscle syndromes

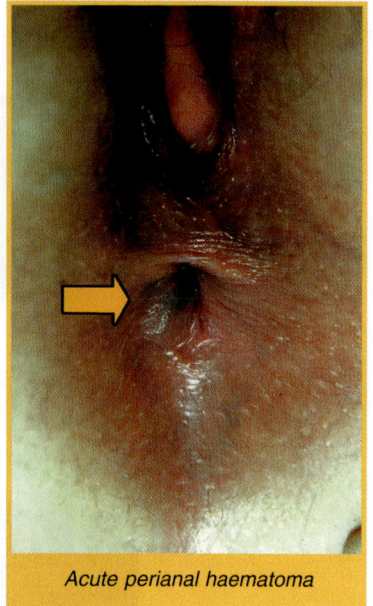

Acute perianal haematoma

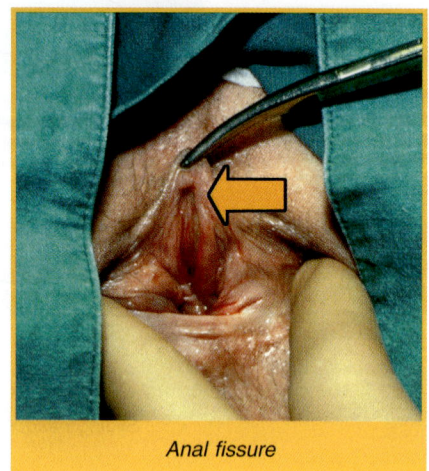

Anal fissure

Key Objective

- Perform visual inspection, palpation, and ano-rectal examination in all patients presenting with anal pain.

General/Specific Objectives

- Through efficient, focused data gathering:

  - Differentiate between the causes of anal pain.

  - Establish whether tenesmus (an uncomfortable sense of incomplete evacuation leading to frequent, painful straining) is present.

- Interpret the critical clinical and laboratory findings which were key in the processes of exclusion, differentiation and diagnosis:

  - Based on inspection, palpation and ano-rectal examination, differentiate the cause of anal pain.

- Conduct an effective plan of management for a patient with anal pain:

  - Select patients with perirectal abscess for urgent surgical treatment.

  - Counsel patients with haemorrhoids and anal fissure in the conservative treatment options including *sitz* baths, stool softeners and secondary preventive measures such as strict avoidance of constipation.

  - Select patients in need of specialised care.

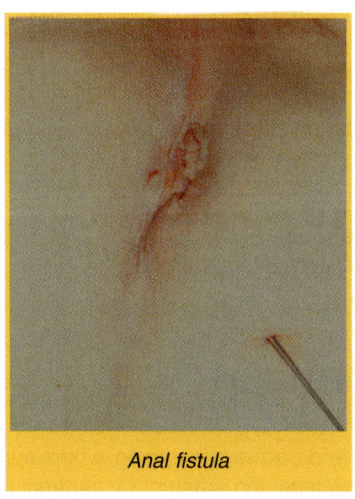

Anal fistula

003F Acute Abdominal Pain in Children

Overview

Acute abdominal pain in children may result from intra-abdominal inflammation or obstruction. Thorough clinical evaluation is usually the most important step in the diagnosis of abdominal pain so that directed management can be initiated.

Causes

1) Right lower quadrant / Left lower quadrant

   a) Appendicitis, constipation

   b) Mesenteric lymphadenitis

   c) Inflammatory bowel disease (IBD)

   d) Inguinal hernia (incarcerated)

2) Generalised

   a) Peritoneal inflammation (ruptured viscus, bacterial peritonitis)

   b) Bowel (infantile colic, gastroenteritis, bowel obstruction (intussusception, constipation))

   c) Psychosomatic

   d) Extra-abdominal (referred pain – pneumonia)

Key Objective
- Select patients with abdominal pain who require emergency treatment, medical or surgical.

General/Specific Objectives
- Through efficient, focused data gathering:

   - Elicit clinical findings which are key to establishing the most likely source of the pain.

- Interpret critical clinical and laboratory findings which were key in the processes of exclusion, differentiation, and diagnosis:

   - Select laboratory and diagnostic imaging, where appropriate, to determine whether conditions requiring emergency treatment are present.

   - Interpret abdominal X-rays.

- Conduct an effective plan of management for children with acute abdominal pain:

   - Select patients who require emergency surgery and those who require emergency medical care.

- Outline the initial plan of management in infants with acute intestinal obstruction.

- Outline a plan of management for common causes of abdominal pain (e.g. infantile colic) with the child's interest as the focus.

- Outline a plan of management for a child with acute abdominal pain using support from parents, family, and community services.

- Select patients in need of specialised care and/or further investigation.

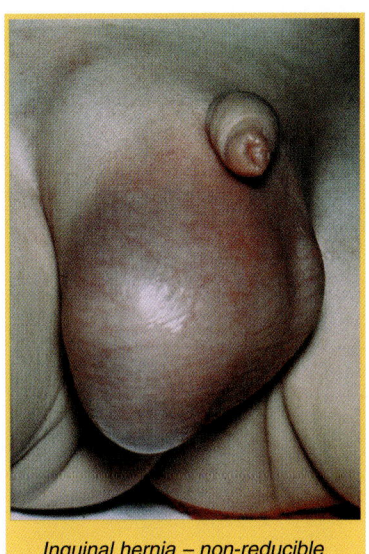

Inguinal hernia – non-reducible

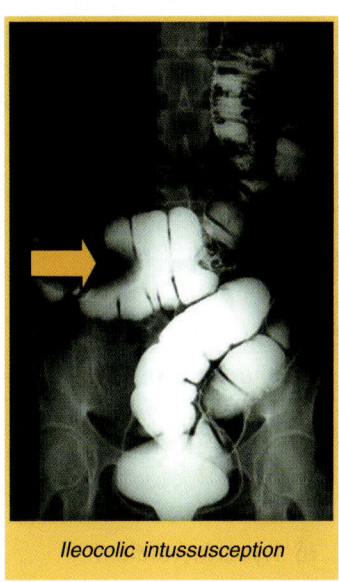

Ileocolic intussusception

004A Hypercalcaemia

Overview

Hypercalcaemia may be associated with an excess of calcium in both extracellular fluid and bone (e.g. increased intestinal absorption), or with a localised or generalised deficit of calcium in bone (e.g. increased bone resorption). This differentiation is important for both diagnostic and management reasons. Hypercalcaemia in adults requires investigation to identify the cause. Primary hyperparathyroidism (HPT) is a common cause and is differentiated from other causes such as bone malignancy by high serum parathormone.

Most patients with hypercalcaemia due to primary HPT have or will develop symptoms, the most important of which are changes in the mental state, lethargy, constipation, thirst, urinary frequency and nocturia. Surgery is indicated in the majority of patients with established primary HPT – the commonest cause is a single parathyroid adenoma. Hypercalcaemia can cause severe anatomic injury to the kidneys and, if severe, patients may develop hypercalcaemic crisis.

Causes

1) Increased bone resorption

   a) Malignancy

   b) Primary HPT

   c) Secondary/Tertiary HPT

   d) Hyperthyroidism

   e) Immobilisation

   f) Paget disease of bone

2) Increased intestinal absorption

   a) Increased intake (e.g. milk alkali syndrome)

   b) Vitamin D-mediated (e.g. granulomatous diseases such as sarcoidosis)

3) Diminished excretion (familial hypocalciuric hypercalcaemia, drugs)

4) Miscellaneous

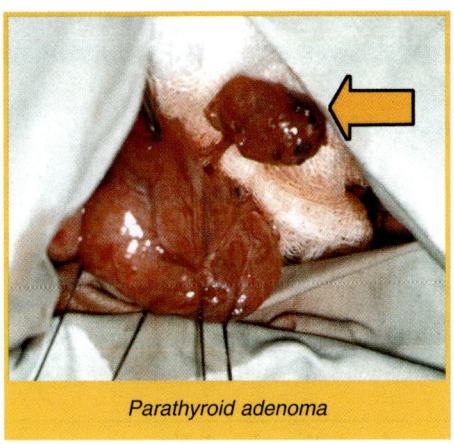

Parathyroid adenoma

Key Objective

- Formulate a management plan for hypercalcaemia consistent with its causal conditions.

General/Specific Objectives

- Through efficient, focused data gathering:

    - Outline a diagnostic and management plan for a patient with hypercalcaemia.

    - Outline laboratory tests and diagnostic imaging findings in relation to the common causes and contrast the findings in primary HPT, secondary HPT, cancer and Paget disease.

    - Outline embryological development of parathyroids and the relevance to sites of parathyroid adenomas.

    - Differentiate hypercalcaemia caused by increased intake from that of excess bone resorption.

- Interpret the critical clinical and laboratory findings which were key in the processes of exclusion, differentiation and diagnosis.

- Conduct an effective plan of management for a patient with hypercalcaemia:

    - Select patients in need of specialised care.

004B Hypocalcaemia

Overview

Hypocalcaemia is an important and potentially serious complication from a variety of causes. Tetany, seizures, and papilloedema may occur in patients who develop acute hypocalcaemia. Early recognition of symptoms of paraesthesiae is important in diagnosis and treatment in order to prevent these complications in patients at risk.

Causes

1)   Loss of calcium from the circulation

      a) Hyperphosphataemia (renal insufficiency)

      b) Pancreatitis

      c) Osteoblastic metastases

      d) Drugs (ethylene diamine tetra-acetic acid (EDTA), citrate)

      e) Rhabdomyolysis

      f) Respiratory (overbreathing) or metabolic alkalosis

2)   Decreased vitamin D production or action

      a) Renal failure

      b) Rickets/Rachitis

      c) Malabsorption

3)   Decreased parathyroid hormone (PTH) production or actions

      a) After thyroid/parathyroid surgery

      b) Autoimmune

      c) Diminished response

4)   Hypomagnesaemia

Key Objectives

- Early recognition and treatment of hypocalcaemia in patients at risk.

- Calculate a corrected calcium concentration in the presence of hypoalbuminaemia before initiating any other investigation.

General/Specific Objectives

- Through efficient, focused data gathering:

  - Differentiate hypocalcaemia caused by hyperphosphataemia/hypomagnesaemia from that of diminished production or action of PTH or vitamin D.

- Interpret the critical clinical and laboratory findings which were key in the processes of exclusion, differentiation and diagnosis:

  - Contrast laboratory findings in the various conditions causing hypocalcaemia.

- Conduct an effective plan of management for a patient with hypocalcaemia:

  - Formulate a management plan for acute hypocalcaemia associated with either tetany or seizures.

  - Select patients in need of specialised care.

004C Hypophosphataemia / Fanconi Syndrome

Overview

Of hospitalised patients, 10–15% develop hypophosphataemia, and a small proportion have sufficiently profound depletion to lead to complications (e.g. rhabdomyolysis).

Causes

1) Gastro-intestinal

a) Decreased dietary intake / Vomiting (prolonged, severe)

b) Decreased absorption (chronic diarrhoea, steatorrhoea, vitamin D malabsorption)

c) Antacids (binding of ingested and secreted phosphate)

2) Renal losses

a) Hyperparathyroidism (HPT) (also associated with diminished vitamin D)

b) Osmotic diuresis (salt, glucose)

c) Primary (isolated, Fanconi syndrome)

3) Redistribution (intracellular shift)

a) Re-feeding (stimulated by insulin)

b) Respiratory alkalosis, acute

c) 'Hungry-bone' syndrome

Key Objectives

• Appreciate that the likely causes are gastrointestinal, renal or redistributive.

• Select the most conservative form of therapy, since intravenous (IV) phosphate salts are potentially hazardous.

General/Specific Objectives

• Through efficient, focused data gathering:

  - Diagnose the cause of hypophosphataemia.

• Interpret the critical clinical and laboratory findings which were key in the processes of exclusion, differentiation and diagnosis:

  - If no cause is clinically apparent, differentiate between **redistribution**, **gastrointestinal** and **renal** causes by measuring fractional urinary phosphate excretion.

- Conduct an effective plan of management for a hypophosphataemic patient:
  - State that most patients **will not** require therapy other than repair of the underlying causes.
  - Recognise that phosphate is a major intracellular anion and cellular energy store component; and is a necessary additive in prolonged parenteral nutritional therapy.
- Select patients with vitamin D deficiency for replacement with vitamin D.

Overview

The hydrogen ion content of arterial blood is normally kept blandly alkaline at about 40 nanomolar ([H$^+$] between 36 and 44 nmol/L, which coincidentally equals a range of pH from 7.44 to 7.36), by combined renal and respiratory regulatory mechanisms together with extracellular and intracellular buffer systems.

Major adverse consequences may occur with severe acidaemia and alkalaemia despite absence of specific symptoms (the range of extracellular hydrogen ion content compatible with life is approximately 20–200 nmol/L. This 10-fold change is expressed in the pH notation as a change of one pH unit, e.g. from 7.8 to 6.8). The reversible reaction $H^+ + HCO_3^- \rightleftharpoons H_2CO_3 \rightleftharpoons H_2O + CO_2$ forms the basis of renal and respiratory control. The diagnosis of acid-base disorders depends on recognition of the clinical setting and appropriate laboratory studies. It is crucial to distinguish acidaemia and alkalaemia due to metabolic causes from those due to respiratory (gaseous) causes; especially important is detecting the presence of both. Management of the underlying causes and not simply of the change in hydrogen ion concentration is essential.

Causes

1) 005A Metabolic acidosis

   a) Addition of acid (high anion gap)
- ❏ Endogenous acids (lactic acidosis, ketoacidosis, renal failure)
- ❏ Exogenous acids (methanol, ethylene glycol, salicylate, etc.)

   b) Loss of alkali/base (normal anion gap)
- ❏ Gastrointestinal bicarbonate loss (e.g. diarrhoea, small bowel or pancreatic fistula)
- ❏ Renal bicarbonate loss (e.g. renal tubular acidosis, interstitial nephritis)

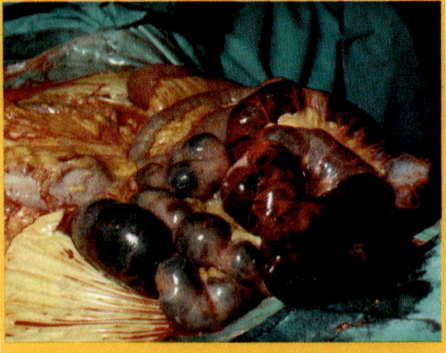

Serum / Plasma	
Sodium	138 mmol/L
Potassium	5.5 mmol/L
Chloride	113 mmol/L
Bicarbonate	⇓ 15 mmol/L
Urea	⇑ 11.5 mmol/L
Creatinine	⇑ 140 μmol/L
Lactate	⇑ 3.2 mmol/L
Arterial pH	⇓ 7.28
P_aCO_2	⇓ 30 mm Hg
P_aO_2	⇓ 70mm Hg

Mesenteric ischaemia and serum chemistry – metabolic (lactic) acidosis

2) 005B Metabolic alkalosis

a) Addition of alkali/base

- ❏ Milk-alkali syndrome

b) Loss of acid

- ❏ Gastrointestinal loss of acid (gastric loss in vomiting, pyloric stenosis)
- ❏ Renal loss of acid (e.g. diuretics)
- ❏ Associated with potassium loss (e.g. Conn syndrome – primary aldosteronism)

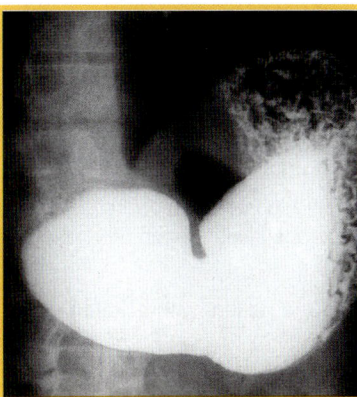

Serum / Plasma

Sodium	⇩ 129 mmol/L
Potassium	⇩ 2.9 mmol/L
Chloride	⇩ 85 mmol/L
Bicarbonate	⇧ 39 mmol/L
Creatinine	120 μmol/L
Arterial pH	⇧ 7.49
P_aCO_2	41 mm Hg
P_aO_2	100mm Hg

Pyloric stenosis and serum chemistry – hypochloraemic hypokalaemic metabolic alkalosis

3) 005C Respiratory (gaseous) acidosis (due to decreased alveolar ventilation, usually with attendant hypoxia)

a) Pulmonary causes of underventilation (e.g. chronic obstructive pulmonary disease (COPD), upper airway obstruction, atelectasis and sputum retention, pneumonia, interstitial lung disease, pulmonary fibrosis, etc.)

b) Neuromuscular causes (e.g. wound pain, drugs, cerebral trauma and coma, encephalitis, bulbar palsy, myasthenia, muscle paralysis)

4) 005D Respiratory alkalosis (due to increased alveolar ventilation from overbreathing)

a) Psychogenic overbreathing from anxiety state

b) Miscellaneous (e.g. fever, drugs, salicylate, central nervous system (CNS) disorders)

5) 005E Mixed acid-base disorders

Key Objectives

- In relevant clinical situations, determine the possibility of an acid-base disorder by examining laboratory parameters of: [H^+], P_aCO_2, [HCO_3^-], and anion gap.

- Diagnose and treat the causal condition in conjunction with appropriate additional measures to correct the abnormality and restore or maintain renal and respiratory functions.

General/Specific Objectives

- Through efficient, focused data gathering:

  - Diagnose the precipitating cause of acidaemia/alkalaemia expeditiously.

- Interpret critical clinical and laboratory findings which were key in the processes of exclusion, differentiation and diagnosis:

  - Select and interpret appropriate investigations for various patients with acidaemia/alkalaemia in order to identify the primary abnormality and the adequacy of the associated secondary 'compensation' (e.g. renal failure with acidotic breathing, pyloric stenosis with secondary renal effects, etc.).

- Conduct an effective plan of management for a patient with acidaemia/ alkalaemia:

  - Outline general supportive measures.

  - Outline specific management for patients in each of the main groups.

  - Select patients who need specialised care and/or consultation.

Overview

Abnormalities of serum lipid levels in Australian society due to dietary and other lifestyle factors are very common. Secondary causes are relatively uncommon. Abnormal lipid levels comprise one of the risk factors for arterial disease, particularly coronary artery disease (CAD).

Identification is by screening of well adults, those with other risk factors and patients with suspected or established CAD. Interpretation of results and their classification is complex depending on the lipid profile found and the presence of other risk factors. Levels can be modified by lifestyle changes and drug therapy, although the use of lipid lowering agents to reduce risk is expensive.

Causes

1) Hypercholesterolaemia (elevated low-density lipoprotein (LDL))

a) **Primary causes**
- ❑ Polygenic (most common)
- ❑ Familial hypercholesterolaemia (rare)

b) **Secondary causes**
- ❑ Hypothyroidism
- ❑ Obstructive liver disease
- ❑ Nephrotic syndrome
- ❑ Drugs (such as cyclosporine, thiazides)

2) Hypertriglyceridaemia

a) **Primary causes**
- ❑ Dietary
- ❑ Familial hypertriglyceridaemia

b) **Secondary causes**
- ❑ Obesity
- ❑ Diabetes mellitus
- ❑ Chronic renal failure
- ❑ Moderate ethanol use

3) Low high-density lipoprotein (HDL)

a) **Obesity**

b) **Cigarette smoking**

c) **Inactivity**

Key Objectives

- Identify persons at risk of CAD who would benefit from serum lipid reduction.

- Conduct an effective management plan for a patient with abnormal serum lipids, which includes behavioural change and possible drug therapy, according to their overall risk of CAD.

General/Specific Objectives

- Understand the principles of population screening.

- Identify patients with secondary causes of lipid abnormalities.

- Interpret and integrate lipid profile with other risk factors for CAD.

- Specify lipid levels (especially LDL cholesterol) to be attained by treatment, including a long term followup plan.

- Be aware of the range of therapeutic agents which lower serum lipids, their indications, costs and side-effects.

007 Abnormal Liver Function Tests

Overview

Thorough investigation can distinguish benign reversible liver disease requiring no treatment from potentially life-threatening conditions requiring immediate therapy. Drugs, alcohol and infection (hepatitis) are the commonest causes. Liver function tests may also assist in making the decision on whether some form of intervention is required.

Causes

1) Isolated hyperbilirubinaemia

a) **Unconjugated or indirect**
- ❏ Haemolysis and ineffective erythropoiesis
- ❏ Defects in transport into the hepacytes or intracellular conjugation:
  - Gilbert disease
  - Neonates
  - Crigler-Najjar syndrome

b) **Conjugated or direct – defect in transport out of the hepatocyte**
- ❏ Rotor syndrome, Dubin-Johnson syndrome

2) Hepatocellular (may lead to cirrhosis)

a) **Alcohol, drugs, toxins (paracetamol, isoniazid)**

b) **Fatty liver and steatohepatitis**

c) **Viral hepatitis**

d) **Metabolic liver disease (haemochromatosis, Wilson disease, etc.)**

e) **Autoimmune chronic hepatitis**

f) **Shock or ischaemia**

g) **Septicaemia**

3) Cholestatic

a) **Intrahepatic**
- ❏ Drugs (oral contraceptives)
- ❏ Infiltrative (amyloid, malignant)
- ❏ Congestive (e.g. heart failure)
- ❏ Autoimmune (primary biliary cirrhosis, sclerosing cholangitis)
- ❏ Granulomatous disease

b) **Extrahepatic (cholestasis from stone or neoplasm, stricture, atresia)**

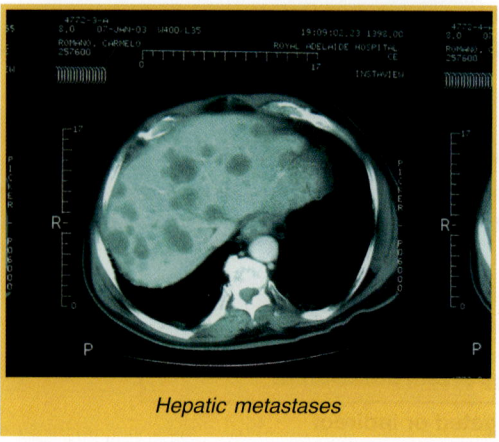

Hepatic metastases

Key Objectives

- Discuss abnormal laboratory tests in the context of the clinical presentation, and select patients requiring medical or interventional management.

- Understand the effects of various toxins (e.g. drugs, alcohol, sepsis) on the liver.

- Understand the liver's role in storage, synthesis and metabolism.

General/Specific Objectives

- Through efficient, focused data gathering:

  - Differentiate between the causal conditions for abnormal liver function tests.

  - Identify complications related to the presence of liver disease.

- Interpret the critical clinical and laboratory findings which were key in the processes of exclusion, differentiation and diagnosis:

  - Select diagnostic tests appropriate for the identification of acute and chronic liver diseases.

  - List the indications for abdominal ultrasound and ascitic fluid analysis.

  - List indications for liver biopsy.

- Conduct an effective plan of management for a patient with abnormal liver function tests:

  - Select patients in need of hospitalisation.

  - List indications for active and passive prophylaxis against infective hepatitis.

  - Select patients in need of specialised care.

  - Counsel and educate patients about primary and secondary prevention strategies for viral hepatitis (include public health measures).

  - Understand the role of monitoring liver function in terms of management of a patient's illness.

008A Hypokalaemia

Overview

Potassium is the major intracellular cation. Of a total body potassium of 3,000 mmol in adults, only two percent is in extracellular fluid (60 mmol) at a concentration of around 5 mmol/L. Normal daily intake is also about 60 mmol. Most excretion is in the urine, which is the source of most depletions, but abnormal gastrointestinal losses are also important. Hypokalaemia usually indicates potassium depletion; and is most often discovered on routine analysis of serum electrolytes or electrocardiogram (ECG) results. Symptoms usually develop much later when depletion is quite severe (muscle weakness, paralytic ileus, cardiac arrhythmias and sensitivity to digitalis). Hypokalaemia implies a serum level below 3.5 mmol/L. Potassium deficiency, metabolic alkalosis, hypocalcaemia and hypomagnesaemia are commonly associated.

Causes

1) Increased losses

a) **Renal losses**
   - ❏ Diuretics
   - ❏ Endocrine effects
     - Prolonged steroid therapy
     - Primary hyperaldosteronism (Conn syndrome)
     - Secondary hyperaldosteronism (e.g. renovascular disease)
     - Adrenal hyperplasia
     - Cushing syndrome
     - Ectopic adrenocorticotrophic hormone (ACTH)

b) **Gastrointestinal losses**
   - ❏ Vomiting – vomiting and pyloric stenosis; secondary renal losses occur as well.
   - ❏ Bowel obstructions and prolonged gastrointestinal aspirates
   - ❏ Diarrhoea (villous adenoma of colorectum, laxative abuse, inflammatory bowel disease (IBD), enteric fistula)

2) Decreased intake (e.g. anorexia nervosa, malnutrition)

3) Redistribution (familial periodic paralysis)

Key Objective

- Assess intake and shift of potassium into cells, select renal loss as the category into which most problems fall, but remember gastrointestinal causes of loss.

General/Specific Objectives

- Through efficient, focused data gathering:

  - Differentiate between renal and gastrointestinal losses as causative lesions.

- Interpret the critical clinical and laboratory findings which were key in the processes of exclusion, differentiation and diagnosis:

  - Outline how urinary electrolytes assist in the elucidation of excess losses of potassium.

- Conduct an effective plan of management for a hypokalaemic patient based on sound principles:

  - Outline indications and guidelines for intravenous (IV) potassium therapy.

008B Hyperkalaemia

Overview

Hyperkalaemia (serum [K^+] greater than 5.5 mmol/L) may produce serious side-effects and may also be indicative of the presence of serious associated medical conditions. Dangerous hyperkalaemia (greater than 6 mmol/L) is rare if renal function is normal, despite significant release of intracellular potassium into the extracellular phase in response to the stress of injury, acidosis, sepsis and any catabolic state. Hyperkalaemia is seen when renal failure and shock interfere with renal handling of potassium.

Causes

1) Reduced urinary excretion in renal failure and shock

    a) Decreased glomerular filtration rate (GFR) in shock, acute or chronic renal failure

    b) Decreased tubular secretion in adrenal insufficiency

    c) Effects of drugs on tubular function (angiotensin-converting enzyme (ACE) inhibitors, nonsteroidal anti-inflammatory drugs (NSAIDs))

2) Redistribution

    a) Red cell lysis

        ❑ Rhabdomyolysis

        ❑ Crush syndrome / Burns

        ❑ Intravascular haemolysis

        ❑ Tumour breakdown

    b) Metabolic acidosis with normal anion gap

Key Objectives

- Diagnose true dangerous hyperkalaemia (greater than 6.0 mmol/L), a potentially lethal condition for which emergency treatment is the first consideration, from pseudohyperkalaemia, due to cell lysis during collection, and screen for causal conditions.

- Recognise that dangerous effects are confined to the heart, and cause changes as in the electrocardiogram (ECG), arrhythmias and death.

- Recognise principles of emergency (temporary plus definitive) treatment of dangerous hyperkalaemia.

General/Specific Objectives

- Through efficient, focused data gathering:

    - Distinguish between life-threatening hyperkalaemia and pseudohyperkalaemia utilising ECG.

    - Recognise signs of dangerous hyperkalaemia on ECG.

    - Distinguish between causes of hyperkalaemia by ruling out redistribution or intake problems quickly, and concentrating on the more common renal causes.

- Interpret the critical clinical and laboratory findings which were key in the processes of exclusion, differentiation and diagnosis:

    - Identify patients with renal failure.

- Outline an effective emergency treatment plan for a dangerously hyperkalaemic patient:

    - Select patients in need of specialised care and dialysis.

    - Understand principles of haemodialysis and peritoneal dialysis.

008C Hypomagnesaemia

Overview

Although hypomagnesaemia occurs in only about 10% of hospitalised patients, the incidence rises to over 60% in severely ill patients. Hypomagnesaemia may be responsible for otherwise puzzling clinical features in patients with prolonged illness. Clinical features are mainly neuromuscular. Magnesium, like potassium, is a predominantly intracellular cation and is poorly absorbed orally, so replenishment is best by intravenous (IV) supplementation.

Causes

1) Gastrointestinal

    a) Marked decrease in dietary intake

    b) Diarrhoea, acute/chronic; malabsorption and steatorrhoea, short gut

    c) Acute pancreatitis

2) Renal loss

    a) Diuretics (loop, thiazide, hypercalcaemia)

    b) Volume expansion

    c) Tubular dysfunction (alcoholics, aminoglycosides, amphotericin, cisplatin, cyclosporin, acute tubular necrosis (ATN) in diuretic phase, primary)

Key Objectives

- Determine which patients are likely to be hypomagnesaemic since magnesium levels are not measured routinely.

- Evaluate patients with ventricular arrhythmias for possible hypomagnesaemia, especially during ischaemic events and if diuretics were prescribed.

General/Specific Objectives

- Through efficient, focused data gathering:

    - Diagnose the cause of hypomagnesaemia.

- Interpret the critical clinical and laboratory findings which were key in the processes of exclusion, differentiation and diagnosis:

    - If no cause is clinically apparent, differentiate between gastrointestinal and renal causes by measuring urinary magnesium excretion.

- Conduct an effective plan of management for a hypomagnesaemic patient:

    - Recognise that cellular uptake of magnesium is slow, and repletion requires sustained correction.

    - Select potassium-sparing diuretics as an adjunct to management in patients with diuretic-induced hypomagnesaemia if diuretic therapy cannot be stopped.

009A Hyponatraemia

Overview

Serum sodium levels comprise the major determinant of extracellular fluid osmolality and are normally held constant within a range of 135–145 mmol/L by regulatory mechanisms acting via sensitive hypothalamic osmoreceptor feedback, utilising stimulation of antidiuretic hormone (ADH) by increased osmolality or vice versa. Causes of increased ADH secretion, apart from hypertonicity of body fluids, include volume depletion, stress, drugs and inappropriate sources of ADH from cerebral injury, tumours or burns. The syndrome of inappropriate ADH secretion (SIADH) is seen quite commonly in the setting of chest infections and other lung conditions and is an idiosyncratic reaction of a number of drugs, particularly thiazide diuretics.

Hyponatraemia implies only a fall in the concentration of serum sodium and may be associated with water gain, sodium depletion or often both.

Hyponatraemia (serum [Na$^+$] less than 135 mmol/L) is often detected in asymptomatic patients because serum electrolytes are measured almost routinely. Minor abnormalities often are transient and need no treatment. In adults or children with hyponatraemia, the cause is usually iatrogenic, and the hyponatraemia dilutional rather than depletional. Normally any fall in body fluid osmolality due to water overload is countered by the excretion of excess water by the kidneys. Poor renal function with poor concentrating power diminishes the ability to cope with excess water, which is also a feature of the early period after major surgery.

Causes

1) Hypo-osmolar hyponatraemia

a) **Water gain**

❏ **Iatrogenic** excess water administration (particularly after operations and in children)

❏ SIADH with decreased water excretion

b) **Sodium depletion**

❏ Renal or extrarenal **sodium and water loss with water replacement in excess of electrolytes** (enteric losses and fistulae, renal losses)

❏ Addison disease

c) **Oedema states**

2) Non–hypo-osmolar hyponatraemia – associated with hyperglycaemia or azotaemia

Key Objectives

- Recognition that hyponatraemia may mean water gain, sodium depletion or a mixture of both.

- Recognition that minor abnormalities are often transient and need no treatment.

- Identification of the main process is important because this will affect need for and choice of therapy, and rate of correction.

- Recognition that water retention is spread over the whole body, and marked intracellular oedema has its most severe effects on essential functions causing mental confusion and ultimately coma.

General/Specific Objectives

- Through efficient, focused data gathering:

  - Determine whether an increase in water relative to sodium exists thereby expanding volume of cells or the change in sodium concentration is artefactual or caused by hyperglycaemia.

  - Differentiate between sodium depletion and water gain by assessment of volume status and/or the presence of an oedema state.

- Interpret critical clinical and laboratory findings which were key in the processes of exclusion, differentiation, and diagnosis:

  - Interpret urinary electrolyte concentrations.

  - Interpret plasma and urinary osmolality.

- Conduct an effective plan of management for a patient with hyponatraemia:

  - Outline a therapeutic approach based on the underlying process.

  - Select the patients with hyponatraemia in need of specialised care or consultation.

N.B. *When serum sodium concentration is measured by flame photometry or other methods requiring major dilution of plasma, hyperlipidaemia or hyperproteinaemia may cause pseudohyponatraemia (iso-osmotic). If sodium concentration is measured with a sodium selective electrode on undiluted plasma (most laboratories today), a true sodium concentration is obtained, and this type of 'pseudohyponatraemia' no longer exists.*

009B Hypernatraemia

Overview
Hypernatraemia is often iatrogenic with solute administration in excess of the water required to excrete it. Thirst is a significant warning sign of hyperosmolar states in the conscious patient. Hypernatraemia is usually associated with inability to respond to thirst by drinking water. Hypernatraemia is thus most likely to be encountered at the extremes of life in the very young and in the very old, in comatose patients and in those depending on tube or parenteral intravenous (IV) feeding.

Causes

1) Sodium gain (relative solute excess)

    a) Excessively concentrated enteric or IV feeding solutions

    b) Primary hyperaldosteronism (Conn syndrome)

2) Water depletion (true dehydration)

    a) Water intake insufficient, inability of unconscious or incapacitated patient to respond to thirst

    b) Excess renal water loss – osmotic diuresis, diabetes insipidus

    c) Excess insensible water loss – fever, overbreathing, burns

Key Objectives
- Recognition that hypernatraemia is almost always caused by a combination of water loss with diminished ability to respond to thirst.

- Recognition of importance of careful monitoring of use of parenteral or enteral feeding solutions in incapacitated patients to avoid hyperosmolar hyperglycaemic hypernatraemic coma.

- Recognise that correction of the hypernatraemic state requires restoring the water deficit to relieve and to reverse the hyperosmolar state, and restoring normal urine output instead of continuing osmotic solute diuresis.

General/Specific Objectives
- Through efficient, focused data gathering:

  - Determine the underlying cause of water loss and/or diminished thirst.

  - Determine the severity of the problem by assessment of patient's volume status.

- Interpret critical clinical and laboratory findings which were key in the processes of exclusion, differentiation, and diagnosis:

    - Evaluate urinary osmolality results in order to differentiate between causes of water loss.

- Conduct an effective plan of management for a patient with hypernatraemia:

    - Outline a therapeutic approach based on the underlying process.

    - Discuss potential side-effects of rapid replacement of water losses.

    - Select the patients with hypernatraemia in need of specialised care or consultation.

Overview

Because abnormalities of white blood cells occur commonly in both asymptomatic as well as acutely ill patients, every clinician will need to evaluate patients for this common problem. Most important to understand are the causes and clinical implications of neutropenia and neutrophilia.

Causes

1)   Leucopenia

a) Neutropenia

❏ Decreased marrow production

- Drug-induced (alkylating agents, antimetabolites, antibiotics (sulphonamides, penicillins, cephalosporins), anti-thyroid drugs (carbimazole, propylthiouracil), anticonvulsant drugs (phenytoin, carbamazapine, sodium valproate), anti-inflammatory drugs (phenylbutazone, gold, diflunisal, penicillamine, naproxen), antidepressants (amitriptyline, dothiepin, mianserin), antimalarial drugs (maloprim, fansidar, chloroquine))

- Nutritional deficiency (vitamin B_{12}, folate)

- Sepsis
    - Viral (hepatitis, human immunodeficiency virus (HIV), influenza)
    - Bacterial (typhoid, tuberculosis (TB))

- Hypersplenism
    - Immune: rheumatoid arthritis (Felty syndrome); systemic lupus erythematosus (SLE)
    - Nonimmune: severe portal hypertension

- Marrow infiltration
    - Malignancy: haematologic (acute and chronic leukaemia); non-haematologic (carcinoma lung)

- Cyclic neutropenia

b) Lyphocytopenia

❏ Drug-induced (glucocorticoids, cytotoxics)

❏ Infections (HIV, TB)

❏ Tumour-associated (lymphoma)

❏ Acute illness (sepsis, myocardial infarction (MI))

❏ Chronic illness (uraemia, congestive cardiac failure (CCF), SLE)

❏ Marrow infiltration (*vide supra*)

c) **Combined neutropenia and lyphocytopenia**

- ❏ Marrow infiltration (*vide supra*)
- ❏ Drug-induced (cytotoxics)
- ❏ Aplastic marrow (idiopathic, benzene, irradiation)

2) Leucocytosis

a) **Neutrophilia**

- ❏ Inflammation
  - • Infective – bacterial
  - • Noninfective
    - - Tissue necrosis / Infarction / Trauma of burns
    - - Autoimmune disorders: SLE/vasculitis
    - - Gout
- ❏ Neoplasia
  - • Myeloproliferative neoplasms, other malignancies
- ❏ Drugs (glucocorticoids, lithium)
- ❏ Acute stress or haemorrhage
- ❏ Post-splenectomy
- ❏ Leukaemoid reactions (white cell count (WCC) greater than 50.0 x 10^9/L – normal range 4.0 – 11.0 x 10^9/L)
  - • Severe sepsis
    - - Acute (septicaemia)
    - - Chronic (TB)
  - • Malignancy
  - • Severe haemolysis
  - • (Chronic myeloid leukaemia is a myeloproliferative disorder ***not*** a leukaemoid reaction)

b) **Lymphocytosis**

- ❏ Infections (viral, TB, pertussis, other)
- ❏ Acute and chronic lymphocytic leukaemia
- ❏ Other (adrenal insufficiency)

Key Objective
- • Interpret the clinical setting in which the leucocyte abnormality occurs as this will often suggest the correct diagnosis and direct further investigation.

General/Specific Objectives

- Through efficient, focused data gathering:

  - Distinguish between chronic conditions requiring non-urgent evaluation and acute life-threatening illnesses requiring admission to hospital.

- Interpret critical clinical and laboratory findings important in formulating a differential diagnosis:

  - Interpret the differential leucocyte count.

  - List the indications for bone marrow aspiration and biopsy.

- Conduct an effective plan of management for a patient with white blood cell abnormalities:

  - Diagnose or exclude infection first as the cause of the leucocyte abnormality.

  - Select patients for specialised care, including those with a neutrophil count of less than 1.0×10^9/L.

  - Counsel and educate patients with chronic leucocyte abnormalities.

011A   *Paediatric Emergencies*

Overview
Although paediatric emergencies such as the ones listed below are discussed with the appropriate condition, the care of the patient in the paediatric age group demands special skills.

Causes

1)   Respiratory emergencies

(see #126 Wheezing/Respiratory Difficulty/Stridor)

a) **Upper respiratory tract disorders** (see #126A Upper Respiratory Tract Disorders)

b) **Lower respiratory tract disorders** (see #126B Lower Respiratory Tract Disorders)

2)   Infectious emergencies

(see #040 Fever and Chills (Adult and Paediatric) and #102B Childhood Communicable Disease With or Without Skin Rash)

3)   Cardiovascular emergencies

a) **Arrhythmias** (see #072 Palpitations (Abnormal Electrocardiogram (ECG) / Arrhythmia))

b) **Congestive heart failure** (see #032A With Diffuse Chest X-Ray Abnormality)

4)   Fluid and electrolyte emergencies

a) **Dehydration / Volume depletion** (see #098 Shock/Hypotension and #009B Hypernatraemia)

b) **Hyperkalaemia** (see #008B Hyperkalaemia)

5)   Neurological emergencies

a) **Seizures** (see #095 Seizures (Epilepsy))

b) **Febrile seizure**

6)   Abdominal emergencies

a) **Abdominal pain** (see #003E Anal Pain)

b) **Abdominal distension** (see #001 Abdominal Distension/Ileus)

7) Trauma

(see #018 Burns and #113 Trauma/Accidents/Prevention)

8) Poisoning

(see #079 Poisoning)

9) Environmental emergencies (hypothermia / heat stroke)

(see #040D Hypothermia and #040E Hyperthermia)

Key Objectives

- Recognise and manage effectively infants and children with life-threatening paediatric emergencies.

- Describe the differences between paediatric and adult medicine and their effect on emergency management.

General/Specific Objectives

- Through efficient, focused data gathering:

    - Elicit symptoms and signs in a focused fashion for the assessment of an infant/child in an urgent/emergent situation.

    - Perform physical examination and blood pressure (BP) measurement and determine whether the patient is in shock.

- Interpret critical clinical and laboratory findings which were key in the processes of exclusion, differentiation and diagnosis.

- Conduct an effective plan of management for an infant/child in an urgent/ emergent situation:

    - Recognise special features of paediatric airway management.

    - List sites for intravenous (IV) access in the paediatric population.

    - Select patients in need of referral to intensive care units.

    - Outline initial management in a paediatric patient with seizures including febrile seizures.

    - Outline initial management in a paediatric patient with acute sepsis.

011B   Crying/Fussing Child

Overview
A young infant whose only symptom is crying/fussing, challenges the doctor to distinguish between the various causes, some of which can be serious.

Causes

1)   Infections (systemic/focal)

2)   Gastrointestinal/Intra-abdominal conditions

    a) Infection

    b) Inflammation

    c) Intussusception

    d) Constipation/Anal fissure

    e) Diarrhoea

3)   Trauma (neglect / child abuse / fracture)

4)   Psychologic / Functional / Hunger / Discomfort / Boredom / Irritability

Key Objective
*   Differentiate paediatric emergencies, including intussusception, from conditions not requiring emergency treatment.

General/Specific Objectives
*   Through efficient, focused data gathering:

    -   Elicit a history of patient's previous behaviour, oral intake of food and drink, vomiting, diarrhoea or constipation, and any medications received.

    -   Assess the parent-child emotional interaction.

- Perform a full physical examination in order to identify the cause of the illness with a focus on searching for sites of infection, intra-abdominal conditions, increased intracranial pressure, cardiac and respiratory disorders.

- Differentiate serious from benign causes, and determine if a life-threatening situation exists.

• Interpret critical clinical and laboratory findings which are key in the processes of exclusion, differentiation and diagnosis:

- Select investigations (when appropriate) to differentiate between acute and benign disease.

• Conduct an effective plan of management for a crying/fussing child:

- Counsel caregivers of crying/fussing children without organic disease.

- Select children who require followup for additional investigation and management.

- Select patients in need of referral.

011C Hypotonia / Floppy Infant

Overview

Children with decreased resistance to passive movement differ from those with weakness and hyporeflexia. They require detailed, careful neurologic evaluation. Management programmes, often life-long, are multidisciplinary and involve patients, family and community.

Causes

1) Central causes

    a) 'Benign congenital hypotonia'

    b) Cerebral malformations (holoprosencephaly); neurodegenerative (leucodystrophy)

    c) Seizures, trauma (subarachnoid or subdural haemorrhage)

    d) Hydrocephalus / Increased intracranial pressure

    e) Infectious causes (e.g. encephalitis, abscess, meningitis)

    f) Neoplasms

    g) Hypoxic/Ischaemic encephalopathy

    h) Effects of toxins and drugs

2) Neural disease, peripheral

    a) Anterior horn cell (e.g. progressive spinal muscular atrophy, spinal cord infarction)

    b) Peripheral nerves / Polyneuropathies (trauma)

    c) Myoneural junction (myasthenia gravis, botulism)

3) Muscular disease

    a) Muscular dystrophy

    b) Myotonic dystrophy

    c) Congenital myopathies

    d) Inflammatory myopathies (dermatomyositis / polymyositis)

4) Metabolic/Electrolyte causes (hypokalaemia, hypoglycaemia, etc.)

5) Other genetic causes (trisomy 21, Prader-Willi syndrome, Niemann-Pick disease, Tay-Sachs disease)

Key Objectives

- Determine the presence of conditions amenable to rapid treatment (electrolyte imbalance, seizure, infection, intracranial bleeding, hydrocephalus).

- Differentiate infants with generalised hypotonia from those with weakness and hyporeflexia.

General/Specific Objectives

- Through efficient, focused data gathering:

  - Determine birth history, age and rapidity of onset and progression of symptoms.

  - Determine whether lesion is localised or general, through appropriate observation of posture, together with neurological, muscle and joint examination.

- Interpret critical clinical and laboratory findings which were key in the processes of exclusion, differentiation and diagnosis:

  - Select investigations to differentiate central from neuromuscular causes (e.g. computed tomography (CT) versus serum creatine kinase (CK), electromyelography (EMG), muscle biopsy).

  - Determine which children require genetic studies.

- Conduct an effective plan of management for a floppy infant:

  - Determine whether respiratory status is adequate or intubation is required.

  - Counsel families with afflicted children about management, prognosis and genetic implications.

  - Develop a management plan that involves the family and community resources.

  - Select patients in need of specialised care.

Overview

Anaemia may be the sole manifestation of serious medical disease. Anaemia may be due to blood loss, decreased production or increased destruction of red blood cells. Simple tests may provide important information. Key to an understanding of anaemia is a full blood examination (FBE) (which includes a blood film). This will give an indication as to both the aetiology and the severity of the anaemia, and will guide the direction for further investigation.

Causes

1)   Normocytic

    a) Decreased production (bone marrow disease, reduced erythropoietin, drugs)

    b) Increased destruction

        ❏ Red blood cell (RBC) abnormalities

        ❏ Auto-antibodies

        ❏ Drugs

    c) Blood loss (visible, occult)

    d) Apparent (dilutional anaemia, e.g. of pregnancy)

2)   Microcytic (iron deficiency, chronic blood loss, haemoglobinopathies)

3)   Macrocytic (folate, vitamin B_{12} deficiency, chemotherapy, alcohol abuse)

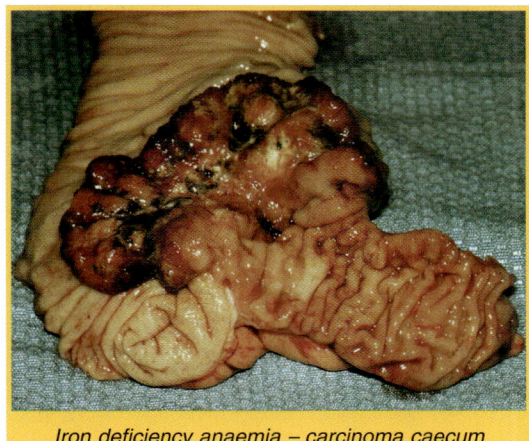

Iron deficiency anaemia – carcinoma caecum

Key Objectives

- Be able to interpret a blood count and film.

- Understand that iron deficiency anaemia may indicate the presence of serious gastrointestinal disease.

- By considering the clinical context, determine if anaemia is present, since all three laboratory indices of anaemia are concentration measurements.

- Interpret the signs and symptoms of anaemia with the understanding that they are dependent on the rapidity with which anaemia developed.

General/Specific Objectives

- Through efficient, focused data gathering:

  - Determine the presence of anaemia and differentiate between the various causes, according to the patient's age.

  - Select a causal classification of anaemias using red cell morphology.

- Interpret critical clinical and laboratory findings which were key in the processes of exclusion, differentiation, and diagnosis:

  - Outline diagnostic plans for an adult presenting with an iron-deficiency anaemia.

- Conduct an effective plan of management for a patient with anaemia:

  - Outline treatment of iron deficiency anaemia.

  - Outline treatment of vitamin deficiency anaemias.

  - Select patients in need of referral for haematological consultation and care (e.g. haemolysis, bone marrow disease).

  - Conduct counselling and education of patients with anaemia caused by nutritional deficiencies and haemoglobinopathies.

Overview

Doctors may be confronted by developmental and behavioural problems of childhood and adolescence and required to liaise with other caregivers.

Causes

Learning disability – differential diagnosis includes:

1) **Global cognitive problem (mental retardation or borderline IQ)**

2) **Sensory impairment (auditory/visual)**

3) **Family emotional disturbance: oppositional defiant / conduct disorder**

4) **Anxiety/Mood disorders**

5) **Developmental coordination disorder**

6) **Dyslexia**

7) **Attention deficit hyperactivity (hyperkinetic) disorder (ADHD)**
   a) Predominantly inattentive
   b) Hyperactive/Impulsive
   c) Combined

8) **Pervasive developmental disorder**
   a) Autistic disorder
   b) Rett disorder/syndrome
   c) Childhood disintegrative disorder
   d) Asperger disorder

9) **Communication and language**

10) **Child abuse or neglect**

11) **Chronic medical disease**

12) **Tic disorder**

13) **Drug or alcohol dependence**

Key Objectives

- Make a clinical assessment of a child's developmental level.

- List the criteria of ADHD.

General/Specific Objectives

- Through efficient, focused data gathering:

  - Determine whether environmental factors in school or family may be contributing to school failure.

  - Determine whether there is a family history for attention deficit or any of the comorbid conditions.

  - Determine whether there is evidence of developmental delay, genetic syndromes, encephalopathies, or poisoning (e.g. alcohol, lead).

- Interpret critical clinical and laboratory findings which were key in the processes of exclusion, differentiation and diagnosis:

  - Select patients who require further investigation or psychological testing.

- Conduct an effective plan of management for a patient with school failure:

  - Select patients in need of specialised care.

  - Along with other caregivers, outline a management plan which includes (when appropriate):

    * Parent, child and teacher education and other educational interventions.

    * Structured educational and recreational activities.

    * Behavioural management strategies.

    * Psychological counselling.

    * Medication.

  - Discuss the use of medication (amphetamine derivatives) in the treatment of ADHD.

014 Behaviour Disorder

(See also #026 Development Disorder / Developmental Delay)

Overview
Clinicians are usually the initial caregivers to be confronted by the developmental and behavioural problems of childhood and adolescence, which can lead to impaired social, academic and occupational functioning. The behaviour disorders are more common in males, eating disorders are more common in females. The early diagnosis of autism is particularly difficult.

Causes

| 1) | Attention deficit hyperactivity (hyperkinetic) disorder (ADHD) |

| 2) | Oppositional defiant / Conduct disorder |

| 3) | Eating disorders (anorexia nervosa / bulimia, pica, rumination disorder) |

| 4) | Sleep disorders (nightmares, sleep terror disorder, sleepwalking, enuresis) |

| 5) | Tic disorders (Tourette syndrome, motor or vocal tic disorders) |

| 6) | Autism |

Key Objective
- Determine whether the patient has a behaviour disorder or some other underlying medical condition, mood disorder or a comorbid developmental disability.

General/Specific Objectives

- Through efficient, focused data gathering, which includes assessment of family history, context and culture:

  - Determine whether the patient requires consultation with a psychiatrist/ psychologist for oppositional defiant or conduct disorder.

  - Determine whether criteria for anorexia/bulimia are present (on history and physical examination).

  - Determine whether a patient with a tic disorder requires referral to a paediatrician, neurologist, or child psychologist.

  - Determine whether a patient with a sleep disorder requires further investigation or specialist referral.

- Interpret critical clinical and laboratory findings which were key in the processes of exclusion, differentiation and diagnosis:

  - Select patients requiring further investigation.

- Conduct an effective plan of management for a patient with behaviour disorder:

  - Discuss indications for hospital admission in a patient with an eating disorder.

  - In a patient with an eating disorder, outline a management plan including (when appropriate) psychotherapy (individual and family), behaviour modification techniques, nutritional therapy, and medication.

Overview

A bleeding tendency can manifest with cutaneous and/or systemic features. It may signify a drug-induced disorder, a problem of haemostasis or a vessel abnormality. Taking a detailed history (including a family history) is essential.

Causes

1) Platelet problem

a) **Decreased number**
- Decreased production (e.g. leukaemia)
- Increased destruction
- Abnormal sequestration

b) **Abnormal function**
- Congenital
- Acquired
  - Drugs (aspirin)
  - Renal disease

2) Coagulation factor problem

a) **Congenital**
- Factor VIII deficiency
- von Willebrand disease
- Factor IX deficiency

b) **Acquired**
- Liver disease
- Anticoagulants
- Disseminated intravascular coagulation (DIC)
- Vitamin K deficiency
- Inhibitors
- Drugs (heparin-induced thrombocytopenia)
- Massive blood transfusion

3) Vessel problem

a) **Congenital (collagen disorders)**

b) **Acquired (steroids, vasculitis)**

Key Objectives

- Understand the role of a clinical history in determining the cause of a bleeding disorder.

- Be aware of the appropriate clinical signs and tests that will help to determine the underlying cause of a bleeding disorder.

General/Specific Objectives

- Through efficient, focused data gathering:

    - Differentiate between platelet problems, coagulation factor problems, and vessel problems.

- Interpret critical clinical and laboratory findings which were key in the processes of exclusion, differentiation, and diagnosis:

    - Select investigative tests appropriate for platelet, coagulation, and vessel problems.

    - Contrast the results and their interpretation.

    - Select 'at risk' families for investigation of potentially affected children.

- Conduct an effective plan of management for a patient with bleeding tendency or bruising:

    - Select platelet transfusions, vitamin K, and plasma derivatives in the management of patients with bleeding disorders according to the diagnosis made.

    - Formulate a management plan for the reversal of the anticoagulant effect of heparin, warfarin or aspirin.

    - Select patients in need of specialised care.

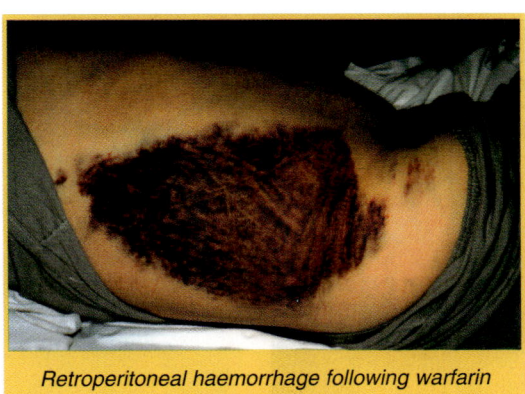

Retroperitoneal haemorrhage following warfarin

Overview

Occult gastrointestinal bleeding may be due to serious gastrointestinal disease (carcinoma of the colon or stomach). Screening the stool for occult blood in high-risk groups may increase diagnostic yield.

Bright red blood unmixed with the stool noticed at the time of defaecation is usually due to a benign anorectal cause, but other associated serious pathology must be excluded.

Acute lower gastrointestinal bleeding with fresh blood and clots independent of defaecation is usually colonic and associated with colonic diverticula. Localisation of the bleeding source can be difficult.

Melaena (a black tarry stool), with or without haematemesis, almost invariably signifies significant upper gastrointestinal haemorrhage.

Causes

1) Upper gastrointestinal bleeding with melaena

(see #048 Haematemesis/Melaena)

2) Lower gastrointestinal bleeding

a) Colorectal cancer/polyp

b) Anorectal disease (haemorrhoids, anal fissure, acute or chronic)

c) Colonic diverticulosis

d) Angiodysplasia

e) Enterocolitis (ischaemic, infectious, inflammatory bowel disease (IBD), nonsteroidal anti-inflammatory drugs (NSAIDs))

f) Other (small bowel neoplasms, Meckel diverticulum)

3) Occult blood in stool

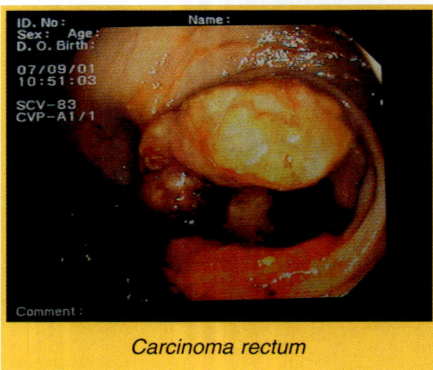
Carcinoma rectum

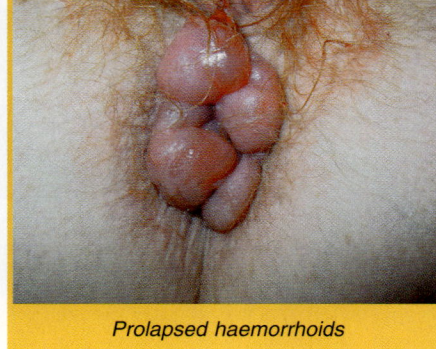
Prolapsed haemorrhoids

Key Objective

- List the three key steps in the management of the separate presentations of lower gastrointestinal bleeding as: resuscitation and assessment; localisation; and diagnosis and treatment.

General/Specific Objectives

- Through efficient, focused data gathering:

    - Define the relationship between bleeding and defaecation.

    - Undertake an appropriate examination to determine the cause of the bleeding.

    - List and diagnose the most likely cause of blood in the stool.

    - Identify patients requiring urgent assessment and treatment.

    - List and diagnose the presence of associated medical conditions predisposing to the development of colorectal cancer.

- Interpret critical clinical and laboratory findings which were key in the processes of exclusion, differentiation and diagnosis:

    - List advantages and disadvantages for anoscopy, rectoscopy, sigmoidoscopy, colonoscopy versus barium studies, radionuclide imaging, and angiography in patients with blood in the stool and the appropriate time to perform these.

    - Select asymptomatic patients in need of screening for colorectal cancer.

    - Outline the diagnostic value and limitations of contrasting haematochezia (fresh blood in stool) and melaena.

- Conduct an effective plan of management for a patient with blood in stool:

    - Select patients in need of immediate therapy.

    - Contrast diagnostic and management plans for patients with persisting acute lower gastrointestinal haemorrhage with plans for evaluation of intermittent passage of bright blood unmixed with the stool.

    - Evaluate patients in a cost-effective manner.

    - Outline the assets and limitations of screening using faecal occult blood testing.

    - Select patients in need of specialised care.

017A Male (Gynaecomastia)

Overview

Physiologic gynaecomastia is common in the newborn, in adolescence, and in males over 50 years of age. In pathologic gynaecomastia, a definite aetiology is found in the minority; but a careful drug history is important to detect a treatable cause, as is clinical screening for occult malignancy. An underlying feature is increased oestrogen to androgen ratio.

Causes

1) Physiologic gynaecomastia

a) **Newborn**

b) **Adolescence**

c) **Ageing (50–80 years; decreased testosterone or increased binding globulin)**

2) Pathologic gynaecomastia

a) **Deficient production or action of testosterone**
- ❏ Anorchia
- ❏ Defects in testosterone synthesis
- ❏ Orchitis
- ❏ Renal failure

b) **Increased oestrogen production**
- ❏ Testicular tumours
- ❏ Other tumours producing human chorionic gonadotropin (hCG)
- ❏ Klinefelter syndrome
- ❏ Hyperthyroidism
- ❏ Liver disease
- ❏ Obesity
- ❏ Malnutrition/Starvation

c) **Drugs**
- ❏ Oestrogens/Oestrogen-like (oral contraceptive pill (OCP), digitalis)
- ❏ Anabolic steroids in body-builders
- ❏ Inhibitors of testosterone synthesis or action (spironolactone, cimetidine, flutamide)
- ❏ Other drugs (methyldopa, captopril, tricyclics)

d) **Idiopathic**

Key Objectives

- Differentiate between gynaecomastia and breast cancer.

- Differentiate between gynaecomastia and pseudogynaecomastia (fat deposition without glandular proliferation).

General/Specific Objectives

- Through efficient, focused data gathering:

  - Differentiate patients with gynaecomastia due to physiologic or pathologic causes.

- Identify patients who require further investigation.

- Interpret the critical clinical and laboratory findings which were key in the processes of exclusion, differentiation and diagnosis:

  - Select and interpret laboratory tests in the investigation of gynaecomastia.

  - Select and interpret imaging tests and cytology/histology in the investigation of gynaecomastia.

- Conduct an effective plan of management for a patient with gynaecomastia:

  - Diagnose patients with physiologic gynaecomastia who require no specific therapy.

  - Diagnose patients with drug-induced gynaecomastia who would benefit from withdrawal of the drug.

  - Identify patients requiring surgery.

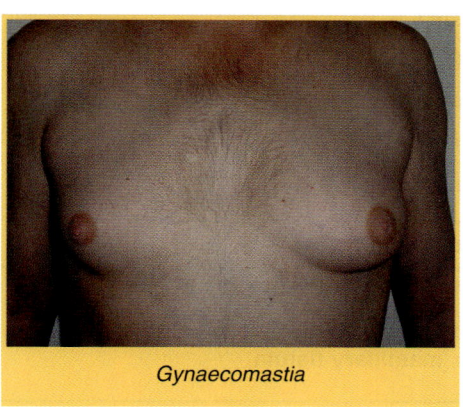

Gynaecomastia

017B   Female (Breast Lump / Prevention of Cancer / Screening)

Overview

Breast cancer is the most common cancer in women. One in 13 Australian women will develop breast cancer in their lifetime. Screening women over 50 years and other high-risk groups by regular two-yearly mammography improves survival and identifies small preclinical lesions. A small but significant proportion of patients have familial cancer in whom genetic screening and counselling may be helpful.

Causes

1)   Breast carcinoma (the most important, although not the most common cause of a breast lump)

a) **Non-invasive**
- ❏ Ductal carcinoma-*in-situ* (DCIS)
- ❏ Lobular carcinoma-*in-situ* (LCIS)

b) **Invasive**
- ❏ Invasive ductal carcinoma
- ❏ Invasive lobular carcinoma
- ❏ Others (tubular, medullary, papillary, mucinous)

2)   Diffuse nodularity – fibrocystic change

3)   Discrete benign breast lumps ('dominant lumps')

a) **Localised fibrocystic change**

b) **Gross cysts**

c) **Galactoceles**

d) **Fibroadenomas**

e) **Traumatic fat necrosis**

f) **Mammary duct ectasia**

4)   Breast infections

a) **Associated with lactation – lactational mastitis / breast abscess**

b) **Not associated with lactation – mammary duct ectasia, subareolar abscess, mamillary fistula**

5)   Rarer causes – phyllodes tumour (usually benign – and only locally invasive, occasionally true sarcoma)

Key Objectives

- Ability to perform a standardised clinical breast examination, ensuring correct patient comfort and positioning, and appropriate technique.

- Ability to distinguish normal from abnormal and suspicious findings.

- Understanding risk factors for development of breast cancer in women.

- Understanding the investigations for mammography and breast ultrasound and the appropriateness of each for different clinical situations and age groups.

- Understanding the principles of management of breast cancer by surgery and adjuvant means.

General/Specific Objectives

- Through efficient, focused data gathering:

  - Determine which women are at high risk for breast cancer.

- Interpret critical clinical and laboratory findings, which were key in the processes of exclusion, differentiation and diagnosis.

- Identify groups based on age or other pre-existing risk factors for regular screening mammography; outline benefits and drawbacks of screening programmes.

- Identify families in whom genetic screening and counselling may be considered; outline the benefits and drawbacks of genetic screening.

- Counsel and educate patients on the role of breast self-examination.

- Conduct an effective diagnostic/management plan for a patient presenting with a breast lump:

  - Outline an algorithm for diagnosis of a patient presenting with a breast lump. Which patients do NOT require surgery?

  - Outline the indications for percutaneous fine needle aspiration cytology (FNAC) and core biopsy in patients with breast pathology.

  - Outline the indications for surgery, radiotherapy, hormonal antihormonal therapy, and chemotherapy in women with breast cancer.

  - Outline the indications for breast-conserving surgery in women with breast carcinoma.

  - Counsel women with risk factors for the development of breast cancer on the utility of screening.

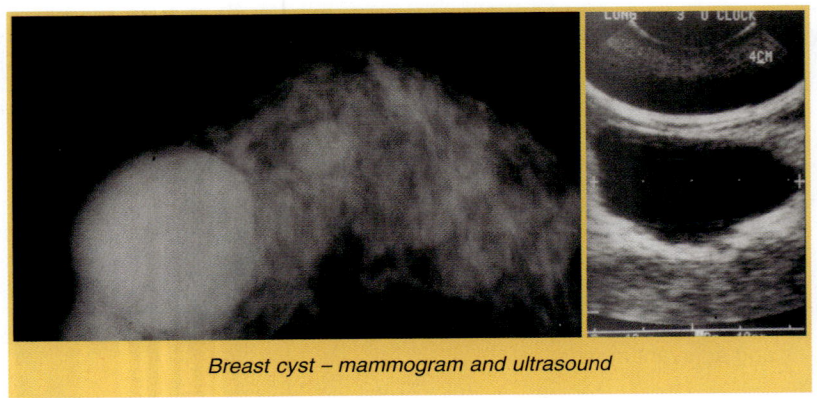

Breast cyst – mammogram and ultrasound

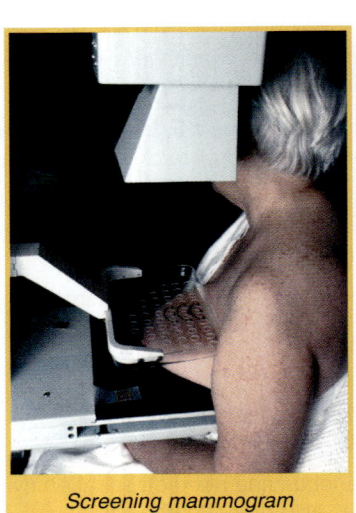

Screening mammogram

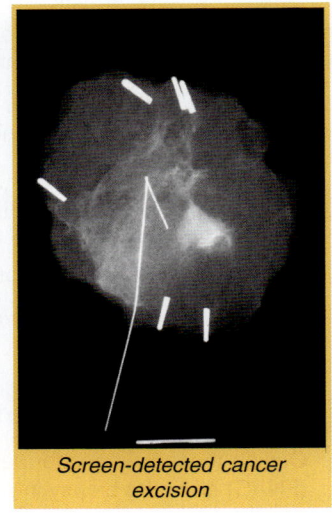

Screen-detected cancer excision

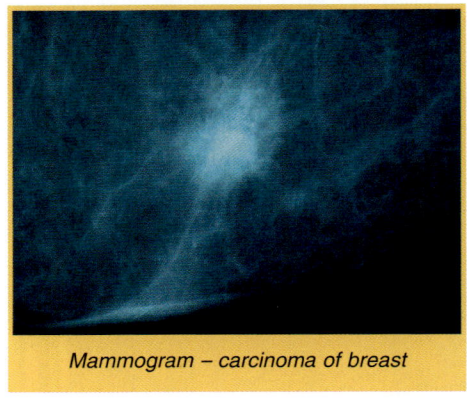

Mammogram – carcinoma of breast

017C Nipple Discharge / Galactorrhoea

Overview

Nipple discharge is a common symptom of concern to the patient. Spontaneous discharges are of more significance than those evoked only by squeezing, as are bloody discharges from a single duct. In the absence of an accompanying lump, the cause is almost always benign. Although milky breast secretions may be noticeable (and are normal) in 25% of previously pregnant women, spontaneous persistent galactorrhoea may reflect underlying breast or endocrine disease and requires investigation.

Causes

1) Nipple discharge

    a) **Bloody:** breast neoplasm, usually benign duct papilloma

    b) **Serous, green, yellow-brown:** usually benign fibrocystic change

    c) **Toothpaste, worms:** mammary duct ectasia

2) True galactorrhoea (fat droplets present)

    a) **Autonomous prolactin production**

        ❑ Pituitary tumours (micro- or macro-adenoma)

        ❑ Ectopic production of prolactin (bronchogenic or renal cell cancer)

    b) **Enhanced prolactin release**

        ❑ Hypothyroidism

        ❑ Sucking reflex

    c) **Failure to inhibit release of prolactin**

        ❑ Pituitary stalk section or compression by mass lesion

        ❑ Drugs (phenothiazines, methyldopa, opiates)

    d) **Idiopathic (most common cause)**

Key Objectives

- Identify patients with nipple discharge requiring surgery.
- Differentiate between nipple discharge and galactorrhoea.
- Differentiate physiological from pathological galactorrhoea.

General/Specific Objectives

- Through efficient, focused data gathering:

  - Identify patients with spontaneous or evoked, unilateral or bilateral, single or multiple duct discharges and different types of discharge.

  - For galactorrhoea, determine which patients have menstrual irregularities or visual field defects since they are likely to have an underlying disease.

- Interpret critical clinical and laboratory findings which were key in the processes of exclusion, differentiation and diagnosis:

  - Select and interpret laboratory tests and diagnostic imaging in patients with nipple discharge/galactorrhoea.

- Outline an effective plan of diagnosis and management for a patient with nipple discharge:

  - Determine which patients are likely to have a breast neoplasm.

  - Outline the role of surgery in patients with nipple discharge

  - List the medications which can cause galactorrhoea.

  - Outline the role of bromocriptine and other dopamine agonists in the management of patients with hyperprolactinaemia and galactorrhoea.

  - Counsel and educate patients with chronic galactorrhoea how the galactorrhoea may be minimised.

017D   Breast Pain (Mastalgia)

Overview
Breast pain is a very common symptom in women. It is rarely caused by malignant disease, and pain severity varies widely. Mastalgia is most common between the ages of 30–50 years; it is unusual after the menopause, apart from those patients on hormone replacement therapy (HRT). Pain may be cyclical or non-cyclical, bilateral or unilateral. Pain is a feature of acute infections (mastitis / breast abscess) complicating lactation.

Causes

1)	**Cyclical mastalgia and nodularity (two-thirds)**

2)	**Non-cyclical mastalgia**

3)	**Focal mastitis/abscess**

4)	**Extramammary causes (costochondritis / Tietze syndrome, musculoligamentous strain, etc.)**

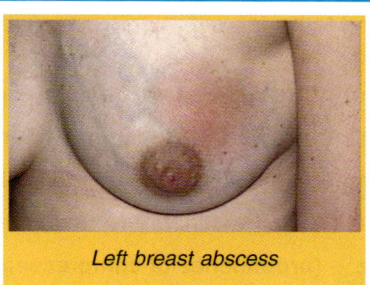

Left breast abscess

Key Objectives
- Exclude focal treatable lesions (inflammations, infections, neoplasms).

- Arrange treatment according to severity and with appropriate reassurance as to benign aetiology.

General/Specific Objectives
- Through efficient, focused data gathering:

  - Identify focal or diffuse infective mastitis and treat appropriately with antibiotics, expression or drainage.

- Interpret critical clinical and laboratory findings which were key in the process of exclusion, differentiation and diagnosis.

  - Select appropriate investigations in a patient with mastalgia.

- Conduct an appropriate step-wise plan of management for a patient with mastalgia.

017E   Breast – Skin Changes

Overview

Skin changes involving the breast, nipple and areola may indicate tethering or invasion from an underlying carcinoma. Physical examination should be meticulous to identify suspicious features.

Causes

1)   Nipple and areola

    a) Paget disease – underlying duct carcinoma

    b) Simple dermatitis/eczema

    c) Benign squamous papilloma of nipple, accessory nipple(s)

    d) Enlarged/Inflamed sudoriferous gland (Montgomery follicle)

    e) Retraction – significant if recent and fixed (underlying carcinoma)

2)   Skin of breast

    a) Skin dimple and tethering over carcinoma (may only be evident on raising arms)

    b) 'Peau d'orange' – due to dermal oedema (neoplastic or inflammatory)

    c) Subcutaneous 'string' from lymphangitis (Mondor disease)

    d) Intertrigo (common beneath pendulous large breasts)

    e) Mamillary sinus/fistula (secondary to mammary duct ectasia)

    f) 'Pseudolipoma' – (prominence of compressed fat overlying a deeper carcinoma)

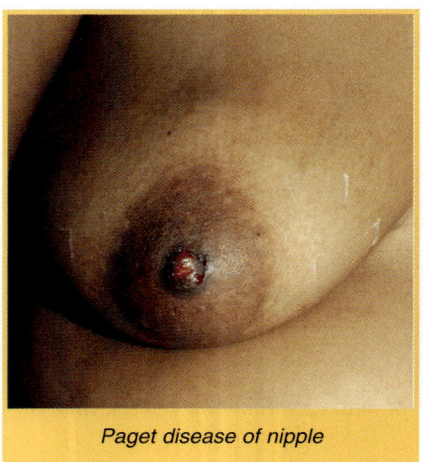

Paget disease of nipple

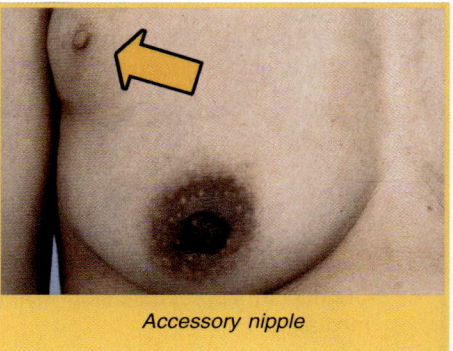

Accessory nipple

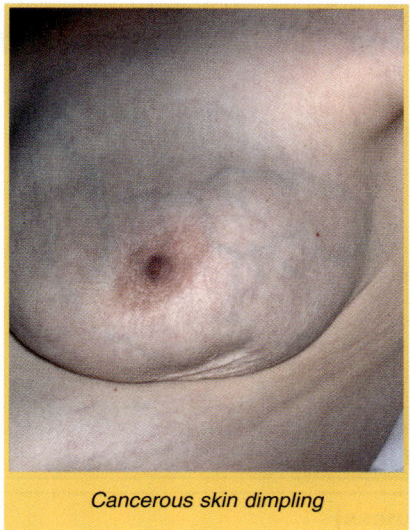

Cancerous skin dimpling

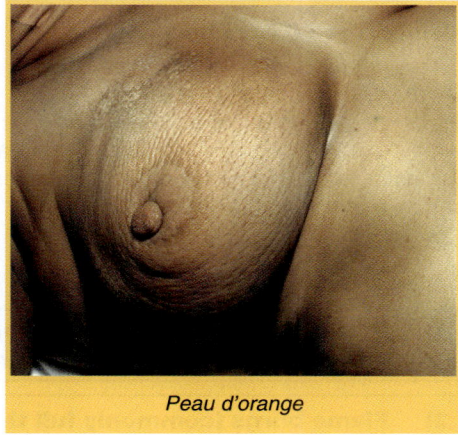

Peau d'orange

(See also #113C Burn Injuries)

Overview

Burns range from minor cutaneous wounds to massive life-threatening traumas, and remain a frequent cause of accidental death, and of gross burn morbidity. Many domestic and industrial accidents are preventable. Public education concerning risks and their avoidance is of major importance.

Causes

1) **Scalds (hot water spills are commonly partial thickness, molten metal spills cause full thickness localised burns)**

2) **Flame burns (commonly full thickness)**

3) **Burns from radiant heat and hot objects**

4) **Electrical burns (high amperage and voltage electrical burns add risks of electrocution)**

5) **Chemical burns (cause additional damage by continuing contact)**

6) **Requiring special care**

   a) Partial thickness (second degree) and full thickness (third degree) greater than 10% body surface area (BSA) in patients aged less than 10 and more than 50 years or greater than 20% any age

   b) Second and third degree greater than 15% BSA require intravenous (IV) replacement; greater than 20% BSA require urinary catheter

   c) Second and third degree on face, hands, feet, genitalia, perineum, major joints

   d) Third degree greater than 5% BSA

   e) Electrical burns (including lightning) and chemical burns

   f) Circumferential burns

   g) Burns plus other serious illness

Key Objectives

- Perform assessment and initial treatment of burn patients according to emergency management of severe trauma (EMST) protocol: primary survey, secondary survey, etc.

- Diagnose burns according to:

  - Percentage BSA involved ('rule of nines', modified in children).

  - Depth of skin injury.

  - Partial thickness burns (first and second degree) – erythema, blistering, moist exudates, soft, painful to pinprick, circulation present.

  - Full thickness burns (third and fourth degree) – dull white, opaque, brown and charred, visible thrombosed veins, dry, firm, painless to pinprick, no capillary response.

- Outline effective management plans for:

  - The burned patient.

  - The burn wound.

General/Specific Objectives

- Through efficient, focused data gathering:

  - Determine the BSA affected first, since depth is difficult to determine initially.

  - After 24 hours, determine depth of skin injury (first degree to fourth degree).

  - Determine whether there are other associated clinical problems or other trauma.

  - Determine patient's tetanus immunisation status.

  - Determine whether inhalation injury has caused respiratory distress.

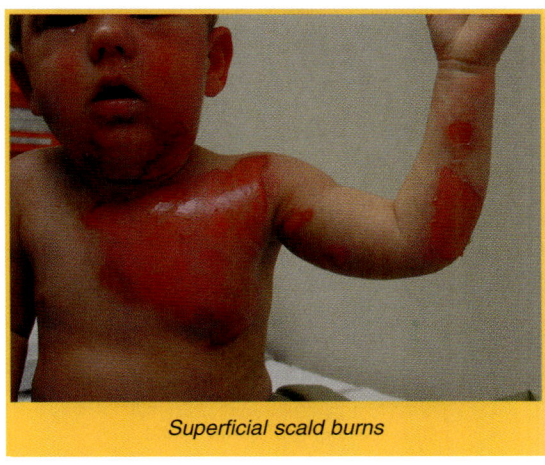

Superficial scald burns

- Interpret critical clinical and laboratory findings which were key in the processes of exclusion, differentiation and diagnosis:

  - Determine whether carbon monoxide poisoning has occurred by measuring carboxyhaemoglobin.

- Conduct an effective plan of management for a patient with severe burns:

  - Outline initial management in a burn patient who will require referral including stopping further burn injury, covering of burn area, and resuscitation with oxygen, IV fluids, and physiologic monitoring.

  - Outline initial topical antibacterial treatment.

  - Discuss mechanism of injury of electrical burns and need for cardiac and renal monitoring.

  - Select patients in need of specialised care.

- Outline an appropriate initial plan of IV fluid replacement (e.g. %BSA x kg weight x 2 ml fluid in first 24 hours – one-third first 4 hours, one-third next 8 hours, one-third next 12 hours).

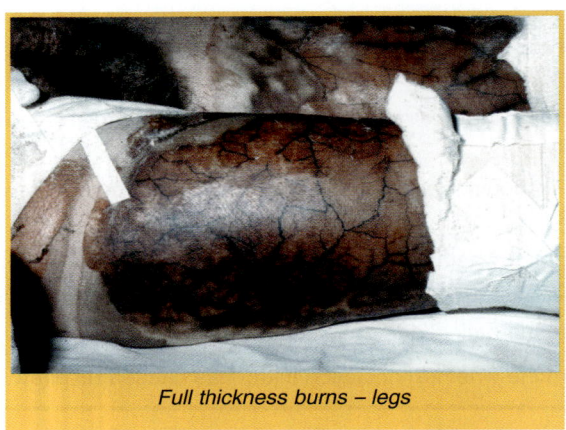

Full thickness burns – legs

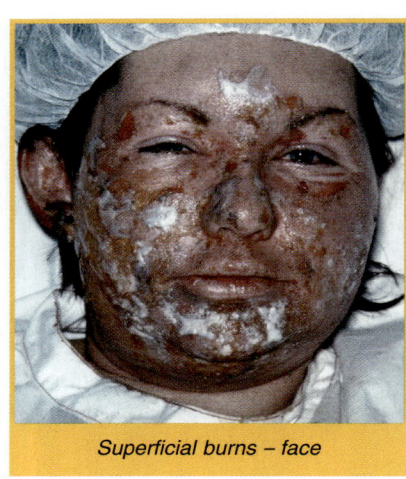

Superficial burns – face

Overview

Most cases of cardiac arrest occur secondary to a cardiac arrhythmia. The ability to perform and manage cardio-pulmonary resuscitation effectively is a pre-requisite for all medical graduates.

Causes

1) Tachyarrhythmias (marked)

    a) Ventricular fibrillation/tachycardia

    b) Atrial fibrillation/flutter

2) Bradyarrhythmias / Asystole

    a) Sinus bradycardia / Arrest / Sick sinus syndrome

    b) Third degree block (slow/absent escape rhythm)

3) Acute vascular occlusion

    a) Myocardial infarction (MI)

    b) Obstruction of cardiac filling

       ❏ Pulmonary embolus (massive)

       ❏ Acute cardiac tamponade

       ❏ Tension pneumothorax

    c) Mechanical heart valve blockage

4) Cardiac/Vascular ruptures

    a) Type I dissecting aortic aneurysm

    b) Ventricular rupture

    c) Mitral papillary muscle rupture with torrential mitral regurgitation

5) Vasodepressor collapse

    a) Neurocardiogenic collapse

    b) Hypersensitive carotid sinus syndrome

    c) Marked orthostatic hypotension

Key Objective

- Be confident and competent in your ability to manage a cardio-pulmonary arrest.

General/Specific Objectives

- Conduct an effective plan of management for a patient with cardiac arrest / respiratory arrest:

  - Evaluate the status of the airway and provide respiratory support as indicated.

  - Demonstrate the techniques of cardiopulmonary resuscitation (CPR) according to the age of the patient.

- Through efficient, focused data gathering:

  - Identify and interpret quickly the signs of impending and actual cardiac and/or respiratory arrest.

  - Differentiate between the possible causes of the cardiac and/or respiratory arrest.

- Interpret critical clinical and laboratory findings which were key in the processes of exclusion, differentiation and diagnosis:

  - Select and interpret appropriate investigations for patients presenting with cardiac and/or respiratory arrest, including electrocardiography, chest X-ray, serum electrolytes, and blood gases.

  - If the resuscitation attempt was not successful, communicate, with sensitivity, the news of death to family members and discuss the possibility of an autopsy if indicated; if resuscitation is successful, communicate with sensitivity, the news to the family and answer all pertinent questions.

Overview

Chest pain may be central or peripheral. Central chest pain is a common presentation of cardiac disease, but it may also be due to disease of the lungs, gastrointestinal tract or a musculoskeletal disorder. Coronary artery disease (CAD) is a potential life-threatening disease. Doctors must recognise the manifestations of CAD and the key characteristics that help to distinguish cardiac pain from other causes of chest pain.

Causes

1) Ischaemic heart disease

    a) Acute myocardial infarction (MI)

    b) Angina pectoris (stable, unstable, microvascular, coronary spasm)

2) Mitral valve prolapse

3) Aortic dissection

    a) Hypertensive

    b) Cystic medial necrosis, Marfan syndrome, Ehlers-Danlos syndrome

    c) Connective tissue disease

    d) Syphilis

4) Pericarditis

    a) Infective
- Viral (Bornholm disease)
- Bacterial

    b) Noninfective
- Post-myocardial infarction
- Post–coronary artery bypass graft (CABG)
- Uraemic
- Connective tissue disease

5) Pulmonary causes (embolism, pneumonia, pleuritis, pneumothorax, etc.)

6) Chest wall origin

    a) Costochondritis (Tietze syndrome)

    b) Herpes zoster

a) **Anxiety, hyperventilation syndrome**

b) **Cardiac neurosis**

Key Objectives

- Know the key characteristics that help to distinguish cardiac and non-cardiac sources of chest pain.

- Differentiate between MI and other forms of CAD early, in order to take advantage of potential life-saving therapy.

General/Specific Objectives

- Through efficient, focused data gathering:

    - Differentiate cardiac pain from other types of visceral pain.

    - Differentiate MI from unstable and stable angina.

- Interpret critical clinical and laboratory findings which were key in the processes of exclusion, differentiation, and diagnosis:

    - Select and interpret electrocardiograms (ECGs) and cardiac enzymes, and discuss newer biochemical markers (such as troponin).

    - Select and interpret diagnostic imaging of the chest.

- Conduct an effective plan of management for a patient with chest pain:

    - Outline initial management of stable and unstable angina, acute MI, and other causes of chest discomfort.

    - List indications and contraindications of thrombolytic therapy and list potential complications.

    - Select patients in need of specialised care and/or consultation.

    - Counsel patients with chest pain caused by life-threatening conditions and counsel their families.

    - Identify the coronary risk factors and define a plan of management for these where appropriate.

    - State the long term management of patients after MI, including secondary prevention strategies.

    - Select cost-effective investigative and therapeutic modalities.

    - Discuss primary and secondary preventive strategy education for patients with ischaemic heart disease.

Overview

Patients with altered level of consciousness account for five percent of hospital admissions. Causes range from those which are rapidly treatable and recoverable, to those causing severe morbidity and mortality. Management of prolonged coma requires expert and intensive nursing and medical care and monitoring for changing levels of consciousness.

Causes

1) Metabolic encephalopathy

    a) Drugs or toxins (e.g. alcohol)

    b) Electrolyte abnormalities (hyponatraemia/hypernatraemia, hypercalcaemia, hypoglycaemia)

    c) Liver or renal failure

    d) Hypertensive encephalopathy

    e) Hypoxaemia/Hypercapnia

    f) Sepsis (systemic)

2) Structural brain damage

    a) Hemispheric (haemorrhage, ischaemia/infarction, neoplastic, traumatic)

    b) Brainstem (haemorrhage, ischaemia/infarction, neoplastic, traumatic)

3) Infectious

    a) Central nervous system (CNS) (meningitis, encephalitis)

    b) Non-CNS (sepsis)

4) Miscellaneous

    a) Seizure (post-ictus)

    b) Myxoedema

5) Malingering

Key Objective

- Diagnosis and management of coma relies on the knowledge of the potential causes, an interpretation of simple clinical signs and the efficient use of diagnostic tests.

General/Specific Objectives

- Through efficient, focused data gathering:

  - Determine the most likely cause for, and seriousness, of coma by means of physical examination leading to rational investigation.

  - Conduct a clinical assessment of the level of consciousness.

- Interpret critical clinical and laboratory findings which were key in the processes of exclusion, differentiation and diagnosis:

  - Select and interpret laboratory investigations for patients suspected of metabolic encephalopathy.

  - Select diagnostic imaging appropriate for comatose patient.

- Conduct an effective plan of management for a patient with coma/impaired consciousness:

  - Define level of consciousness utilising the Glasgow Coma Scale.

  - Select patients in need of immediate therapy and perform initial treatment.

  - Select patients in need of specialised care.

  - Outline potential issues of importance in the ethical management of the incompetent patient, including those of consent for treatment and advanced directives.

  - Conduct assessment for suspected brain death prior to referring patient to neurological specialist for the definitive diagnosis of brain death.

Overview

Delirium is a common and serious problem, particularly in the elderly, the hospitalised and postoperative patients. It represents a disturbance of consciousness and cognitive impairment with reduced ability to focus, sustain, or shift attention (The Diagnostic and Statistical Manual 4 – Text Revision (DSM-IV-TR)). This disturbance tends to develop over a short period of time (hours to days) and tends to fluctuate during the course of the day. It is often associated with a disturbance of both the sleep-wake cycle and psychomotor behaviour. It may be superimposed on a dementing process or it may have multiple contributing factors. A clear understanding of the differential diagnosis enables rapid and appropriate treatment.

Causes

1) Systemic

a) Intoxication/Withdrawal

- ❏ Drugs (opiates, psychotropics, anticholinergics, corticosteroids, cannabis, alcohol, amphetamines, hallucinogens)
- ❏ Withdrawal (alcohol, opiates, psychotropics)
- ❏ Poisoning / Toxins / Heavy metals

b) Metabolic

- ❏ Hypoxaemia
- ❏ Electrolyte disturbances (hyponatraemia/hypernatraemia, hypercalcaemia)
- ❏ Hypoglycaemia
- ❏ Organ failure (uraemia, hepatic encephalopathy, hypoxaemia, hypercarbia, heart failure)
- ❏ Hypertensive encephalopathy
- ❏ Hypoalbuminaemia
- ❏ Porphyria
- ❏ Thiamine deficiency

c) Miscellaneous

- ❏ Systemic sepsis, pneumonia, urinary tract infections (UTIs), encephalitis, acquired immune deficiency syndrome (AIDS)
- ❏ Postoperative states (residual anaesthetics, stress, sleep deprivation, cataract surgery, fat embolism, anaemia)
- ❏ Endocrinopathies (thyroid, adrenal)
- ❏ Burns/Electrocution
- ❏ Hyperthermia

a) **CNS infections**

b) **Acute vascular events (stroke, migraine, vasculitis, carotid stenosis)**

c) **Neoplasm and paraneoplastic processes**

d) **Epilepsy**

e) **Post–electroconvulsive therapy**

f) **Post–head injury**

Key Objective

- Differentiate delirium due to general medical conditions from dementia, drug intoxication or withdrawal, psychotic disorders, personality disorders or malingering and factitious disorder.

General/Specific Objectives

- Through efficient, focused data gathering (which will frequently involve interviewing other informants):

  - Determine which patients are at risk for the development of delirium.

  - Diagnose the underlying causes for delirium.

  - Contrast delirium and dementia (a potent risk factor for delirium); categorise a sudden change in behaviour in a patient with dementia as possible delirium superimposed on dementia.

- Interpret critical clinical and laboratory and mental state findings which were key in the processes of exclusion, differentiation and diagnosis:

  - Select and interpret laboratory investigations in a patient with delirium.

  - List the indications for radiological imaging of the brain in a patient with delirium.

- Conduct an effective plan of management for a patient with confusion/delirium:

  - Outline the initial emergency management of patients with delirium including protection of the patient from self-inflicted harm, harm to others and methods to reduce disorientation and anxiety.

  - Describe the specific management of patients with delirium due to hepatic encephalopathy, metabolic abnormalities and drugs.

  - Select patients in need of specialised care.

  - Inform and support relatives.

Overview

Cyanosis is the physical sign of hypoxaemia, but at times is difficult to detect (cyanosis must be sought carefully, under proper lighting conditions). Hypoxaemia (low partial pressure of oxygen in blood), when detected, may be reversible with oxygen therapy after which the underlying cause requires diagnosis and management.

Causes

1) Central cyanosis

a) Lung disease

- ❏ Upper airway obstruction
- ❏ Pulmonary embolism
- ❏ Interstitial
  - Infectious
  - Inorganic dust (silicosis, asbestosis, coal, metals, etc.)
  - Associated with other diseases (sarcoid, vasculitis, etc.)
  - Chronic pulmonary oedema
  - Idiopathic pulmonary fibrosis / fibrosing alveolitis
  - Lymphangitic carcinomatosis
- ❏ Chronic obstructive airways disease

b) Cyanotic heart disease

- ❏ Eisenmenger syndrome (pulmonary hypertension with right-to-left shunt)
- ❏ Fallot tetralogy (ventricular septal defect (VSD); right ventricular outflow obstruction; overriding aorta; right ventricular hypertrophy)
- ❏ Transposition of great vessels
- ❏ Total anomalous pulmonary venous drainage, truncus, single ventricle

2) Peripheral cyanosis

a) Low cardiac output

b) Local flow diminished (arterial/venous obstruction)

3) Localised cyanosis

Key Objectives

- Define cyanosis, hypoxaemia, and hypoxia (insufficient levels of oxygen in tissues to maintain cell function).

- Contrast pathophysiology of central and peripheral cyanosis.

General/Specific Objectives

- Through efficient, focused data gathering:

  - Differentiate central cyanosis from peripheral and localised cyanosis.

  - Contrast respiratory causes and cyanotic congenital heart disease.

- Interpret critical clinical and laboratory findings which were key in the processes of exclusion, differentiation, and diagnosis.

- Conduct an effective plan of management for a patient with cyanosis/hypoxaemia/hypoxia:

  - Outline an initial plan of management which includes treatment of the underlying condition along with oxygen administration.

  - List the adverse effects of oxygen treatment.

  - List useful outcome criteria for a trial of long term use of oxygen in patients with chronic hypoxaemia.

023 Cyanosis/Hypoxaemia / Hypoxia

023A   Cyanosis / Hypoxia / Apnoea in Children

Overview
Evaluation of cyanosis and hypoxia in children depends heavily on the age of the child. Cyanosis is an ominous finding, especially in the older child, and differentiation between peripheral and central is essential in order to mount appropriate management.

Causes of cyanosis or hypoxaemia

1)   Neonatal

a) **Central**
- ❏ Cyanotic congenital heart disease
  - Increased pulmonary blood flow (transposition, truncus arteriosus, total anomalous pulmonary venous return, hypoplastic left heart)
  - Obstruction to pulmonary blood flow (tricuspid, pulmonary atresia)
- ❏ Respiratory insufficiency
  - Pulmonary (respiratory distress syndrome, sepsis, aspiration, diaphragmatic hernia)
  - Central nervous system (CNS) (maternal sedative, asphyxia, intracranial haemorrhage, hypoglycaemia)

b) **Peripheral vascular ('physiologic acrocyanosis', sepsis, cardiogenic/ septic shock, thrombosis, vasomotor instability)**

2)   Infant and child

a) **Central**
- ❏ Decreased oxygenation of haemoglobin
  - Respiratory (pneumonia, cystic fibrosis, embolus, aspiration / foreign body, CNS depression)
  - Cardiac disease – cyanotic congenital heart disease, severe congestive cardiac failure (CCF) from any cause
- ❏ Abnormalities of haemoglobin (methaemoglobinaemia)

b) **Peripheral**
- ❏ Vascular problem (Raynaud disease, sepsis)
- ❏ Obstruction (superior vena cava syndrome, deep venous thrombosis (DVT))
- ❏ Hyperviscosity (polycythaemia)

Key Objectives

- Differentiate between peripheral and central cyanosis since generalised cyanosis is more consistent with primary heart disease or respiratory insufficiency.

- Appreciate that if the process causing peripheral cyanosis is severe enough (e.g. sepsis), generalised cyanosis may occur.

General/Specific Objectives

- Through efficient, focused data gathering:

  - Elicit maternal history of illness or sepsis in pregnancy, gestational age, delivery complications, presence of meconium, suction of infant, Apgar score, family history of congenital heart disease.

  - Determine the vital signs, age of infant (ductus arteriosus usually closes by third day), whether the infant is alert and active, if the infant is able to feed, and the presence of respiratory distress (tachypnoea, grunting, costal margin flaring or retraction).

  - Perform examination of the newborn for evidence of respiratory distress, congestive heart failure or shock, signs of CNS depression, whether the cyanosis is central or peripheral.

  - Elicit history in the older child of acute versus chronic or recurrent cyanosis, history of lung disease or heart disease, history of foreign body or aspiration, fever, upper respiratory symptoms, exposure to medications, dyes, chemicals.

  - In the older child, focus examination first on respiratory distress and obtundation of neurologic disease; determine whether hypotension or bradycardia is present (ominous signs).

- Interpret critical clinical and laboratory findings which were key in the processes of exclusion, differentiation and diagnosis:

  - Select laboratory investigations including diagnostic imaging, electrocardiogram (ECG), and blood tests.

  - Explain the interpretation of hyperoxia test (arterial blood gas from a site distal to the ductus on room air and 100% oxygen).

- Conduct an effective plan of management for a patient with cyanosis / hypoxia / apnoea in children:

  - Outline initial management including cardio-respiratory monitoring.

  - Explain the benefit of 'knee-chest' position in a child with cyanosis and tetralogy of Fallot.

  - Select patients in need of specialised care.

Overview

Dementia is an acquired, progressive impairment of cognitive function characterised by memory impairment, accompanied by other intellectual and personality changes, in the setting of full consciousness. Dementia is a common problem, with most cases being irreversible, the commonest cause being Alzheimer disease (more than 50% of cases). Progress may be temporarily arrested or modified with specific treatments, and potentially treatable causes must be sought.

Causes

1) Primary dementias (Alzheimer disease, Lewy body dementia, Niemann-Pick disease, fronto-temporal dementia)

2) Vascular

   a) Multi-infarct

   b) Vasculitis / Autoimmune diseases

   c) Focal subcortical strokes

3) Toxic

   a) Alcohol, drugs and narcotics

   b) Heavy metals / Dialysis dementia

   c) Organic toxins

   d) Carbon monoxide

4) Brain trauma (head injury, boxing, hypoxia)

5) Chronic infections (HIV, syphilis, Creutzfeldt-Jakob disease, herpes simplex, malaria)

6) Mass lesions and/or neoplasms

   a) Primary and secondary tumours, carcinomatous meningitis, paraneoplastic encephalitis

   b) Chronic subdural haematoma

   c) Normal pressure hydrocephalus

7) Movement disorders

   a) Parkinson disease

   b) Huntington chorea

   a) Hypothyroidism/Hyperthyroidism

   b) Hypoparathyroidism/Hyperparathyroidism (HPT)

   c) Hypoglycaemia/Hyperglycaemia (chronic)

   d) Hypopituitarism

   e) Pyridoxine, vitamin B_{12} and thiamin deficiency

9) Depressive pseudodementia

Key Objective
- Assess and identify treatable and reversible causes of cognitive dysfunction, including the early stages of Alzheimer-type dementia.

General/Specific Objectives
- Through efficient, focused data gathering involving other informants as well as the patient:
  - Establish the history of onset and progression of symptoms and current level of functioning including daily living activities.
  - Conduct a baseline mental status assessment, including a Folstein Mini–Mental State Examination (MMSE) and tests of frontal lobe functioning.
  - Using the MMSE, differentiate depression or delirium from dementia.
  - Perform a comprehensive physical examination including neurological, cardiovascular and endocrine systems and sensory impairments.
  - Categorise possible causes of dementia, and perform screening investigations.
- Interpret critical clinical and laboratory findings which were key in the processes of exclusion, differentiation, and diagnosis:
  - Identify and treat correctable conditions.
  - Know the indications for centrally acting cholinergic agents.
  - Determine the need for antidepressant or antipsychotic medication, or psychiatric referral.
  - Assess and determine the role of the family or primary carer in the support of the patient. Break the news sensitively.
  - Determine whether occupational and social or other therapy referral and assessment is needed after considering the availability of community resources.

- Conduct an effective plan of management for a patient with dementia with memory/behaviour disturbances:

    - Outline management based on the patient's current and future levels of disability, taking into account the wishes of the patient, the primary carer/family, and available community resources.

    - Financial, legal and vehicle driving issues need to be considered.

    - Appreciate the indications, risk and benefits of the various psychotropic agents which may be of value with specific symptoms.

    - Counsel and educate patients, carers and families about the natural history of the disease and future care options.

    - Continue to provide support and advice to carers.

    - Consider end of life decisions and anticipate death and bereavement issues.

Overview

A call requesting assistance in the delivery room following the birth of a newborn may be 'routine' or because the neonate is apparently depressed and requires resuscitation. For any type of call, the doctor needs to be prepared to manage potential problems.

Causes

1) Respiratory problems

(see #023A Cyanosis/Hypoxia / Apnoea in Children)

a) **Birth asphyxia or central nervous system (CNS) depression (maternal drugs)**

b) **Meconium aspiration**

c) **Sepsis**

d) **Pneumothorax**

2) Severe anaemia (erythroblastosis fetalis and secondary hydrops fetalis)

3) Seizures

4) Congenital malformations including congenital heart disease / birth injury

5) Shock – including that due to feto-maternal haemorrhage

6) Other (hypothermia, hypoglycaemia, small for dates neonate)

Key Objective

- Elicit selective maternal history, determine fetal vital signs, rapidly assess for possible causes of the neonate's condition and initiate supportive measures for the infant.

General/Specific Objectives

- Through efficient, focused data gathering:

  - Elicit a maternal history including maternal illnesses, maternal use of drugs, previous high-risk pregnancies, infections during pregnancy or now, how long have membranes been ruptured, mother's blood type and Rh status, evidence of polyhydramnios or oligohydramnios, gestational age, any meconium, etc.

  - Identify significant causes of cardiorespiratory depression in the newborn.

- Interpret critical clinical and laboratory findings which were key in the processes of exclusion, differentiation and diagnosis:

  - Outline the appropriate investigation of various causes of a 'depressed' newborn and interpret the results.

- Conduct an effective plan of management for a 'depressed' newborn:

  - Differentiate management of respiratory failure in the presence and absence of thick meconium.

  - Select patients in need of specialised care and initiate respiratory and circulatory support prior to transfer of the infant for special care.

  - Counsel and provide explanation to family of the neonate's condition.

(See also #014 Behaviour Disorder)

Overview
A clinician is expected to assess development in an infant in order to diagnose developmental delay.

Causes

1) Global delay

a) Environment (neglect, understimulation)

b) Chromosome disorders (e.g. trisomy 21)

c) Genetic syndromes

d) Mental retardation, central nervous system (CNS) abnormalities

e) Inborn errors of metabolism / Hypothyroidism

2) Speech delay

a) Isolated speech delay

b) Sensory impairment (auditory/visual)

c) Autistic spectrum disorders (infantile autism)

3) Motor delay (Duchenne disease, cerebral palsy)

Key Objectives
- Using knowledge of normal child development, determine which children have evidence of developmental delay.
- Determine whether the delay is global, isolated to speech/language or motor delay, or includes abnormal social interaction.

General/Specific Objectives
- Through efficient, focused data gathering:
  - Determine whether there is chronic illness, family history of developmental delay, or risk factors for mental retardation.
  - Determine whether there was a congenital infection or HIV infection.
  - Determine whether there were factors predisposing to speech delay (e.g. ototoxic drugs, recurrent otitis, mastoiditis).
  - Perform a developmental assessment to confirm or disprove developmental delay.

- Interpret critical clinical and laboratory findings which were key in the processes of exclusion, differentiation and diagnosis:

  - Determine if there is reason to suspect child abuse or neglect.

  - List indications for referral for audiology assessment and referral to speech and language pathologist.

- Conduct an effective plan of management for a patient with development disorder / developmental delay:

  - Select children in need of specialised care.

  - Once a diagnosis of global delay is made outline for parents, along with other caregivers, a management plan which includes (when appropriate) medical care, multidisciplinary services, family support, child placement, and academic support.

  - In a child with speech/language developmental delay, outline with the assistance of specialised caregivers, a management plan which includes (when appropriate) speech therapy, amplification devices, family support, and educational modification.

027A   Acute Diarrhoea

Overview
Diarrhoeal diseases represent the second most common cause of death worldwide and the leading cause of childhood death. Acute diarrhoea is defined as more than two to three stools per day for up to three weeks. Chronic diarrhoea lasts over four weeks. International travellers frequently suffer from acute attacks of diarrhoea in areas where sanitation and hygiene are poor due to a variety of bacteria, viruses and parasites.

Causes

1) **Dietary indiscretion**

2) **Laxatives (osmotic diarrhoea – e.g. magnesium sulphate, lactulose)**

3) **Infectious**

   a) Viral (rotavirus, cytomegalovirus (CMV), AIDS)

   b) Travellers' diarrhoea
   - *Escherichia coli*, enterotoxigenic
   - *Escherichia coli*, enteroadherent
   - *Shigella, Salmonella*
   - Protozoa (Amoebae, *Giardia lamblia*)

4) **Food poisoning**

   a) *Staphylococcus aureus*

   b) *Escherichia coli*

   c) *Shigella, Salmonella*

   d) *Campylobacter, etc.*

5) **Post-antibiotic (e.g. *Clostridium difficile* pseudomembranous colitis)**

6) **Ischaemic**

7) **Inflammatory (exudative diarrhoea)**

   a) Inflammatory bowel disease (IBD)

Key Objectives
- Define the patient's precise diarrhoea with respect to the number of bowel actions per day, the consistency, colour and volume of stools and the presence of other symptoms including blood, mucus or undigested food in the faeces.
- Determine the time of onset and progress over time.

General/Specific Objectives
- Through efficient, focused data gathering:
  - Differentiate infectious diarrhoea from IBD and other causes of acute diarrhoea.
- Interpret critical clinical and laboratory findings which were key in the processes of exclusion, differentiation, and diagnosis:
  - Select and interpret appropriate investigations for patients with acute diarrhoea.
- Conduct an effective plan of management for a patient with blood in stool:
  - Outline management of patients with acute diarrhoea with attention to public health concerns.
  - Select patients in need of specialised care and/or consultation.
  - Be aware of preventive measures to avoid traveller's diarrhoea and be able to provide advice to travellers on steps to be taken in the event of contracting a diarrhoeal illness.

027B Chronic Diarrhoea

Overview

Patients with inflammatory bowel disease (IBD), especially ulcerative colitis, are at risk for a variety of serious complications; patients with fatty stools suffer from malabsorption of nutrients. An organised approach to the investigation of patients with chronic diarrhoea will result in early diagnosis and avoidance of serious nutritional deficiencies and/or serious complications.

Causes

1) Osmotic

   a) Malabsorption
- ❏ Small bowel disease (gluten-sensitive enteropathy (coeliac disease), bile acid malabsorption, small bowel diverticulosis, neoplasms (villous adenoma, lymphoma, carcinoma), Whipple disease, etc.)
- ❏ Pancreatic disease (chronic pancreatitis, cystic fibrosis)
- ❏ Drugs
- ❏ Bowel resection

   b) Specific food intolerance (lactase deficiency, fructose intolerance)

2) Secretory

   a) Inflammatory/Exudative
- ❏ Bleeding
  - • Ulcerative colitis
  - • Chronic bacterial infection
- ❏ Non-bleeding
  - • Crohn disease
  - • AIDS, tuberculosis (TB)
  - • Neoplasms (villous adenoma, lymphoma)

   b) Endocrinopathies (carcinoid, Zollinger-Ellison syndrome, VIPomas)

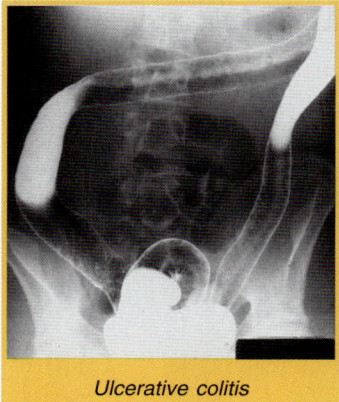

Ulcerative colitis

3) Motility (bacterial overgrowth, diabetic neuropathy, scleroderma, short gut, etc.)

4) Irritable bowel syndrome

5) Spurious diarrhoea (faecal impaction)

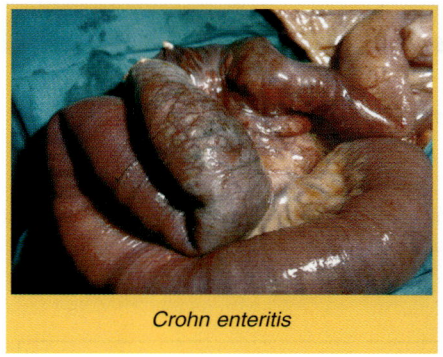

Crohn enteritis

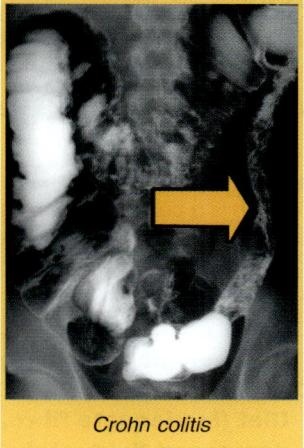

Crohn colitis

Key Objectives
- Differentiate true diarrhoea from spurious diarrhoea associated with faecal impaction.
- Differentiate osmotic from secretory diarrhoea, and malabsorptive diarrhoea from inflammatory causes.

General/Specific Objectives
- Through efficient, focused data gathering:
  - Diagnose patients with irritable bowel syndrome.
  - Determine whether motility problems might be present.
- Interpret critical clinical and laboratory findings which were key in the processes of exclusion, differentiation, and diagnosis:
  - Select and interpret investigations for malabsorptive conditions.
  - Select and interpret investigations for inflammatory bowel conditions.
- Conduct an effective plan of management for a patient with chronic diarrhoea:
  - Outline plan of management for patients with chronic diarrhoea, including the prevention and treatment of related complications (e.g. patients with gluten-sensitive enteropathy, pancreatic insufficiency, vitamin and mineral deficiencies).
  - Select patients in need of specialised care and/or consultation with other healthcare professionals.
  - Conduct education and counselling of patients with malabsorption and IBD.

027C Constipation/Encopresis, Paediatric

Overview

Constipation is a common problem in children. It is important to differentiate functional from organic causes in order to develop appropriate management plans.

Causes

1)	**Psychologic/Developmental delay / Bedridden**

2)	**Diet (inadequate fibre, excessive cow milk, undernutrition, decreased fluid intake)**

3) Anatomic

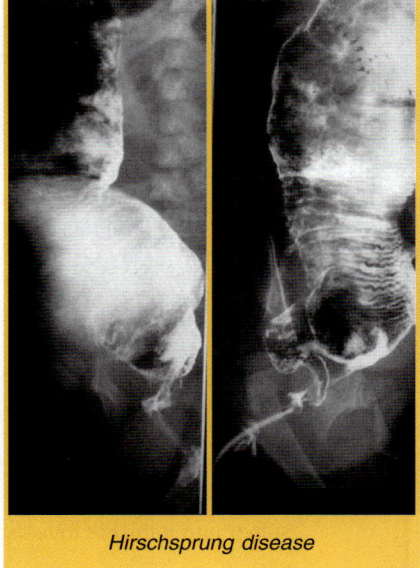

Hirschsprung disease

    a) Hirschsprung disease

    b) Anal stenosis / Atresia / Imperforate anus

    c) Mechanical obstruction/ malrotation

    d) Absent/Abnormal abdominal musculature ('prune belly')

4) Endocrine / Metabolic

    a) Hypothyroid

    b) Hypercalcaemia/Hypokalaemia

5) Neuromuscular

    a) Cerebral palsy

    b) Spinal cord disorders / Meningomyelocele

    c) Peripheral nerves (to gut)

    d) Systemic striated / Enteric smooth myopathy

6) Medications

Key Objectives

- Determine whether the constipation should be investigated to exclude a serious organic cause or should be managed symptomatically.

- Select patients with stool soiling or encopresis in need of investigation and management.

General/Specific Objectives

- Through efficient, focused data gathering:

    - Identify clinical features that help to distinguish functional from organic causes of constipation.

    - Perform rectal examination on a child with minimal discomfort.

    - Evaluate the social and psychologic effects of chronic constipation and chronic encopresis.

- Interpret critical clinical and laboratory findings which were key in the processes of exclusion, differentiation and diagnosis:

    - List appropriate investigation for chronic constipation.

- Conduct an effective plan of management for a patient with constipation:

    - Outline initial and long term therapy for constipation and encopresis, including diet and education.

    - Identify children who require special, as opposed to conservative management.

027D   Diarrhoea, Paediatric

Overview

Diarrhoea is defined as frequent, watery stools and is a common problem in infants and children. In most cases, it is mild and self-limited. However, the potential for hypovolaemia and electrolyte disturbance is ever present and may lead to significant morbidity or even mortality.

Causes

1)   Acute

- a) **Viral gastroenteritis (rotavirus, Norwalk, adenovirus, influenza, enterovirus)**
- b) **Bacterial colitis (*Salmonella, Shigella, Yersinia, Campylobacter, Escherichia coli*)**
- c) **Other infections (*Clostridium difficile,* giardiasis, amoebiasis, parasites)**
- d) **Food poisoning**

2)   Malabsorption

- a) **Lactase deficiency**
- b) **Cystic fibrosis**
- c) **Coeliac disease**
- d) **Primary immunodeficiencies (including HIV)**

3)   In the neonate (milk protein intolerance, necrotising enterocolitis, overfeeding)

4)   Other (drugs, laxative abuse, inflammatory bowel disease (IBD), etc.)

Key Objective

- Determine the presence, degree and type of dehydration/volume depletion and investigate the possibility of electrolyte abnormalities (see #009 Abnormal Serum Sodium Concentration, #008 Abnormal Serum Potassium Concentration / Magnesium).

General/Specific Objectives

- Through efficient, focused data gathering:

  - Elicit a history including previous weight, urine output, and associated symptoms; examine vital signs, mucous membranes, skin turgor, temperature of extremities, and fontanelle in infants, as well as clubbing, wheezing, abdominal examination, etc.

  - Determine whether others have developed diarrhoea and whether the onset was the same day as the ingestion of the same food or 24 hours to days later.

  - Elicit a history of onset and duration of diarrhoea, stool pattern, aggravating and alleviating factors, stool description, fever or associated symptoms, diet history and travel history, etc. in order to diagnose the aetiology of diarrhoea.

- Interpret critical clinical and laboratory findings which were key in the processes of exclusion, differentiation and diagnosis:

  - Select blood and stool investigations in patients with diarrhoea; interpret electrolyte abnormalities.

  - Outline investigation of chronic diarrhoea.

- Conduct an effective plan of management for a young patient with diarrhoea:

  - Outline treatment for the underlying cause of the diarrhoea.

  - Select patients who require referral to a nutrition expert (e.g. malabsorption, coeliac disease).

  - Outline supportive management for patients with volume and/or electrolyte disorders.

  - Discuss nutritional rehabilitation in a malnourished patient.

  - Discuss the use of community resources for parental support.

  - Notify the local public health authority if appropriate.

027E   Adult Constipation

Overview
Constipation is the infrequent passage of stools or of stools that are harder and more difficult to pass than the individual's normal bowel pattern. Low-fibre diets and lack of activity may worsen constipation. Chronic constipation often follows the habitual ignoring of the stimulus to defaecate. Constipation is an important symptom of colon cancer; colonic malignancy is one of the most common causes of mechanical intestinal obstruction.

Causes

1)   Simple constipation

   a) **Low dietary fibre**

   b) **Functional (environment/diet or fluid consumption / activity level change)**

2)   Disordered motility

   a) **Irritable bowel syndrome**

   b) **Diverticular disease / 'Obstipation' / Faecal impaction**

   c) **Idiopathic slow transit**

3)   Secondary constipation

   a) **Local ano-rectal problems (anal fissure/stricture/haemorrhoids)**

   b) **Drugs (opioid analgesics, chronic laxatives, cough medicine, iron, calcium, calcium channel blockers, other antihypertensive drugs, etc.)**

   c) **Prolonged immobilisation**

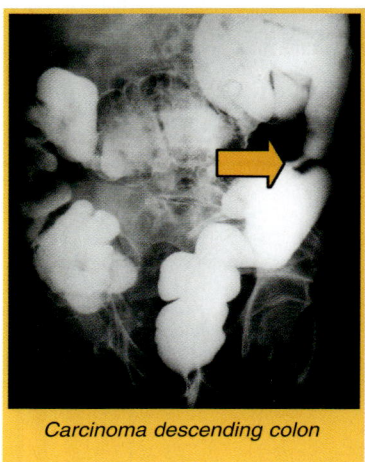

Carcinoma descending colon

d) **Bowel tumours (rectal, colonic)**

e) **Metabolic disorders / Pregnancy (diabetes, hypercalcaemia, hypothyroidism)**

f) **Neurological disorders (Hirschsprung disease, spinal cord disease)**

g) **Bowel obstruction** (see #001 Abdominal Distension / Ileus)

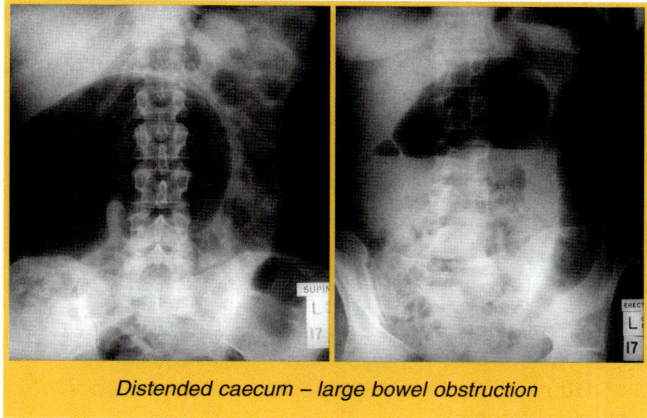

Distended caecum – large bowel obstruction

Key Objectives

- Appreciate that constipation is usually related to influences of diet and activity.

- Appreciate when constipation should be investigated for a serious cause or should be managed symptomatically.

General/Specific Objectives

- In a patient with constipation:

  - Be able to take an appropriate history and undertake a relevant physical examination.

  - Remember to do a rectal examination.

- Appreciate the likelihood that the patient's symptoms may be due to malignancy.

- Understand the place of investigations in diagnosis and management.

- Interpret critical clinical and laboratory findings which were key in the processes of exclusion, differentiation, and diagnosis:

  - Select and interpret investigations including stool for occult blood, and select patients in need of examination by endoscopy or diagnostic imaging.

- Conduct an effective plan of management for a patient with constipation:

  - Outline a plan of management for simple constipation and for constipation due to disordered motility.

  - Select patients in need of specialised care.

Overview

Disorders of eye movement usually present with diplopia. Monocular diplopia (diplopia persisting with occlusion of vision to the other sound eye) is almost always indicative of relatively benign optical problems whereas binocular diplopia is due to ocular misalignment. Once restrictive disease or myasthenia gravis is excluded, the major cause of binocular diplopia is a cranial nerve lesion. Careful clinical assessment is necessary for appropriate management.

Causes

1) Monocular diplopia (refractive error, keratoconus, cataract, functional)

2) Binocular diplopia

    a) Oculomotor nerves

        ❑ Third nerve (ischaemia, especially diabetes-associated, aneurysm, tumour, trauma)

        ❑ Fourth nerve (ischaemia, especially diabetes-associated, trauma)

        ❑ Sixth nerve (ischaemia, especially diabetes-associated, tumour, subdural haematoma, trauma)

        {in children consider also postviral inflammation, brain stem tumour}

    b) Myoneural junction (myasthenia gravis)

    c) Extraocular muscles restriction/entrapment

        ❑ Exophthalmos

        ❑ Orbital inflammation

        ❑ Orbital tumour

        ❑ Fracture of the orbital floor ('blowout' fracture)

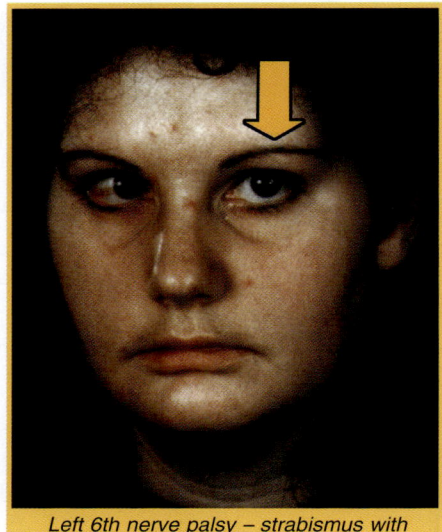

Left 6th nerve palsy – strabismus with diplopia on left lateral gaze

Key Objectives

- Determine whether the rare condition of monocular diplopia is present or the diplopia is binocular (resolves with occlusion of vision to either eye).

- Determine whether the cause of binocular diplopia is a cranial nerve lesion, which may be the first presentation of a life-threatening condition.

General/Specific Objectives

- Through efficient, focused data gathering:

    - Determine whether restrictive disease, oculomotor nerve palsy or myasthenia gravis is the likely cause of diplopia; determine whether one pupil is dilated in a patient with third nerve palsy (suggestive of aneurysm in circle of Willis).

    - Determine whether doubling of images occurred suddenly (acute event such as ischaemia) or is gradually worsening (progressive process such as tumour or inflammation).

- Interpret critical clinical and laboratory findings which were key in the processes of exclusion, differentiation, and diagnosis:

    - Describe the mechanism of development of the 'down and out' eye in a third nerve lesion.

    - Describe findings expected in fourth and sixth nerve lesions.

    - Describe the value of the Tensilon test for myasthenia gravis.

    - List indications for angiography or computed tomography (CT) / magnetic resonance imaging (MRI).

- Develop an effective plan of management and referral for patients with diplopia.

Overview

True vertigo (an episodic sensation of rotation of the body or its surroundings) must be distinguished from dizziness or pseudovertigo (light-headedness, giddiness, faintness, unsteadiness) because it indicates the presence of localised, rather than generalised, pathology. Some causes of vertigo are serious. Others can be chronic and difficult to treat.

Causes

1) True vertigo

a) **Peripheral (labyrinth or acoustic nerve)**
- ❏ Motion sickness
- ❏ Benign positional vertigo
- ❏ Acute labyrinthitis
- ❏ Vestibular neuronitis
- ❏ Ménière disease
- ❏ Acoustic neuroma (Schwannoma)
- ❏ Chronic otitis media
- ❏ Alcohol
- ❏ Drugs prescribed or self-administered
- ❏ Illicit drugs
- ❏ Trauma
- ❏ Wax in ear canal

b) **Central (brainstem or cerebellum)**
- ❏ Vertebrobasilar insufficiency
- ❏ Cerebellar artery syndrome
- ❏ Infarct
- ❏ Tumour (primary or secondary)
- ❏ Migraine
- ❏ Multiple sclerosis
- ❏ Head injury

2) Dizziness (pseudovertigo)

a) **Postural hypotension**

b) **Hyperventilation**

c) **Syncope/Pre-syncope including vaso-vagal attack**

d) **Cardiac arrhythmias**

e) **Aortic stenosis**

f) **Acute myocardial infarction (MI)**

g) Head injury

h) Hypoglycaemia

i) Alcohol and drugs

j) Anaemia

k) Psychogenic

l) Idiopathic (particularly in the elderly)

Key Objectives

- Determine whether patients complaining of dizziness have true vertigo or pseudovertigo.

- Differentiate between central and peripheral causes for true vertigo.

- Identify and counsel patients with other causes of dizziness.

General/Specific Objectives

- Use of directed history-taking and regional examination, particularly neurological examination and special office tests.

- Order and interpret the appropriate investigations used in the diagnosis of patients with dizziness/vertigo.

- Conduct an effective plan of management for a patient with dizziness/vertigo:

  - Determine which patients with vertigo require urgent investigation and management.

  - Describe the symptomatic management of patients with benign causes of vertigo.

  - Counsel and educate patients with benign causes of dizziness/vertigo.

  - Select patients in need of specialised care.

Overview

Doctors are frequently faced with patients dying from incurable disease. In such circumstances, the most important roles of the doctor are to improve the quality of remaining life by alleviating suffering by the patient, thereby facilitating a 'good death'; and to provide comfort and empathetic and compassionate support to patients and their families.

Key Objective

- When caring for a dying patient, doctors must listen to what the patient says are the primary concerns, and should formulate a management plan that ensures adequate control of: pain; relief of anxiety and depression; respect for patient autonomy and control; maintenance of human dignity and privacy. The plan should not prolong life pointlessly; and should avoid isolation of the patient from family and loved ones.

General/Specific Objectives

- Through empathetic and efficient data gathering:

    - Discuss with patients their wishes for care in their final days.

    - For patients who are currently incompetent, insensible or unable to express their wishes, determine whether an advanced directive was previously written or expressed.

- Implement an effective plan of management for a dying patient which includes:

    - Selecting analgesic dosages that are adequate for pain control and alleviating dyspnoea in those who forego mechanical ventilation, even if by doing so death is hastened.

    - Discussing with patients their wishes for care, including resuscitation, well in advance of their death.

    - Discussing the role of an advanced directive and the impact this has on clinicians.

    - Providing or arranging for psychosocial, emotional, practical, legal and spiritual support to the patient and family.

    - Selecting patients in need of referral to other health professionals and ensuring access to information and expertise of whatever kind is necessary.

    - Educating patients and their families about the nature of the causal condition and the process of dying.

    - Promoting active coping strategies when appropriate.

- Gently facilitating and acknowledging the expression of feelings, particularly anticipatory grief; and alleviating fear and depression with appropriate treatments.

- Being sensitive to the burden of care borne by others.

- Encouraging the strengthening of relationships with loved ones.

- Remembering the relevance of funerals as life-enhancing experiences.

Overview

Dysphagia is a significant symptom that, if appropriately approached, will enable doctors to distinguish between a benign or malignant cause. With more effective therapy for gastro-oesophageal reflux disease and an increase in the incidence of oesophageal cancer, the symptom of dysphagia is now more frequently an indication of malignant oesophageal obstruction. Mechanical dysphagia thus represents carcinoma until proved otherwise. Physical signs are usually few and appropriate endoscopic/radiologic investigation is essential.

Dysphagia should be distinguished from the anxiety disorder globus hystericus (globus disorder), which is the sensation of a constant irritating lump in the throat without swallowing difficulty.

Causes

1) **Oropharyngeal dysphagia (peritonsillar abscess, pharyngitis, cancer, pharyngeal pouch)**

2) **Oesophageal dysphagia**

   a) **Mechanical obstruction**

      ❏ Carcinoma (squamous cell, adenocarcinoma)

      ❏ Other causes (stricture (reflux oesophagitis, corrosives), paraoesophageal hiatus hernia, foreign body, goitre, upper oesophageal web (sideropenic dysphagia))

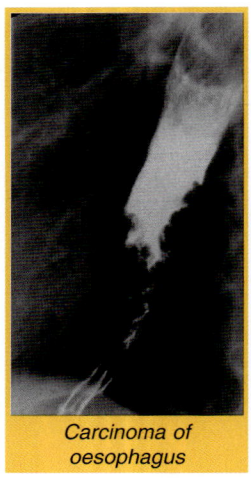

Carcinoma of oesophagus

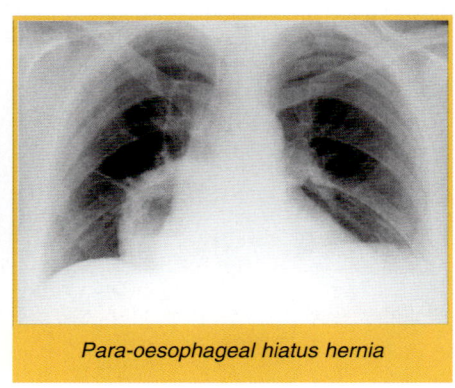

Para-oesophageal hiatus hernia

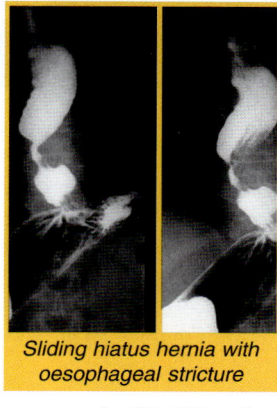

Sliding hiatus hernia with oesophageal stricture

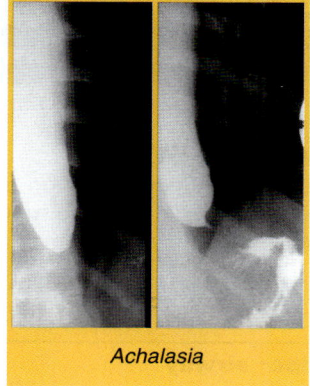

Achalasia

b) Neuromuscular/Motility disorder

- ❏ Intermittent (oesophageal spasm)
- ❏ Progressive
    - Achalasia
    - Central nervous system (stroke, Parkinson disease, amyotrophic lateral sclerosis, poliomyelitis, multiple sclerosis, pseudobulbar palsy)
    - Cranial nerves (diabetes, laryngeal nerve palsy)
    - Skeletal muscle disease (poliomyelitis, dermatomyositis, scleroderma)

Key Objectives

- Contrast difficulty initiating swallowing (coughing, choking, nasal regurgitation), from food sticking after being swallowed, and then dysphagia involving only solid food from dysphagia of both solid and liquid food, and whether intermittent or progressive.
- Distinguish between oropharyngeal and oesophageal dysphagia.
- Distinguish between difficulty in swallowing and pain on swallowing.

General/Specific Objectives

- Through efficient, focused data gathering:
    - Determine whether symptomatology is intermittent or progressive, whether weight loss (late sign) is a problem, and whether any neurologic symptom or aspiration coexists.
    - Determine the presence of coughing, choking, drooling, or regurgitation.
- Interpret critical clinical and laboratory findings which were key in the processes of exclusion, differentiation, and diagnosis:
    - Select patients in need of specialised investigative procedures (e.g. endoscopy); if not available, select diagnostic imaging.
- Conduct an effective plan of management for a patient with dysphagia:
    - Select patients in need of specialised care and/or referral.

Overview

Shortness of breath may be due to a variety of causes. It is imperative to identify rapidly the aetiology in order to mount, if required, an immediate and long term management programme to minimise complications and excessive morbidity.

Causes

1) Upper airway

  a) Stridor

2) Lower airway

  a) Obstructive (asthma, chronic obstructive lung disease, inhaled foreign body)

  b) Non-obstructive (interstitial lung disease, restrictive lung disease)

3) Cardiac causes

  a) Left heart failure

  b) Aortic stenosis

4) Pneumothorax

5) Pulmonary embolism

6) Pleural effusion

7) Psychogenic

8) Severe anaemia

9) Metabolic acidosis

10) Central nervous system (CNS)

11) Musculoskeletal

Key Objectives

- Differentiate dyspnoea from tachypnoea, hyperpnoea or hyperventilation.

- Differentiate cardiac from pulmonary, neuromuscular or other causes of dyspnoea.

- Develop management programmes to treat the immediate problem and involve the patient, the family and community resources in the overall care of chronic patients.

General/Specific Objectives

- Through efficient, focused data gathering:

    - Differentiate between the causes of cardiac pulmonary oedema.

    - Differentiate between the various causes of pulmonary oedema and pulmonary infiltrations.

    - Diagnose the various causes of life-threatening dyspnoea.

- Interpret critical clinical and laboratory findings which were key in the processes of exclusion, differentiation and diagnosis:

    - Appropriately select and interpret lung imaging.

    - Appropriately select and interpret cardiac-related investigations.

- Conduct an effective plan of management for a young patient with dyspnoea:

    - Outline initial management for patients with acute dyspnoea of cardiac, pulmonary, or other origins.

    - Select patients in need of specialised care and referral to other healthcare professionals or institutions.

    - Select those patients in need of hospitalisation.

    - Conduct appropriate education of patients including secondary prevention strategies.

032A With Diffuse Chest X-Ray Abnormality

Overview

Shortness of breath has many causes. Prompt recognition of the diagnosis and initiation of therapy can limit associated morbidity and mortality.

Causes

1) Cardiac causes – pulmonary oedema

a) **Cardiomyopathy**
   - ❏ Ischaemic
   - ❏ Dilated (idiopathic, alcoholic, haemochromatosis)

b) **Hypertensive heart disease**

c) **Restrictive cardiomyopathy (amyloid, sarcoid)**

d) **Valvular heart disease**

e) **Diastolic dysfunction (hypertension, ischaemia, infiltrative disease)**

f) **Increased cardiac output (anaemia, arteriovenous (AV) malformation, hyperthyroid)**

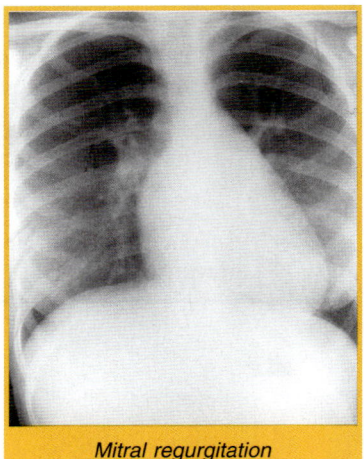

Mitral regurgitation

2) Pulmonary Causes

a) **Infectious Pneumonia**
   - ❏ Bacterial, including tuberculosis (TB)
   - ❏ Atypical
   - ❏ Fungal, including *Pneumocystis carinii*
   - ❏ Viral, including HIV

b) **Inhalational/Environmental 'pneumoconiosis' (inorganic, organic)**

c) **Vasculitis (Wegener granulomatosis, Goodpasture syndrome)**

d) **Pulmonary fibrosis, sarcoidosis, scleroderma**

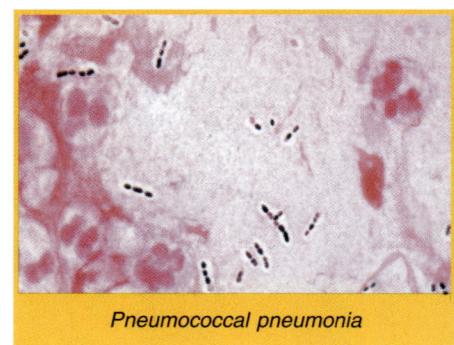

Pneumococcal pneumonia

e) **Neoplastic (lymphangitic carcinomatosis)**

f) **Drugs/Radiation (amiodarone, bleomycin, *beta*-blockers, nitrofurantoin)**

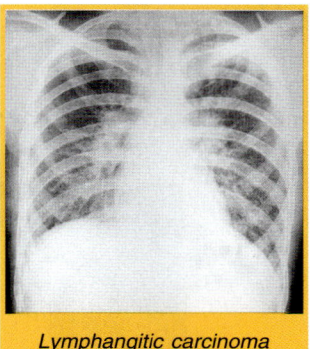
Lymphangitic carcinoma

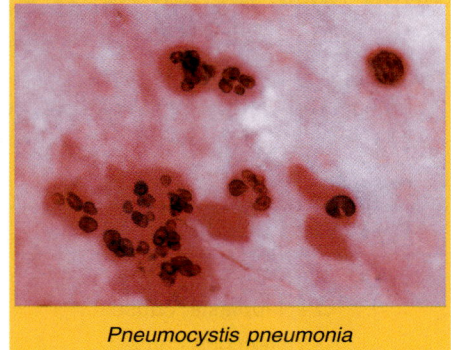
Pneumocystis pneumonia

Key Objectives

- Differentiate true cough from upper airway clearing, saliva from sputum or haemoptysis, and true dyspnoea from tachypnoea, hyperpnoea, and hyperventilation.

- If initial evaluation indicated that a chest X-ray was necessary, differentiate between cardiac disease, pulmonary disease, and neuropsychiatric disease.

General/Specific Objectives

- Through efficient, focused data gathering:

  - Differentiate between causes of cardiac pulmonary oedema.

  - Differentiate between causes of pulmonary disease.

  - Diagnose acute, life-threatening dyspnoea.

- Interpret critical clinical and laboratory findings which were key in the processes of exclusion, differentiation, and diagnosis:

  - Select and interpret lung imaging.

  - Select and interpret heart-related investigations.

- Conduct an effective plan of management for a patient with cough and/or dyspnoea with diffuse chest X-ray abnormality:

  - Outline initial management for patients with acute dyspnoea of cardiac, pulmonary, or neuropsychiatric origin.

  - Select patients in need of specialised care and referral to other healthcare professionals.

  - Select patients requiring hospitalisation.

  - Conduct appropriate education of patients including secondary prevention strategies.

032B With Pleural Chest X-Ray Abnormality

Overview

Pleural effusions are common and may represent local or systemic disease.

Causes

1) Pleural effusion

a) **Exudative**
- ❏ Neoplastic causes
- ❏ Infectious causes
  - • Parapneumonic
  - • Empyema (bacterial, fungal, tuberculous)
- ❏ Pulmonary emboli
- ❏ Collagen-vascular diseases (rheumatoid, lupus pleuritis)
- ❏ Gastrointestinal causes (ruptured oesophagus, pancreatitis)

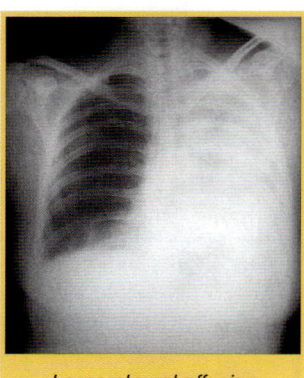
Large pleural effusion

b) **Transudative**
- ❏ Congestive heart failure
- ❏ Cirrhosis
- ❏ Nephrotic syndrome
- ❏ Pulmonary emboli

2) Pleural thickening

a) **Chronic infections (tuberculosis (TB))**

b) **Neoplastic (mesothelioma)**

c) **Inflammatory (chronic asbestos exposure)**

3) Pneumothorax

a) **Spontaneous**
- ❏ Primary
- ❏ Secondary (secondary to chronic obstructive pulmonary disease (COPD))

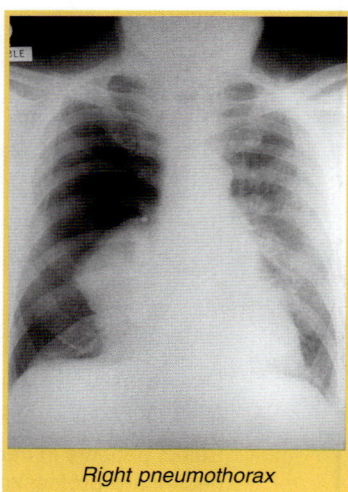
Right pneumothorax

b) **Traumatic**

c) **Tension**

Key Objectives

- Conduct an examination of the thorax and demonstrate how to detect a pleural effusion or a pneumothorax; identify life-threatening tension pneumothorax requiring urgent treatment.

- Differentiate between causes of pleural effusion on the basis of analysis results from pleural fluid.

General/Specific Objectives

- Through efficient, focused data gathering:

  - Differentiate between a pleural effusion and a pneumothorax.

  - Perform intercostal needle thoracentesis as initial life-saving procedure for tension pneumothorax; arrange for subsequent intercostal tube thoracentesis.

- Interpret critical clinical and laboratory findings which were key in the processes of exclusion, differentiation and diagnosis:

  - Interpret the findings of a chest X-ray.

  - Perform (under supervision) and interpret the findings of a thoracocentesis and intercostal catheter insertion; appreciate hazards of procedure and methods of prevention of complications.

  - Discuss the indications for computed tomography (CT) scanning in patients with a pleural effusion.

- Conduct an effective plan of management for a patient with dyspnoea and/or cough with pleural chest X-ray abnormality:

  - Identify patients in need of immediate management for pneumothorax.

  - Discuss the medical and surgical management for patients with pleural effusion.

  - Select patients in need of specialised care.

032C With Fever

Overview
Cough with fever may signify pneumonia that can result in rapid deterioration of health. Prompt management of patients with pneumonia may be life-saving.

Causes

1) Infectious causes

    a) **Bronchitis (bacterial or viral)**

    b) **Pneumonia**

       ❏ Bacterial (typical, atypical)

       ❏ Viral (including severe acute respiratory syndrome (SARS) viral pneumonia)

       ❏ Tuberculous or fungal

    c) **Upper respiratory tract infections (URTIs)**

2) Inflammatory causes (e.g. pulmonary vasculitis)

3) Pulmonary embolus

4) Neoplastic causes

    a) **Primary**

    b) **Secondary**

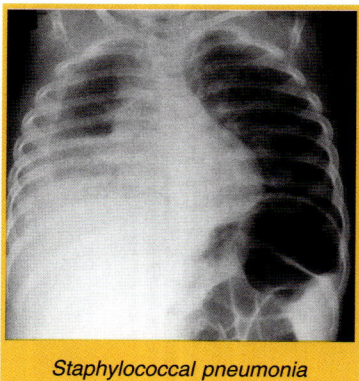

Staphylococcal pneumonia

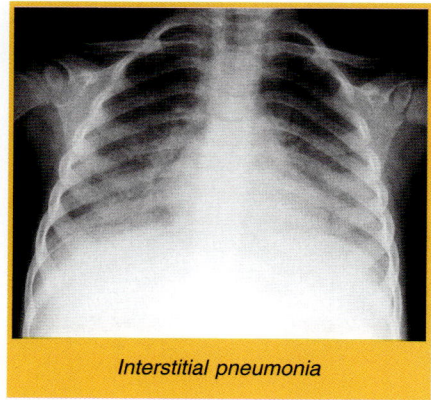

Interstitial pneumonia

Key Objective

- Determine which patients with dyspnoea, cough and fever are likely to have serious pulmonary disease and require immediate investigation and prompt management.

General/Specific Objectives

- Through efficient, focused data gathering:

- Diagnose the cause of dyspnoea, cough and fever.

- For patients with pneumonia, elicit risk factors which predispose such patients to specific organisms.

- Determine which patients are at risk for fungal pneumonia or tuberculosis (TB).

- Interpret critical clinical and laboratory findings which were key in the processes of exclusion, differentiation and diagnosis:

  - Order and interpret the results of a chest X-ray in patients with cough and fever.

  - Order and interpret the results of microbiological cultures and viral serology if appropriate.

- Conduct an effective plan of management for a patient with dyspnoea and/or cough with fever:

  - Assess the severity of the illness and discuss the indications for hospitalisation and referral to specialised care.

  - Discuss the indications for anti-microbial therapy and select the most appropriate antibiotic based on the likelihood of infection with specific micro-organisms.

  - Discuss the treatment and followup of patients with TB.

  - Discuss the preventive and public health measures related to pulmonary infections including TB.

032D *With Local Chest X-Ray Abnormality*

Overview

Dyspnoea and cough with an abnormal chest X-ray are indicative of significant pathology. Accurate interpretation of the chest X-ray is critical for making a diagnosis.

Causes

1) Infectious causes

a) Pneumonia
- ❏ Bacterial (typical, atypical)
- ❏ Viral
- ❏ Tuberculous
- ❏ Fungal
- ❏ Parasitic (hydatid cyst)

b) Lung abscess (bacterial or tuberculous)

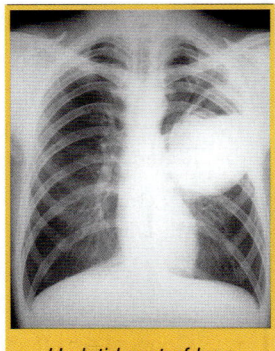

Hydatid cyst of lung

2) Neoplasm

a) Benign (hamartoma, granuloma)

b) Malignant
- ❏ Primary (small cell, non-small cell lung cancer)
- ❏ Secondary (metastases, lymphoma)

3) Interstitial lung disease

(see #032A With Diffuse Chest X-Ray Abnormality)

a) Inhalational/Environmental
- ❏ Inorganic (silicosis, asbestosis, coal worker's pneumoconiosis, etc.)
- ❏ Organic (extrinsic allergic alveolitis)

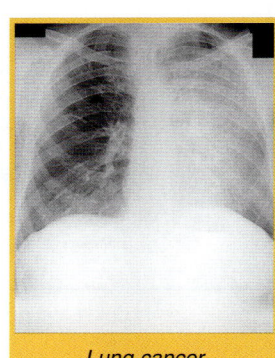

Lung cancer

b) Collagen vascular diseases (systemic lupus erythematosus (SLE), rheumatoid arthritis (RA), ankylosing spondylitis and polymyositis)

c) Drug/Radiation induced (amiodarone, bleomycin, nitrofurantoin)

d) Idiopathic (pulmonary fibrosis, sarcoidosis)

e) Vasculitis (Wegener granulomatosis)

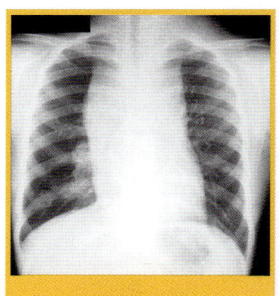

Lymphoma

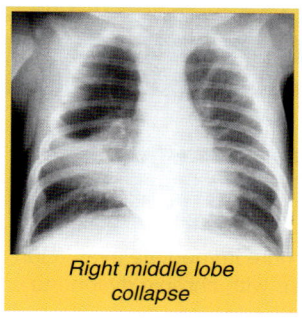
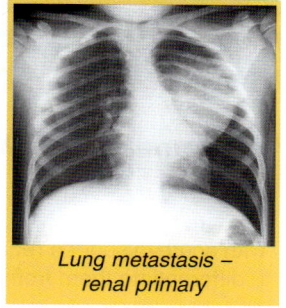

Right middle lobe collapse

Lung metastasis – renal primary

4) Mediastinal masses

    a) **Anterior (thymomas, lymphoma, thyroid mass, teratoma)**

    b) **Middle and posterior (unlikely to present with dyspnoea/cough)**

5) Miscellaneous

    a) **Atelectasis / Pulmonary collapse**

    b) **Loculated pleural effusion**

Key Objective
- Differentiate patients with infectious or neoplastic causes for their dyspnoea and/or cough and chest X-ray abnormality.

General/Specific Objectives
- Through efficient, focused data gathering:
  - Diagnose the cause of dyspnoea and/or cough and localised chest X-ray abnormality.
  - Determine the most likely cause for interstitial lung disease.
  - In patients with pulmonary nodules, describe risk factors and clinical features favouring malignancy.
- Interpret critical clinical and laboratory findings which were key in the processes of exclusion, differentiation and diagnosis:
  - List indications for chest computed tomography (CT) scan in patients with dyspnoea, cough and a localised X-ray abnormality.
  - Discuss investigation for patients with a pulmonary nodule.
  - Describe chest X-ray features of pulmonary nodules favouring malignancy.
- Conduct an effective plan of management for a patient with dyspnoea and/or cough with a local chest X-ray abnormality:
  - Assess the severity of illness and discuss the indications for hospitalisation and referral for specialised care.
  - Describe a management plan based on the mostly likely cause of the chest X-ray abnormality.

032E With Normal Chest X-Ray

Overview

Since patients with acute dyspnoea require more immediate evaluation and treatment, it is important to differentiate them from those with chronic dyspnoea.

Causes

1) Acute dyspnoea

   a) **Exacerbation of obstructive airways disease**

   ❏ Asthma

   ❏ Chronic obstructive pulmonary disease (COPD)

   b) **Pulmonary embolus**

   c) **Early pneumonia**

   d) **Miscellaneous (anxiety, fever, sepsis, salicylate, metabolic acidosis)**

2) Chronic dyspnoea

   a) **Obstructive airways disease**

   ❏ Asthma

   ❏ COPD

   ❏ Bronchiectasis

   b) **Chronic congestive heart failure**

   c) **Neuromuscular disorders (post-poliomyelitis, myasthenia gravis, muscular dystrophy)**

Key Objective

• Differentiate clinically among the causes for acute and chronic dyspnoea.

General/Specific Objectives

• Through efficient, focused data gathering:

   - Differentiate between the different causes for obstructive airways disease.

   - Determine which factors may precipitate dyspnoeic episodes in patients with asthma or chronic obstructive lung disease.

- • Interpret critical clinical and laboratory findings which were key in the processes of exclusion, differentiation and diagnosis:

  - Order and interpret appropriate initial investigations including chest X-ray, arterial blood gas and pulmonary function tests.

  - Outline the diagnostic imaging appropriate for a patient with suspected pulmonary embolus.

- • Conduct an effective plan of management for a patient with dyspnoea and/or cough with a normal chest X-ray:

  - Determine which patients have life-threatening acute dyspnoea and perform immediate management, including intubation if necessary.

  - Discuss the acute and chronic pharmacological management of patients with obstructive airways disease.

  - Select patients in need of hospitalisation and/or specialised care.

  - Counsel and educate patients in strategies for smoking cessation and avoidance of precipitants.

  - Describe the complications of chronic hypoxia and hypercapnia and outline the role of oxygen supplementation in patients with chronic hypoxia.

032F   Cough

Overview

Chronic cough is one of the most common symptoms for which patients seek medical advice. Assessment of chronic cough must be thorough. Patients with benign causes for their cough (e.g. gastro-oesophageal reflux, post-nasal drip, two of the commonest causes) can often be effectively and easily managed. Patients with more serious causes for their cough (e.g. asthma, the other common cause of chronic cough) require full investigation, and management is more complex.

Causes

1)   Chronic cough

a) **Miscellaneous**
- ❏ Post-nasal drip
- ❏ Gastro-oesophageal reflux
- ❏ Drugs (angiotensin-converting enzyme (ACE) inhibitors)
- ❏ Foreign body
- ❏ Chronic sinusitis

b) **Obstructive airways disease**
- ❏ Asthma
- ❏ Chronic bronchitis
- ❏ Bronchiectasis
- ❏ Cystic fibrosis

c) **Congestive heart failure**

d) **Lung neoplasm**
- ❏ Bronchogenic carcinoma
- ❏ Carcinoid tumour

e) **Chronic lung infections**
- ❏ Lung abscess
- ❏ Tuberculosis (TB)

f) **Interstitial lung disease**

2) Acute cough

a) Infectious (upper respiratory tract infection (URTI), bronchitis, pneumonia)

b) Irritant (noxious fumes, smoke)

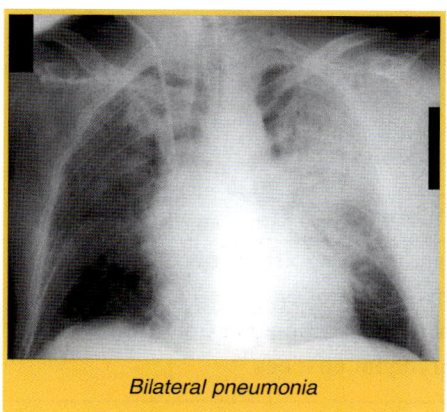

Bilateral pneumonia

Key Objective

- Differentiate patients with chronic cough due to upper or lower respiratory, cardiac or gastrointestinal causes.

General/Specific Objectives

- Through efficient, focused data gathering:

    - Determine whether the patient smokes or takes ACE inhibitors (if not, consider reflux or post-nasal drip).

    - Diagnose the cause of a chronic cough and distinguish those patients with innocuous cough from those with significant disease.

- Interpret critical clinical and laboratory findings which were key in the processes of exclusion, differentiation and diagnosis:

    - Outline value of spirometry before and after broncho-dilators for assessment of chronic cough.

    - Order and interpret a chest X-ray if appropriate.

- Conduct an effective plan of management for a patient with a chronic cough:

    - Prescribe appropriate medications used in the management of chronic cough, with proper attention to their indications, contra-indications and adverse effects.

    - Select patients in need of specialised care.

    - Counsel and educate patients with chronic cough including the provision of strategies aimed at smoking cessation.

032G Dyspnoea / Respiratory Distress, Paediatric

Overview
Respiratory distress is one of the most common paediatric emergencies and can be a life-threatening acute emergency.

Causes

1) Airway problems

    a) 'Croup' (acute laryngotracheobronchitis)

    b) Foreign body aspiration

    c) Laryngeal oedema / Spasm / Epiglottitis

    d) Retropharyngeal abscess

2) Pulmonary problems

    a) Tracheitis/Bronchiolitis

    b) Pneumonia

    c) Asthma/Bronchospasm

3) Cardiac problems

    a) Congestive heart failure (left-to-right shunt, left ventricular failure)

    b) Cardiac tamponade

    c) Pulmonary embolus

4) Pleural problems

    a) Pleural effusion, empyema

    b) Pneumothorax

5) Neurologic problems (opiates, increased intracranial pressure, neuromyopathic)

6) Neonatal conditions

    a) Transient tachypnoea of the newborn

    b) Respiratory distress syndrome (hyaline membrane disease)

    c) Diaphragmatic hernia

    d) Massive ascites

    e) Tracheo-oesophageal fistula

7) Other (e.g. severe scoliosis)

Key Objectives

- Differentiate the child who appears well from a child in distress or in critical condition.

- Evaluate the respiratory rate in the context of age of the child (neonates normally breathe 35–50 times per minute, infants 30–40, elementary school children 20–30, and pre-adolescents 12–20) and describe and explain the quality of the breathing.

- Differentiate dyspnoea from tachypnoea, hyperpnoea or hyperventilation.

General/Specific Objectives

- Through efficient, focused data gathering:

  - Differentiate the child who appears well from a child in distress or in critical condition.

  - Ensure patent airway.

  - Determine presence, duration, and type of onset of respiratory distress, presence of cyanosis.

  - Perform examination for vital signs, retraction, flaring, wheezing, or coughing.

  - Perform examination – cyanosis, upper airway, heart, lungs and other relevant areas.

  - Assess pulse oximetry.

- Interpret critical clinical and laboratory findings which were key in the processes of exclusion, differentiation and diagnosis:

  - Determine presence of hypoxia; select and interpret lung imaging and/ or cardiac investigations.

  - Outline other tests of blood, sputum, electrocardiogram (ECG), echocardiography, etc. as appropriate. Special tests may be required if patient is immuno-compromised.

- Conduct an effective plan of management for a patient in respiratory distress:

  - Outline immediate management of hypoxia; select patients in need of hospitalisation/referral.

  - Discuss potential side-effects of oxygen therapy.

  - Explain choice of antibiotics for pulmonary disorders; discuss use of bronchodilators and steroids if appropriate.

  - Explain advantages/disadvantages of diuretics (e.g. frusemide) in the treatment of cardiac dyspnoea.

  - Counsel patients/parents about secondary prevention strategies.

Overview

Many causes of ear pain exist but **acute otitis media** is by far the most common, especially in children. Diagnosis and treatment of otitis media is usually straightforward but other causes may present more difficult management situations.

Causes

1) Pinna

   a) **Cellulitis/Perichondritis**

   b) **Chilblains**

   c) **Trauma**

2) External auditory meatus and ear canal

   a) **Impacted wax / foreign body**

   b) **Furunculosis**

   c) **Otitis externa**

   d) **Herpes zoster – geniculate herpes (Ramsay Hunt syndrome)**

   e) **Tumour (basal cell carcinoma (BCC), squamous cell carcinoma (SCC), osteoma)**

3) Middle Ear

   a) **Acute otitis media**

   b) **Eustachian obstruction**

   c) **Barotrauma**

   d) **Acute mastoiditis**

   e) **Chronic otitis media and cholesteatoma**

   f) **Penetrating injury**

4) Peri-otic

   a) **Temporomandibular joint (TMJ) dysfunction**

   b) **Impacted wisdom teeth**

   c) **Parotitis**

   d) **Temporal arteritis**

   e) **Erysipelas**

   f) **Pharyngitis/Tonsillitis**

5) Referred Pain

a) Cervical adenitis

b) Upper cervical spine disorder

c) Glossopharyngeal neuralgia

d) Thyroiditis

e) Laryngeal/Pharyngeal tumours

Key Objectives

- Skill in examination of the ear canal and tympanic membrane using an auroscope.

- Identification of diagnostic features of otitis media, and knowledge of the treatment of acute otitis media.

- Identification and management of other causes of ear pain.

General/Specific Objectives

- Through efficient, focused data gathering:

  - Localise the site of pain.

  - Systematically examine structures which may be the source of origin of the pain.

  - Differentiate between localised and referred pain.

- Interpret critical clinical findings and investigations which were key in the process of exclusion, differentiation and diagnosis:

  - Select any necessary investigation which will confirm, exclude or suggest a possible cause of the ear pain.

- Conduct an effective plan of management for a patient with ear pain:

  - Specific treatments for infective causes.

  - Minor procedures for mechanical causes.

  - Select patients in need of specialised care.

034A Generalised Oedema

Overview
Patients frequently complain of generalised swelling or bloating. At times, the swelling may be caused by relatively benign conditions, but at times, serious underlying diseases may be present.

Causes

1)	Idiopathic (cyclical oedema)

2)	Drugs

    a) Causing fluid retention (minoxidil, nonsteroidal anti-inflammatory drugs (NSAIDs), etc.)

    b) Without fluid retention (calcium channel blockers, especially dihydropyridines)

3)	Cardiac failure

4)	Nephrotic syndrome (and/or severe hypoalbuminaemia)

5)	Liver failure

6)	Renal failure

Key Objective
- Differentiate systemic generalised oedema from localised oedema; categorise oedema as *'underfill'* or *'overfill'* based on patient's volume status, since management may be affected.

General/Specific Objectives
- Through efficient, focused data gathering:

  - Differentiate between the various causes of systemic oedema.

- Interpret critical clinical and laboratory findings which were key in the processes of exclusion, differentiation, and diagnosis:

  - Select and interpret laboratory investigations for oedema.

- Conduct an effective plan of management for a patient with generalised oedema:

  - Outline a plan of management for oedema of varying causes.

  - List appropriate dietary interventions.

  - List complications of diuretic use; contrast diuretic use in *'underfill'* versus *'overfill'* oedema.

  - Select patients in need of specialised care and/or consultation.

034B Unilateral Limb Oedema (Swollen Limb)

Overview

The most common causes of unilateral leg oedema are trauma, infection, venous disease and chronic lymphoedema. The ability to reach a diagnosis requires good clinical skills; the most important conditions *not* to miss are **cellulitis** and **deep venous thrombosis (DVT)**.

Causes

| 1) | **Muscle strain, tear, twisting injury to extremity, haematoma** |

| 2) | **DVT** |

    a) **Lower extremity (proximal, calf vein)**

    b) **Upper extremity (effort thrombosis, central venous cannulation, chemotherapy)**

| 3) | **Infection/Inflammation** |

    a) **Cellulitis / Soft tissue / Bone**

    b) **Chronic dermatitis / Cutaneous mucinosis**

| 4) | **Venous insufficiency** |

| 5) | **Lymphatic obstruction / Lymphangitis** |

| 6) | **Baker cyst** |

| 7) | **Infiltrative dermopathy (usually associated with thyroid disease)** |

Key Objectives

- Diagnose proximal lower extremity DVT with accuracy and certainty since untreated, it may lead to pulmonary embolus, and treatment with anticoagulants is associated with significant risk.

- Diagnose cellulitis with accuracy and certainty since early and adequate antibiotic treatment is required to prevent serious complications.

General/Specific Objectives

- Through efficient, focused data gathering:

    - Elicit history of predisposing factors, particularly for DVT and cellulitis. Be aware of the key risk factors for DVT (immobilisation, surgery, obesity, previous episode of thrombosis, varicose veins, trauma, malignancy, postpartum, oestrogen therapy, a thrombophilia or family history of thrombosis).

- Examine extremity for tenderness, presence or absence of pitting oedema, inflammation, discolouration, palpable cord, skin changes, venous ulceration, and especially arterial blood supply.

- Interpret critical clinical and laboratory findings which were key in the processes of exclusion, differentiation, and diagnosis:

  - State that clinical diagnosis of DVT is not sufficiently accurate, and diagnostic tests are indicated to confirm or exclude the diagnosis.

  - Discuss D-dimer measurements, and compression ultrasound and compare to contrast venography.

  - Select duplex ultrasonography Doppler for the diagnosis of chronic venous insufficiency.

- Conduct an effective plan of management for a patient with oedema which is not generalised:

  - Outline primary prevention and management of DVT.

  - Outline the management of cellulitis.

  - Select patients in need of specialised care.

  - List indications, complications and management of anticoagulant therapy.

  - Counsel patients about anticoagulant therapy.

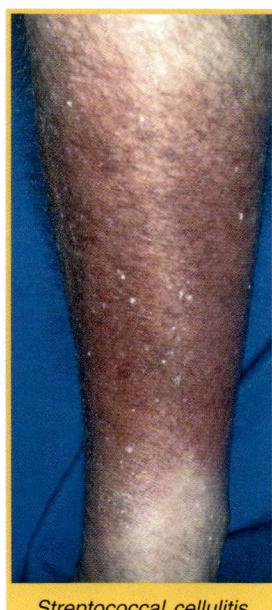

Streptococcal cellulitis

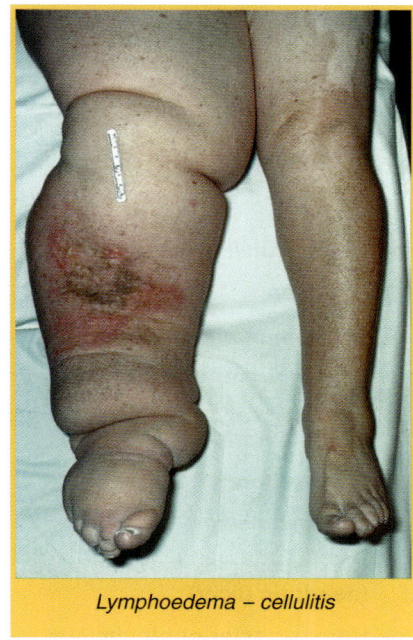

Lymphoedema – cellulitis

Overview

Red eye is a very common complaint, and despite the rather lengthy list of causal conditions, three problems make up the vast majority of causes: **conjunctivitis**, **foreign body**, and **iritis** (**uveitis**). The most common cause is **conjunctivitis**. If unilateral and painful a serious cause is more likely – beware of the unilateral painful red eye!

Causes

1)   Lids / Orbits / Lacrimal system

a) **Foreign body**

b) **Hordeolum ('stye')**

c) **Chalazion (Meibomian cyst)**

d) **Blepharitis**

e) **Cellulitis (anterior, posterior)**

f) **Naso-lacrimal duct obstruction/ dysfunction**

g) **Orbital cellulitis**

'Stye' – infected eyelash

2)   Conjunctiva

a) **Conjunctivitis**

❏   Viral

❏   Bacterial (including gonorrhoea and trachoma in the neonate)

❏   Fungal

❏   Allergic

b) **Pinguecula/Pterygium**

c) **Dry eyes**

d) **Subconjunctival haemorrhage**

Conjunctivitis

3)   Cornea

a) **Corneal abrasion**

b) **Corneal foreign body**

c) **Corneal ulcer**

d) **Herpes simplex keratitis (dendritic ulcer)**

e) **Herpes zoster ophthalmicus**

f) **Fungal keratitis**

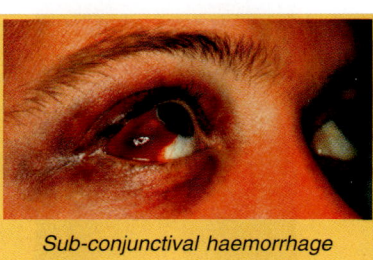

Sub-conjunctival haemorrhage

4) Anterior chamber

a) Acute glaucoma

b) Acute iritis (iridocyclitis, uveitis)

c) Choroiditis

d) Hyphaema

5) Whole eye

a) Penetrating injury

b) Blunt trauma

c) Orbital fracture

d) Chemical injury

Key Objectives

- Identify or exclude serious causes requiring immediate hospitalisation, prompt referral and aggressive treatment.

- For conjunctivitis, define type to determine specific therapy.

General/Specific Objectives

- Through efficient, focused data gathering:

  - Differentiate causal conditions that require prompt referral from those that are less urgent.

- Interpret critical clinical and laboratory findings which were key in the processes of exclusion, differentiation, and diagnosis, *viz* :

  - History-taking essentials.

  - Skills for non-specialist examination of eye.

  - Selection and interpretation of appropriate investigations.

- Conduct an effective plan of management for eye redness:

  - Select patients in need of referral.

- Outline a management plan for the following causes of eye redness:

  - Conjunctivitis, foreign body, acute glaucoma.

036A Infant/Child

Overview

Many infants and children do not follow the expected growth and development paths. It is essential to differentiate the normal from the abnormal patterns.

Causes

1) Prenatal

a) **Placental insufficiency**

b) **Antenatal infections**

c) **Prematurity**

2) Perinatal

a) **Acutely ill neonate – hypoxic ischaemia**

3) Postnatal

a) **Chronic disease**
   - ❏ Cardiac, respiratory, gastrointestinal, neurologic, bone, musculoskeletal

b) **Poor intake**
   - ❏ Maternal-infant bonding
   - ❏ Neglect
   - ❏ Environmental factors (famine)

c) **Excessive utilisation**
   - ❏ Acute or chronic infection

d) **Malabsorption**
   - ❏ Coeliac disease
   - ❏ Cystic fibrosis
   - ❏ Inflammatory bowel disease (IBD)
   - ❏ Malabsorptive enteropathies

Key Objectives

- Identify by comparing to normal growth charts the normal from the abnormally growing and developing child.

- Identify the factors which will give rise to a child who fails to thrive.

General/Specific Objectives

- Through efficient, focused data gathering:

    - Plot growth parameters for any child at regular intervals so as to identify any significant deviation from normal growth curve.

    - Obtain those features on history and physical examination known to be associated with failure to thrive.

    - Diagnose the common causes of failure to thrive at the different age groups.

    - Identify the various social risk factors responsible for failure to thrive.

- Interpret critical clinical and laboratory findings which were key in the processes of exclusion, differentiation and diagnosis:

    - Interpret growth parameters to diagnose failure to thrive.

    - Investigate with minimum but appropriate evaluations the commonly associated problems associated with a child who is failing to thrive.

- Conduct an effective plan of management for a child/infant with a failure to thrive:

    - Conduct a counselling and education programme for caregivers of children with failure to thrive.

    - Conduct an ongoing programme to monitor the progress of such children.

    - Appropriately utilise hospitalisation, consultation with other health professionals and community resources.

    - Explain the social and psychological impact of failure to thrive on the family and child.

036 Failure to Thrive

036B Failure to Thrive in the Elderly

Overview
In an elderly person failure to thrive means the loss of energy, interest and vigour, with or without weight loss. The challenge is to differentiate normal decline of strength with ageing from reversible conditions which may be due to organic disease, environmental factors or psychiatric disorders. Symptoms of serious organic disease are often minimal or even absent in the elderly. Iatrogenic conditions also occur more often in the elderly due to polypharmacy and resultant confusional states. Psychiatric disorders may accompany or be secondary to organic disease, so the search for organic disorders must be thorough before attributing decline to the ageing process or to environmental causes. If clinical assessment does not reveal a cause the most productive investigations in most cases are those which can be attained without invasive procedures.

Causes

1) Organic

    a) Gastrointestinal (poor mastication/swallowing, malabsorption)

    b) Cardiac/Respiratory disease

    c) Metabolic (renal failure, diabetes)

    d) Occult infections (especially urinary tract)

    e) Malignancy – undiagnosed/advanced

    f) Hyper/hypothyroidism

2) Extrinsic / Functional / Social

    a) Medications – especially adverse effects of polypharmacy

    b) Inadequate diet

    c) Loneliness and bereavement

    d) Poverty and isolation (poor mobility)

    e) Elderly abuse or neglect

    f) Alcoholism

3) Psychiatric

    a) Endogenous depression

    b) Confusional states secondary to organic disease including vitamin B_{12} deficiency

    c) Dementia

Key Objectives

- Select the investigations which screen the patient for occult organic causes.

- Conduct an assessment of cognitive function using the Folstein Mini–Mental State Examination (MMSE).

- Calculate the body-mass index (BMI) (= weight (kg)/height (M^2)); recognise that figures outside 22–27 constitute a health risk.

General/Specific Objectives

- Through efficient, focused data gathering:

  - Conduct a review of all body systems.

  - Check the status and management of known continuing health problems.

  - Elicit information about the patient's environment and relationships.

- Interpret critical clinical and laboratory findings which are key in the process of exclusion, differentiation and diagnosis:

  - Select further investigations or specialised care when indicated.

- Conduct an effective plan of management for an elderly patient who is failing to thrive:

  - Treat the identified cause with specific therapy when possible.

  - Counsel the patient and relatives about cause, management and prognosis.

  - List the support services which will improve isolation, nutrition, personal care, medication use, independence and home care.

Overview
Falls are common (30% of people over 65 years; 50% by 80 years) and are associated with functional disability, but they may be preventable. Interventions that prevent falls and their sequelae may delay or reduce the frequency of nursing home admissions.

Causes

1) Factors extrinsic to the patient

    a) **Accidental and environmental factors**

    b) **Medications/Alcohol**

2) Factors intrinsic to the patient

    a) **Age-related changes** (e.g. vision, musculoskeletal, cortical function, etc.)

    b) **Syncope**
       (see #109 Syncope / Pre-Syncope / Loss of Consciousness)

    c) **Dizziness/Vertigo**
       (see #029 Dizziness/Vertigo)

    d) **Gait disturbances / Ataxia** (
       see #042 Gait Disturbances – Ataxia)

3) Other – narcolepsy, cryptogenic, depression

Key Objectives
- In a patient with one or more falls, elicit a description of the fall (obtain collateral information if necessary) and conduct an evaluation of the environment for risk factors.

- Differentiate between causes of falls by determining whether the fall was secondary to factors intrinsic or extrinsic to the patient.

- Appreciate that a minority of falls are caused by a single, specific cause; the remainder are caused by more than a single factor.

General/Specific Objectives
- Through efficient, focused data gathering:

    - Determine whether factors extrinsic to the patient may have caused the fall (drugs, alcohol, environmental hazards such as poor illumination, stairs, clutter, uneven or slippery surface, inappropriate footwear).

    - Determine whether factors intrinsic to the patient may have caused the fall (ataxia, cognitive impairment, impaired vision, gait disturbance, other disease entities).

- Conduct a physical examination and performance evaluation including postural changes in blood pressure (BP), visual acuity, musculoskeletal and neurological function, and footwear. Assess gait and balance.

- Interpret critical clinical and laboratory findings which were key in the processes of exclusion, differentiation, and diagnosis:

  - Conduct an environmental assessment for hazards.

- Conduct an effective plan of management for a patient who has a tendency to fall:

  - Counsel and educate the patient or caregiver about the complications, morbidity, and mortality associated with falls. Describe the sequelae of falls (injury, functional decline, restraints, immobility, death).

  - Treat correctable conditions.

  - Outline a management programme that includes control of risk factors and provision of an active rehabilitation programme that focuses on gait and balance retraining for seniors, with the provision of spectacles and walking aids if appropriate.

  - List possible modifications in the living environment that reduce the risk of falling (e.g. grab rails, sturdy furniture, improved lighting).

  - Select patients in need of specialised care.

Overview

'Fatigue' means weariness from exertion but is used by both patients and doctors synonymously with such terms as tiredness, weariness, lacking energy, listlessness, sleepiness, exhaustion, weakness and being 'run down'. Possible causes are legion, as indicated below.

Accordingly the symptom is not of high diagnostic value unless it is the outstanding feature of a patient's presenting complaint or associated with certain other symptoms such as loss of weight, chest pain, breathlessness, diarrhoea, rectal bleeding. An organic cause will be found in only about one-third of patients with 'fatigue' as their main complaint; many people with heavy domestic or occupational commitments present – not unreasonably – with fatigue.

Of the remainder, about two-thirds will be suffering from a psychological condition. Patients commonly use fatigue to somatise an underlying psychological problem. The challenges are to identify underlying organic causes or associated pathology and manage these appropriately, whilst recognising those patients without physical illness who require more than simple reassurance and advice.

Causes

1) Psychologic

    a) Depression

    b) Anxiety

    c) Somatisation

    d) Bereavement

    e) Lifestyle factors

2) Pharmacologic

    a) Hypnotics

    b) Antihypertensives

    c) Antidepressants

    d) Alcohol

    e) Drug abuse or withdrawal

3) Endocrine/Metabolic

    a) Hypothyroidism

    b) Diabetes mellitus

    c) Adrenal disease (Addison disease, Cushing disease)

    d) Chronic renal failure

    e) Chronic liver failure

    f) Hypercalcaemia

    g) Hypokalaemia

    h) Hypomagnesaemia

4) Cardio-pulmonary

    a) Chronic congestive heart failure

    b) Ischaemic heart disease

5) Infectious

    a) Bacterial endocarditis

    b) Tuberculosis (TB) and other chronic infections

    c) Viral (mononucleosis, hepatitis, HIV, cytomegalovirus (CMV), influenza)

6) Connective tissue disorders

    a) Rheumatoid arthritis (RA) / Polymyalgia

7) Sleep disturbances

    a) Sleep-apnoea

    b) Oesophageal reflux

    c) Chronic pain interfering with sleep

8) Neoplastic-haematologic

    a) Occult malignancy

    b) Anaemia

9) Neuromuscular

    a) Parkinson disease

    b) Multiple sclerosis

    c) Motor neurone disease

    d) Myasthenia gravis

10) Idiopathic

    a) Idiopathic chronic fatigue

    b) 'Chronic fatigue syndrome'

    c) 'Fibromyalgia'

Key Objectives

- Identify underlying organic disease if present.

- For patients whose fatigue does not have an organic basis, determine the cause and provide advice about lifestyle, relationships or environmental changes.

- Select patients who require more formal psychiatric treatment.

General/Specific Objectives

- Take a comprehensive history which includes details of presenting symptoms, past history, family history, social and work history, habits, systems review and current medication.

- Conduct a thorough physical examination, even when finding an abnormality seems improbable.

- Use discrimination in the selection of investigations:

  - Directed at occult organic disease (e.g. anaemia, primary hyperparathyroidism).

  - To followup diagnostic clues found in the history or physical examination.

  - Be familiar with the criteria for the diagnosis of chronic fatigue syndrome.

Overview

Non-reassuring fetal status occurs in 5–10% of pregnancies. Fetal distress, a term also used for this situation, is imprecise and has a low positive predictive value. Thus, when there is concern about fetal status, the newer term should be used.

Causes

1) Utero-placental insufficiency

  a) Placental oedema (diabetes, hydrops)

  b) Placental 'accidents' (abruption, praevia and/or accreta)

  c) Post-dates

  d) Intra-uterine growth restriction

2) Umbilical cord compression

  a) Umbilical cord accidents (prolapse, knot, anomalous insertion of cord)

  b) Oligohydramnios

3) Fetal conditions/anomalies

  a) Sepsis (maternal, fetal, chorioamnionitis)

  b) Fetal congenital anomalies

  c) Prematurity

Key Objective

• Interpret information such as fetal heart rate and acid-base status after considering patient's antepartum information and known risk factors in order to identify non-reassuring fetal status.

General/Specific Objectives

- Through efficient focused data gathering:

    - Identify historical (e.g. hypertension, smoking) and examination risk factors (e.g. fetal size less than expected).

    - List indications for fetal monitoring (antepartum and intrapartum).

    - Diagnose fetal tachycardia (greater than 160 bpm for more than 10 minutes) and fetal bradycardia (fewer than 120 bpm for more than 10 minutes), deceleration patterns, problems of short term variability, reactivity.

- Interpret critical clinical and laboratory findings which were key in the processes of exclusion, differentiation and diagnosis:

    - Describe the measurement of fetal acid-base status (scalp pH, cord pH) and list indications for such assessments.

- Conduct an effective plan of management for a patient whose fetus is in a non-reassuring state:

    - Outline the management of post-term pregnancy.

    - Outline the management of infectious diseases during pregnancy that may impair fetal development.

    - List causes of intra-uterine growth restriction.

    - List options regarding mode of delivery if fetal condition is possibly non-reassuring.

    - While awaiting delivery, outline conservative measures for the management of the mother (e.g. discontinue oxytocin, administer oxygen to the mother, check maternal blood pressure (BP) and treat if necessary, change maternal position to left lateral, volume expansion if problem follows insertion of epidural).

    - Identify the short and long term consequences of fetal non-reassuring status.

    - List risk factors for fetal congenital abnormalities (e.g. chromosomal, associated with teratogens).

    - Counsel parents with psycho-emotional consequences of fetal development problems.

    - Select patients with non-reassuring fetal status for referral since in-depth training and experience in obstetrics are required to manage the condition adequately.

Overview

Fever in children is the most common symptom for which parents seek medical advice. While most causes are self-limited viral infections (febrile illness of short duration), it is important to identify serious underlying disease and/or those other infections amenable to treatment.

Causes

1) Febrile illness of short duration (less than two weeks)

a) **Viral**

❑ With rash (varicella, morbilli, rubella, erythema infectiosum, roseola infantum, Ross River fever, herpes simplex, herpes zoster)

❑ Without rash (common cold, adenoviral, enteroviral, mumps, Epstein-Barr virus (EBV), cytomegalovirus (CMV), influenza, hepatitis A, Murray Valley encephalitis)

b) **Bacterial**

❑ With rash (meningitis, scarlet fever, impetigo)

❑ Without rash (streptoccocal pharyngitis, pneumonia, urinary, meningitis, skin)

c) **Other infectious agents (mycoplasma pneumonia)**

2) Prolonged febrile illness (more than two to three weeks)

(see #040A Fever/Pyrexia of Unknown Origin (PUO))

a) **Familial-hereditary diseases**

b) **Other (malaria, tuberculosis (TB), Hodgkin lymphoma)**

Key Objectives

•   Determine whether the febrile illness is of short duration or is prolonged.

•   Differentiate between acute viral or pyogenic infections, and contrast to prolonged febrile illness.

040A Fever/Pyrexia of Unknown Origin (PUO)

Overview

Fever/Pyrexia of unknown origin (PUO) defines a febrile illness of three weeks or more without an established diagnosis despite extensive investigation.

Causes

1) Infections (approximately one-third of cases)

a) **Systemic**

- ☐ Endocarditis
- ☐ Tuberculosis (TB)
- ☐ Malaria
- ☐ Other infections (e.g. brucellosis, Q fever)

b) **Localised**

- ☐ Abscess
  - • Contiguous spread (e.g. liver, sub-phrenic from hepato-biliary, bowel)
  - • Haematogenous spread (e.g. splenic)
  - • Perinephric/Renal
- ☐ Osteomyelitis
- ☐ Central nervous system (CNS) infections (meningitis, encephalitis)

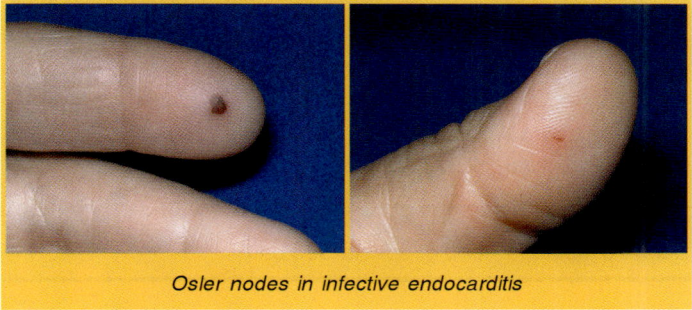

Osler nodes in infective endocarditis

a) Lymphoma/Leukaemia

b) Solid (renal cell, hepatoma/metastases)

3) Multi-system

a) Collagen disease (systemic lupus erythematosus (SLE), rheumatoid arthritis (RA))

b) Granulomatous (sarcoidosis, giant cell arteritis, other vasculitis)

c) Drug reactions

d) Miscellaneous (e.g. factitious)

Key Objectives

- Perform repeated clinical assessments searching for unusual presentations of common conditions.

- Elicit a history of travel, animal exposure, whether the patient may be immunosuppressed, is taking any type of medications (e.g. antimicrobial drugs) or had contact with toxins.

General/Specific Objectives

- Through efficient, focused data gathering:

  - Perform a detailed history and physical examination, especially searching for localising symptoms and signs.

- Interpret critical clinical and laboratory findings which were key in the processes of exclusion, differentiation, and diagnosis:

  - Conduct the minimum diagnostic investigation based on causal conditions most frequently associated with fever of unknown origin.

  - List indications for lumbar puncture, computed tomography (CT) scan of head or spine, serologic testing, or biopsy.

- Conduct an effective plan of management for a patient with fever of unknown origin:

  - State reasons why therapeutic trials without a firm diagnosis are generally counterproductive.

  - Outline a management plan consistent with the underlying causes.

  - Select patients in need of specialised care.

040B Fever in the Immune-Compromised Host / Recurrent Fever

Overview

Patients with certain immunodeficiencies are at high risk for infections, the infective organism and site depending on type and severity of immuno-suppression. Some of these infections are life-threatening.

Causes

1) Defects in cell-mediated immunity (T cells)

    a) Acquired cell-mediated immunity defect (HIV/AIDS, Hodgkin disease, immuno-suppressive therapy, lymphocytic leukaemia)

    b) Inherited cell-mediated immunity defect

2) Defects in humoral immunity (B cells)

    a) Loss (e.g. nephrotic syndrome)

    b) Decreased production (in infancy, transient; myeloma, lympho-proliferative disease)

3) Complement deficiencies (collagen disease, not necessarily associated with infection)

4) Asplenia (splenectomy, congenital absence, sickle cell disease, systemic lupus erythematosus (SLE), etc.)

5) Neutrophil dysfunction (granulomatous disease, uraemia, cirrhosis)

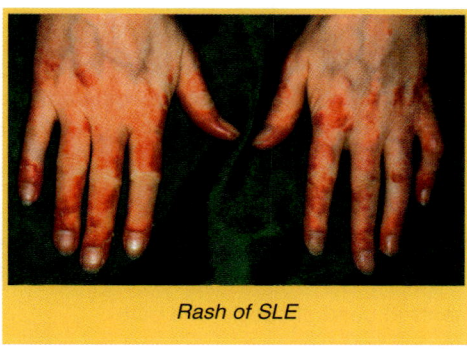

Rash of SLE

(see #010 Abnormalities of White Blood Cells)

7) **Anatomic barriers abnormal (surgery, foreign bodies, burns, desquamating rash)**

Key Objectives

- Determine if patients with fever have isolated febrile episodes or recurrent ones, single or multiple anatomic sites involved in infections, past history of infections and infections in relatives.

- Determine whether possible exposure to HIV occurred.

- Determine if immuno-suppressive or anti-infective medications are being taken or have recently been administered.

General/Specific Objectives

- Through efficient, focused data gathering:

  - Determine whether it is likely the patient with fever is immuno-compromised (e.g. persistent lymphadenopathy).

  - Determine whether the site of infection is single or multiple, and which body systems are likely to be involved (e.g. upper respiratory tract, lungs, skin, gastro-intestinal tract, nervous system).

  - Determine, if possible, the type of infection and/or organism isolated in previous infections.

- Interpret critical clinical and laboratory findings which were key in the processes of exclusion, differentiation, and diagnosis:

  - Select serum protein electrophoresis in a patient suspected of hypogammaglobulinaemia.

  - Select sites from which cultures should be obtained and interpret results.

  - Investigate a patient suspected to have HIV (HIV serology).

  - Select appropriate diagnostic imaging.

  - Contrast the type of organisms likely to cause infection in patients with asplenia or hypogammaglobulinaemia compared to organisms in cell-mediated immune defect.

- Conduct an effective plan of management for an immuno-compromised patient with fever:

  - Outline the initial management of a febrile patient who is immuno-compromised.

  - Select patients in need of specialised care.

  - Discuss indications for intravenous (IV) gamma globulin replacement therapy.

  - Discuss indications for prophylactic pneumococcal vaccination.

040C   Fever in the Neonate (in Child Less than Four Weeks)

Overview
Fever in neonates is serious, and the cause must be immediately identified and treated.

Causes

1)   Infections

a) **Bacterial**
- ❏ Pneumonia
- ❏ Urinary tract
- ❏ Septicaemia
- ❏ Meningitis
- ❏ Omphalitis
- ❏ Osteomyelitis, septic arthritis
- ❏ Conjunctivitis

b) **Toxoplasmosis**

c) **Viral**
- ❏ Cytomegalovirus (CMV)
- ❏ Herpes
- ❏ Rubella
- ❏ Other

2)   Overheating (e.g. in isolette)

Key Objective
- Rapidly assess the neonate to establish a working diagnosis and institute treatment immediately.

General/Specific Objectives
- Through efficient, focused data gathering:
  - Identify the features of a septic neonate.
  - Recognise that fever may be absent in a neonate with sepsis.
  - Identify the risk factors for sepsis in the neonate including maternal, host, immunologic and environmental factors.
  - Identify the causes of fever in the neonate.

- Interpret critical clinical and laboratory findings which were key in the processes of exclusion, differentiation and diagnosis:

  - Outline relevant and cost-effective investigations for a neonate with fever.

  - Contrast the differences in laboratory features in neonates and older infants and children with sepsis.

- Conduct an effective plan of management for a fever in the neonate:

  - Outline resuscitative measures in neonates with sepsis.

  - Outline the management of specific causes of sepsis in the neonate.

  - Perform specific procedures to diagnose cause of neonatal fever.

  - Counsel parents regarding the important issues in the short and long term outcome of neonatal fever.

040D Hypothermia

Overview

Although far less common than is elevation in temperature, hypothermia (central temperature less than 35°C) is of considerable importance because it can represent a medical emergency.

Causes

1)   **Accidental/Immersion hypothermia (exposure to cold)**

2)   **Hypothermia with acute illness (associated with metabolic acidosis, cardiac arrhythmias)**

    a) **Decreased heat production (hypothyroidism, drug overdose, diabetes mellitus, hypoglycaemia, congestive heart failure)**

    b) **Increased heat loss (cirrhosis, uraemia, respiratory failure, drug overdose)**

    c) **Impaired thermoregulation (stroke, drug overdose)**

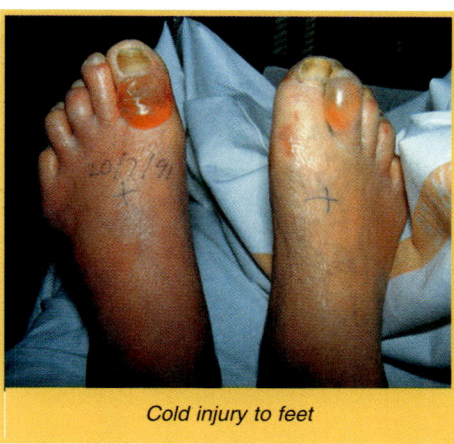

Cold injury to feet

Key Objective
- State that hypothermia is a potential medical emergency and urgent therapy may be necessary.

General/Specific Objectives

- Conduct an effective plan of management for a patient with hypothermia:

    - Outline an emergency management plan.

    - Contrast the advantages and disadvantages of active external re-warming and active core re-warming in accidental hypothermia.

- Through efficient, focused data gathering:

    - In patients with hypothermia secondary to acute illness, determine whether alcohol or other drugs were ingested.

    - Determine whether previous illnesses may have precipitated the hypothermia.

- Interpret critical clinical and laboratory findings which were key in the processes of exclusion, differentiation, and diagnosis:

    - Select, list, and interpret investigations immediately after therapy is initiated.

    - Recognise and prevent the potential hazards of iatrogenic hypothermia (massive transfusion, prolonged surgery, etc.).

    - Select patients in need of specialised care.

040E Hyperthermia

Overview

Hyperthermia is an elevation in core body temperature due to failure in thermo-regulation (in contrast to fever, which is induced by cytokine activation). Although the differential diagnosis is extensive (includes all causes of fever), the three conditions listed below may be associated with severe complications and death.

Causes

1) Heat stroke

    a) Classic

    b) Exertional

2) Neuroleptic malignant syndrome (NMS)

3) Malignant hyperthermia

Key Objective

- Determine the context in which the symptoms developed (e.g. malignant hyperthermia after anaesthetic, NMS after antipsychotics).

General/Specific Objectives

- Through efficient, focused data gathering:

  - Elicit a history of chronic medical conditions that either impair thermoregulation or prevent removal from a hot environment, heavy exercise in high ambient temperatures, anaesthetics, or antipsychotics.

  - Perform examination including rectal temperature, presence of pulmonary oedema, cardiac examination, evidence of bleeding, central nervous system (CNS) dysfunction, muscle tone.

- Interpret critical clinical and laboratory findings which were key in the processes of exclusion, differentiation and diagnosis:
  - Select investigations for the determination of disseminated intravascular coagulation (DIC), rhabdomyolysis, renal or hepatic failure, arrhythmias, pulmonary oedema.
- Conduct an effective plan of management for a patient with severe hyperthermia:
  - Recognise that external cooling may be potentially detrimental.
  - Outline various methods of cooling a hyperthermic patient, and indicate when to stop the cooling process.
  - Outline initial management.

(See also #113 Trauma/Accidents/Prevention and #113B Bone and Joint Injuries)

Overview
Fractures and dislocations are common problems at any age and are related to high-energy injuries (e.g. motor accidents, sport injuries) or, at the other end of the spectrum, simple injuries such as falls (see #037 Falls). Fractures and dislocations in children and young adults tend to be due to motor vehicle and sports injuries whereas in the elderly the cause is more likely to be associated with relatively minor trauma such as a fall.

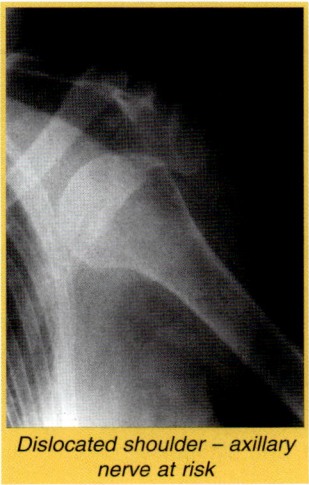

Dislocated shoulder – axillary nerve at risk

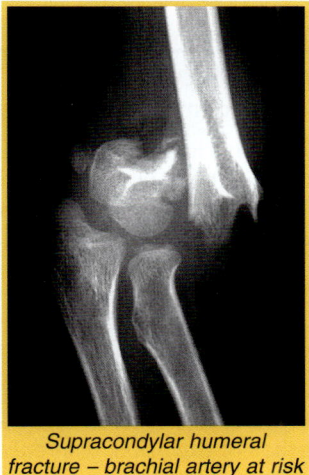

Supracondylar humeral fracture – brachial artery at risk

Causes

1)   **Fractures – traumatic**

2)   **Fractures – pathologic**

   a) **Metabolic bone disease**

   b) **Tumours (benign, malignant, primary, secondary)**

3)   **Fractures – stress**

4)   **Dislocations and fracture/dislocations**

Key Objectives
- In traumatic fractures recognise the importance of differentiating 'open' from 'closed' injuries and the need for early wound closure in the former.

- Appreciate and identify accurately and promptly the potential vascular and neurologic complications of common fractures and dislocations.

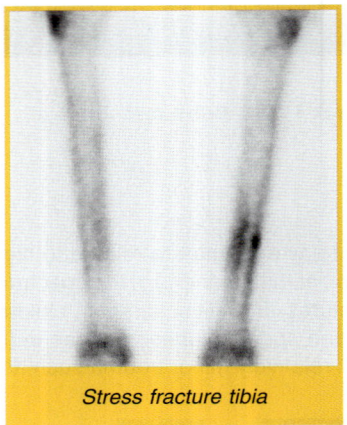

Stress fracture tibia

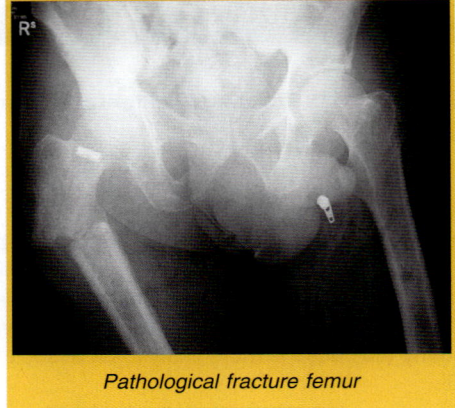

Pathological fracture femur

General/Specific Objectives

- Through efficient, focused data gathering:

    - Determine limb function, local soft tissue changes (closed or open fracture), bone or joint disruption, active and passive range of motion, status of joint above and below suspected long bone fracture.

    - Determine neurologic and vascular status distal to level of injury.

    - If minimal trauma causes a fracture, elicit history of conditions associated with pathologic fractures (metabolic bone disease, tumours), or identify activity that involves highly repetitive low-level stress (e.g. marching, running, ballet dancing).

- Interpret critical clinical and laboratory findings which were key in the processes of exclusion, differentiation, and diagnosis:

    - Select skeletal elements to be included in the diagnostic imaging required, as well as views.

    - List circumstances requiring additional diagnostic imaging such as computed tomography (CT), imaging of opposite side for comparison, joint above and below, bone scan, etc.

    - Outline investigation plan in a patient with a pathologic bone fracture.

- Conduct an effective plan of management for a patient with fractures / dislocations / joint injuries:

    - Recognise differing requirements for management of stable and unstable fractures.

    - List methods to obtain and maintain appropriate reduction.

    - Determine whether closed or open treatment is required and select patients requiring referral.

    - List complications of limb immobilisation and methods of maintaining reduction (e.g. plaster cast).

    - Outline management of specific fractures (e.g. stress fracture, pathological fracture).

Overview

Abnormalities of gait can result from disorders affecting several levels of the nervous system and the type of abnormality observed clinically often indicates the site affected.

Causes

1) Disorders of balance

    a) **Cerebellar ataxia – midline lesions (tumours, haemorrhage, infarct, multiple sclerosis, drugs, toxins)**

    b) **Sensory ataxia**

        ❑ Vestibular
        (see #029 Dizziness/Vertigo)

        ❑ Proprioceptive
        (see #069 Numbness and Tingling)

        ❑ Visual
        (see #120 Visual Disturbance/Loss)

2) Disorders of locomotion

    a) **Weakness disorders**
    (see #122 Weakness/Paralysis/Paresis)

    b) **Parkinsonian gait**
    (see #057 Involuntary Movement Disorders / Tic Disorders)

    c) **Higher level gait disorders (disorders of frontal lobes, basal ganglia, thalamus, midbrain such as stroke, hydrocephalus, dementia, tumours)**

    d) **Antalgic gait (disorders of the musculoskeletal system such as degenerative joint diseases and other arthropathies, deformities of legs, spinal disorders)**

3) Hysterical gait

Key Objective
- Determine whether the gait disturbance occurs more in the dark or light (sensory), whether giddiness or vertigo (vestibular) accompanies the disturbance, presence or absence and distribution of muscle weakness, and whether there is pain, numbness, or tingling in the limbs (sensory).

General/Specific Objectives

- Through efficient, focused data gathering:

  - Differentiate between cerebellar and sensory ataxia.

  - Determine whether there is weakness (difficulty rising from a chair, fatiguability of muscles), stiffness, or pain (trauma to legs, pelvis or spine, arthritis).

- Interpret critical clinical and laboratory findings which were key in the processes of exclusion, differentiation, and diagnosis:

  - Outline initial investigation for a patient with an abnormal gait.

  - Select patients in need of referral for further investigation.

- Conduct an effective plan of management for a patient with gait disturbance/ataxia:

  - Select patients in need of specialised care.

  - Outline a management plan for patients with antalgic gait.

(See also #129A Congenital Malformations)

Overview

Three out of 100 infants are born with a congenital defect or genetic disorder. Many of these are associated with a mental retardation or learning disability. Although early involvement of genetic specialists in the care of children with dysmorphic disorders is prudent, primary care clinicians are at times, required to contribute immediate care, and subsequently, assist with long term management of such patients.

Causes

1)   Teratogenic disorders (fetal alcohol syndrome, cocaine, coumarin)

2)   Chromosomal disorders

    a) **Down syndrome**

    b) **Turner syndrome**

    c) **Fragile X chromosome**

    d) **Klinefelter syndrome**

3)   Genetic syndromes

    a) **Tuberous sclerosis**

    b) **Neurofibromatosis**

    c) **Duchenne muscular dystrophy**

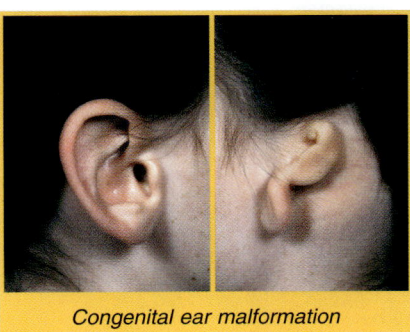

Congenital ear malformation

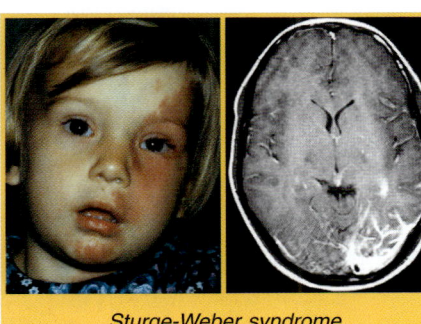

Sturge-Weber syndrome

Key Objective
- Demonstrate empathy for parents' concern, if diagnosis is known, outline probable course/management, and discuss early referral for specialised care, if appropriate.

General/Specific Objectives
- Through efficient, focused data gathering:

    - Formulate a phenotype from relevant family history.

    - Determine exposure, if any, to teratogens in pregnancy.

    - Differentiate chromosome disorders or genetic syndromes in the family from other types of dysmorphic features.

- Interpret critical clinical and laboratory findings which were key in the processes of exclusion, differentiation and diagnosis:

    - List indications for antenatal screening in a subsequent pregnancy.

    - Determine by seeking the advice of a specialist whether any immediate investigation is required prior to referral.

- Conduct an effective plan of management for a patient with dysmorphic features:

    - Explain the alternatives for dealing with the risk of recurrence.

    - Counsel families or refer for genetic counselling if a genetic disorder is identified concerning future risks and prenatal strategies for the prevention of dysmorphic disorders.

    - Discuss with the parents that the long term care will depend on the diagnosis and prognosis, but may involve specialised medical care, multidisciplinary services, family support, and if necessary, academic support and child placement.

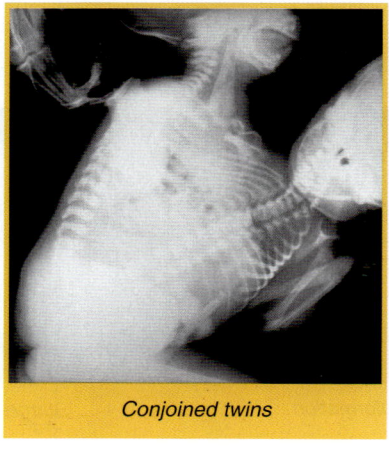

Conjoined twins

043A Genetic Concerns, Screening

Overview

Advances in genetics have increased our understanding of the origin of many diseases. Not infrequently, spouses who are considering becoming parents, or have just conceived, seek medical advice because of concerns they might have. Primary care clinicians and others must provide counselling and referral if further evaluation is necessary.

Causes

1) Chromosome defects

    a) **Numerical (Down syndrome)**

    b) **Structural (*cri-du-chat*)**

2) Mendelian – common causes are listed below

    a) **Dominant**

        ❏ Huntington chorea

        ❏ Familial hypercholesterolaemia

        ❏ Polycystic kidney disease

    b) **Recessive (cystic fibrosis)**

    c) **X-linked**

        ❏ Haemophilia

        ❏ Duchenne muscular dystrophy

3) Multifactorial conditions (neural tube defects)

Key Objective

- Elicit history on the *proband* or *index case* (the clinically affected person who has brought the family to the attention of the clinician) and of each of the *first-degree* relatives (parents, siblings, and offspring of the proband). Formulate a three-generation pedigree.

General/Specific Objectives

- Through efficient, focused data gathering:

  - Elicit history regarding prior obstetrical, medical, and family history, exposure or concerns during current pregnancy, age of mother at date of delivery.

  - Determine whether there are relatives with identical, similar, or associated features, or a problem recognised to be genetically determined: is there consanguinity, what is the ethnic origin of the family? Unexplained early neonatal death may indicate an inherited genetic disorder.

  - Identify/search literature for physical characteristics/hallmark features of genetic conditions.

- Interpret critical clinical and laboratory findings which were key in the processes of exclusion, differentiation and diagnosis:

  - List diagnostic tests available for prenatal diagnosis in a subsequent pregnancy (e.g. amniocentesis, fetal blood sampling); discuss sensitivity, specificity, expense, and risk of such testing.

  - Differentiate between screening tests and diagnostic tests for chromosome disorders and list indications.

  - Select patients who require consultation with a DNA laboratory or geneticist consultant regarding additional investigation and plan this prior to next pregnancy.

- Conduct an effective plan of management for screening genetic concerns/dysmorphic features:

  - Counsel pertinent family members by explaining meiosis, mitosis, and errors leading to aneuploidy.

  - Select patients for referral to genetics specialists, community resources, social support groups, etc.

  - Counsel patients regarding alternative reproductive options (e.g. contraception, therapeutic donor insemination, donor ova, adoption, prenatal diagnosis with/without therapeutic termination of affected fetus, embryo biopsy and assessment within an invitro-fertilisation programme (IVF) (with subsequent transfer of normal embryos only).

044A Hair Disorders

Overview

Symptoms of too little or too much hair are common. Loss of hair and hirsutism may have serious effects on self-esteem. A correct diagnosis is usually possible from systematic history-taking and examination. Hair changes can provide significant hints of underlying systemic disease. A treatable underlying cause may be present; but treatment is poorly effective except when an accompanying local inflammatory disorder is present.

Causes

1) Alopecia (hair loss)

a) Primary

- ❏ Alopecia areata, alopecia totalis, alopecia universalis (poor prognosis)
- ❏ Acute telogen effluvium – pregnancy, surgery, acute illness etc. (good prognosis)

b) Secondary

- ❏ Chronic telogen effluvium
  - • Metabolic and endocrine disorders (thyroid, diabetes, puberty)
  - • Iron and zinc deficiency
  - • Advanced malignancy
  - • Malnutrition
- ❏ Anagen effluvium
  - • Chemotherapy and radiation therapy
  - • Poisoning (thallium, mercury, arsenic)
- ❏ Androgenic alopecia
  - • Male pattern baldness
  - • Female pattern baldness
- ❏ Infections (tinea capitis)

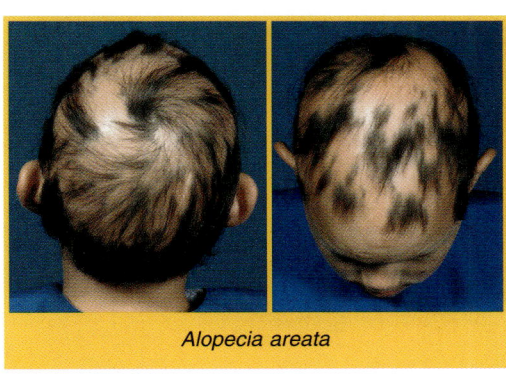

Alopecia areata

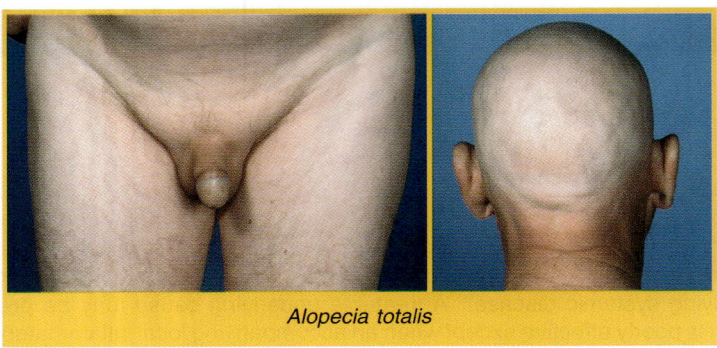
Alopecia totalis

2) Hirsutism

(see #052 Hirsutism and Virilisation)

a) Virilisation absent

- ❏ Idiopathic
- ❏ Familial
- ❏ Drugs (minoxidil, cyclosporine, phenytoin)

b) Virilisation present (clitoromegaly, male habitus, voice deepening)

- ❏ Androgenic excess from ovarian or adrenal source

3) Local inflammation

a) Scaly scalp disorders

- ❏ Dandruff (pityriasis capitis)
- ❏ Seborrhoeic dermatitis
- ❏ Psoriasis

b) Infective hair disorders

- ❏ Folliculitis barbae
- ❏ Tinea capitis
- ❏ Lice (pediculosis) – head, pubic

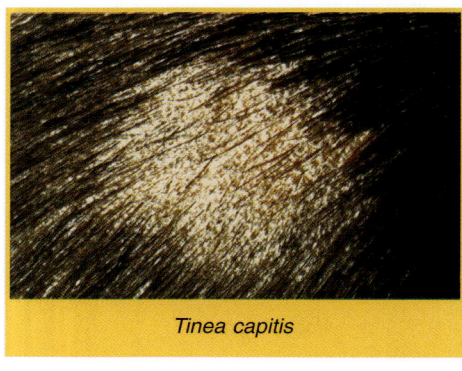
Tinea capitis

Key Objectives

- In patients with alopecia:

  - Identify type of hair loss.

  - Exclude secondary causes and establish whether scarring is present.

- In patients with hirsutism:

  - Determine whether virilisation is present, indicating need for full investigation.

General/Specific Objectives

- Through efficient, focused data gathering:

  - Differentiate between various causes by seeking corroborative evidence.

- Interpret critical clinical and laboratory findings which were key in the processes of exclusion, differentiation, and diagnosis.

- Interpret influences of hair cycles of anagen (the growing phase) and telogen (the resting phase when hair is normally shed).

- Conduct an effective plan of diagnosis and management for a patient with alopecia.

- Conduct an effective plan of diagnosis and management for a patient with other local hair disorders.

044B Nail Disorders

Overview

Nail changes frequently provide significant hints of underlying systemic disease. Changes in colour, surface or shape may be diagnostic.

Local medical and surgical nail disorders may involve nail bed and germinal matrix, nail plate, nail fold sulcus, lateral nail fold, or cuticle.

Causes

1) Nail changes in systemic disease

Nail sign	Condition
a) Colour change	
❏ Nail bed pallor	Anaemia
❏ Blue nails	Cyanosis, Wilson disease
❏ Red nails	Polycythaemia, carbon monoxide poisoning
❏ Yellow nails	Jaundice, tinea, tetracycline, yellow nail syndrome
❏ Brown nails	Nicotine, psoriasis, poisons
❏ White nails – leuconychia	Hypoalbuminaemia ('liver nails')
❏ Black nails	Haematoma, melanoma
❏ Splinter haemorrhages	Infective endocarditis, vasculitis, subclavian artery compression, blood dyscrasias, trauma

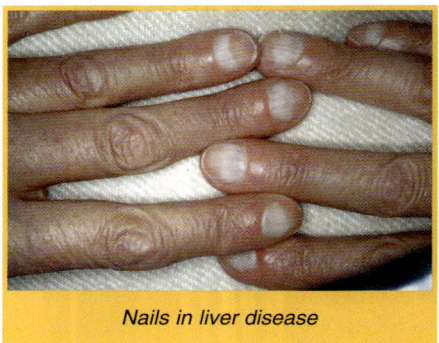

Nails in liver disease

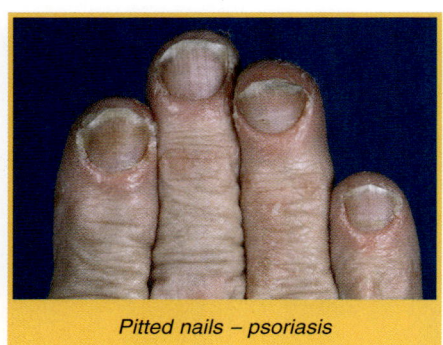

Pitted nails – psoriasis

b) Surface change

- Transverse grooves (Beau lines)   Serious illness or local trauma

- Opaque white transverse bands (Muehrcke or Mees lines)   As above, also hypoalbuminaemia, poisons, chemotherapy

- Pitting   Psoriasis, chronic paronychia

- 'Half and half' nails (white proximal and red distal)   Chronic renal disease, cirrhosis

c) Shape change

- Clubbing   Lung cancer, chronic lung suppuration, cyanotic heart disease, infective endocarditis, ulcerative colitis, thyroid acropathy in Graves disease

- Spoon shaped (koilonychia)   Iron deficiency anaemia, diabetes

- Onycholysis (separation of nail plate from nail bed)   Thyrotoxicosis, psoriasis, trauma

- Nail fold erythema and telangiectasis   Systemic lupus erythematosus (SLE), and other connective tissue disorders

- Hypoplastic   Congenital syndromes

- Onychogryposis (ram-horn nail)   Trauma, fungal infection, ischaemic, idiopathic

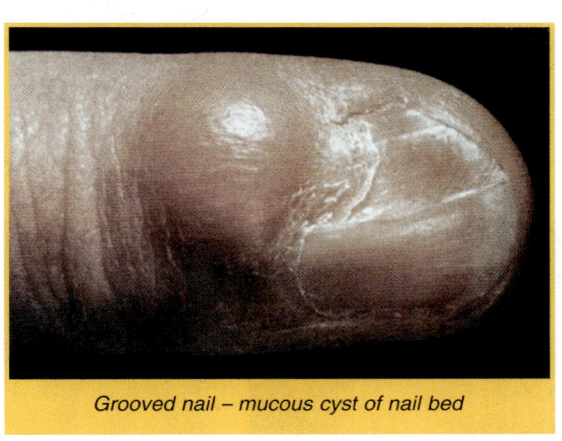

Grooved nail – mucous cyst of nail bed

a) 'Hang nail' – cuticle tear

b) Nail-biting – habit associated with emotional concerns

c) Chipped, engrimed – manual labouring occupations

d) Paronychia ('whitlow') infected nail fold, acute or chronic, bacterial, fungal, herpetic (dishwashers, diabetics and nurses)

e) Onychomycosis – tinea unguim, more frequent in toenails

f) Ingrown toenail – onychocryptosis

g) Mucous cyst of nail bed / nail fold

h) Subungual haematoma or melanoma

i) Glomus tumour – marked tenderness

j) Hereditary pachyonychia

k) Drug effects – minocycline, tetracycline, antimalarials, retinoids, nicotine staining

Key Objectives
- Make nail assessment an integral component of examination of the limbs.
- Differentiate between changes in colour, surface and shape.
- Be alert to nail changes in systemic disease.

General/Specific Objectives
- Through efficient, focused data gathering:
  - Differentiate between various causes by seeking corroborative evidence.
- Conduct an effective plan of management for a patient with a nail disorder.
- Select patients in need of referral.
- Interpret critical clinical and laboratory findings which were key in the process of exclusion, differentiation and diagnosis.

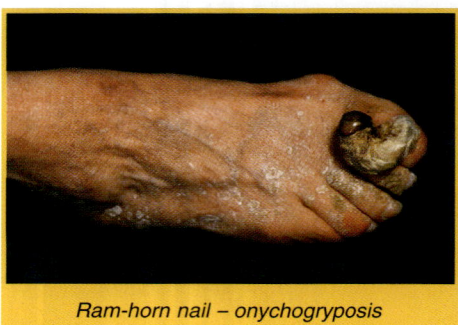

Ram-horn nail – onychogryposis

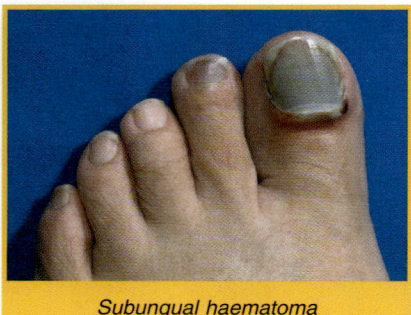

Subungual haematoma

Overview
Most head injuries follow blunt trauma. Fractures of the skull can be open/compound externally in association with scalp wounds, or internally from basal fractures. Cerebral concussion, contusion and laceration represent a spectrum of increasingly severe primary damage. The most important aspect of clinical neurological assessment is level of consciousness, together with abnormal neurological signs. Cerebral compression with progressive clinical deterioration is seen in patients with complications resulting from haematoma formation, cerebral oedema or hypoxic damage. A computed tomography (CT) scan is an essential baseline investigation in the patient with a severe head injury.

Causes

1)	**Blunt or penetrating injuries with or without skull fracture**

2)	**Cerebral concussion, contusion, laceration**

3)	**Cerebral haemorrhage/haematoma (epidural, subdural, subarachnoid, intracerebral)**

4)	**Cerebral oedema/compression**

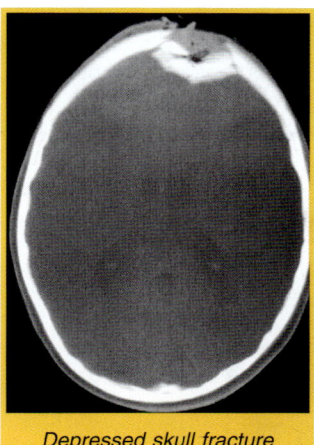

Depressed skull fracture

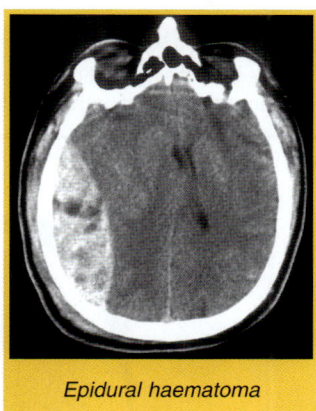

Epidural haematoma

Key Objectives
- Grade level of consciousness on Glasgow Coma Scale using responses of eye opening, best motor response and best verbal response.
- Select CT scan of the head in a patient, whose mental status is depressed or worsening, has focal neurologic deficit, depressed skull fracture, or penetrating head injury.

General/Specific Objectives

- Through efficient, focused data gathering:

  - Elicit history on more than one occasion to detect change in mental status.

  - Perform neurological examination on more than one occasion.

- Interpret critical clinical and laboratory findings which were key in the processes of exclusion, differentiation, and diagnosis:

  - Contrast time course for appearance of abnormal findings on head CT for epidural haematoma from middle meningeal artery injury from epidural or subdural haematoma resulting from venous injury.

  - Order repeat head CT for patient whose neurologic condition deteriorates or fails to improve as expected.

- Conduct an effective plan of management for a patient with head injury:

  - Select patients in need of specialised care.

  - Assess patients with deep non-responsive coma for criteria of brain death by establishing diagnosis of irreversible absence of brain stem reflexes and permanent absence of spontaneous breathing under conditions that exclude the effects of hypocapnia and neuromuscular blocking drugs.

  - In a patient whose head injury has caused brain death but the heart is beating, communicate this information to the transplantation team (or equivalent) if the deceased patient or the family have indicated a desire to donate organ(s).

  - If there is no indication that organ donation has been considered, counsel, with empathy, the family regarding the possibility.

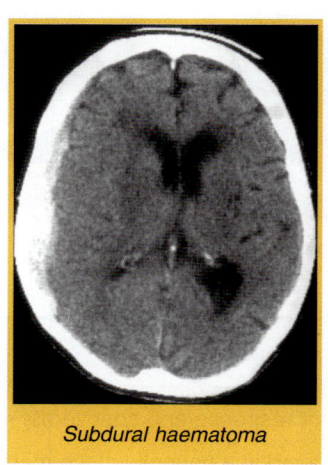

Subdural haematoma

Overview

The differentiation of patients with headaches due to serious or life-threatening conditions from those with benign primary disorders (e.g. tension headaches or migraines) is an important diagnostic challenge. Contrary to popular belief, 'eye strain' is not a common cause of headache.

Causes

1) Migraine

- a) With aura
- b) Without aura

2) Tension-type headache (also headache with medication overuse)

3) Cluster headache

4) Headache associated with vascular disorders

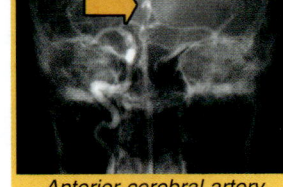

- a) Subarachnoid haemorrhage
- b) Temporal arteritis
- c) Venous thrombosis
- d) Intracranial haematoma (including epidural, subdural)
- e) Severe arterial hypertension

Anterior cerebral artery aneurysm

5) Headache associated with nonvascular intracranial disorder

- a) Elevated cerebrospinal fluid (CSF) pressure (intracranial mass lesion or hydrocephalus)
- b) Intracranial infection (meningitis, abscess, sinusitis)

6) Miscellaneous

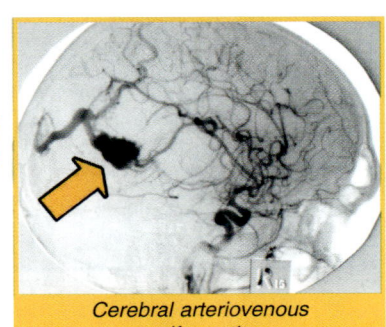

- a) Systemic viral infection
- b) Psychological disorders
- c) Medication use (nitroglycerin) or medication withdrawal (analgesic)
- d) Cervical spondylosis
- e) Poor working ergonomics (computer screen at wrong level, etc.)

Cerebral arteriovenous malformation

213

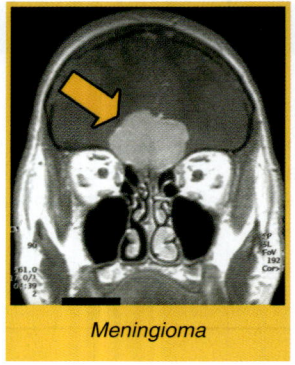

Meningioma

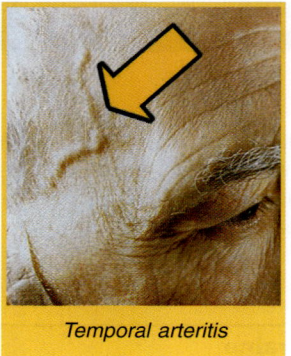

Temporal arteritis

Key Objective
- Elicit the signs and symptoms that help distinguish potentially serious from benign headaches.

General/Specific Objectives
- Through efficient, focused data gathering:

  - Differentiate between the various causes of headaches.

  - Select patients in need of immediate management.

- Interpret critical clinical and laboratory findings which were key in the processes of exclusion, differentiation and diagnosis:

  - Outline and interpret appropriate and cost-effective laboratory and diagnostic imaging tests used in the assessment of patients with headaches.

- Conduct an effective plan of management for a patient with a headache:

  - List the indications and contraindications for the use of various analgesic medications and for the prophylactic use of specific medications.

  - Outline use of analgesics and ergotamine for the purpose of avoiding the development of chronic daily headaches secondary to medication overuse.

  - Select patients in need of specialised care.

  - Provide patient education and counselling regarding the causes and management of headaches.

  - Identify patients with complications related to narcotic therapy and addiction.

Overview

There are many causes for hearing loss, many treatable and/or preventable. In paediatrics, otitis media accounts for 25% of all office visits. Although adults and older children have otitis less commonly, they may be affected by otitis sequelae.

Causes

1) Conductive hearing loss

a) **External ear pathology**

- ❏ Inflammation or infection
- ❏ Obstruction of canal (wax, foreign body, tumour)

b) **Middle ear pathology**

- ❏ Otitis media (acute, serous, chronic)
- ❏ Cholesteatoma
- ❏ Ossicular pathology (otosclerosis, fracture)
- ❏ Tumours (glomus, adenoma)

2) Sensorineural hearing loss (sudden, chronic)

a) **Cochlear (inner ear) pathology**

- ❏ Presbycusis of old-age
- ❏ Loud noise
- ❏ Ototoxic drugs (aminoglycosides)
- ❏ Trauma (temporal bone fracture)
- ❏ Inner ear disease (Ménière disease, autoimmune, etc.)

b) **Retro-cochlear/central pathology**

- ❏ Cerebellopontine angle tumours (acoustic neuroma, meningioma)
- ❏ Infection (meningitis)
- ❏ Multiple sclerosis
- ❏ Vascular occlusion

c) **Congenital**

- ❏ Hereditary, congenital syndromes
- ❏ High-risk birth 'TORCH' infections (*T*oxoplasmosis, *O*ther, *R*ubella, *C*ytomegalovirus, *H*erpes simplex virus), low birth weight, etc.

Key Objectives

- Differentiate between conductive and sensorineural hearing loss by history and tuning fork test.

- Communicate primary prevention strategy (ear noise protection).

General/Specific Objectives

- Through efficient, focused data gathering:

    - Elicit history mindful of the non-specific symptoms of otitis in younger children; examine after wax removal; identify risks of hearing loss (familial, industrial, drugs, at birth).

    - Differentiate conductive and sensorineural hearing loss with a tuning fork test.

- Interpret critical clinical and laboratory findings which were key in the processes of exclusion, differentiation, and diagnosis:

    - Differentiate conductive and sensorineural hearing loss on audiograms.

- Conduct an effective plan of management for a patient with hearing loss / deafness:

    - Select patients in need of specialised care.

    - Outline a management and followup plan for a patient with otitis, selecting appropriate antibiotics.

- Counsel and educate patients about primary prevention of hearing loss (e.g. ear noise protection).

Overview

Haematemesis, although often self-limited, is likely to be large and severe in elderly patients with arteriosclerotic vessels and may be associated with considerable mortality and morbidity without urgent management. Mortality and morbidity is also high in patients with portal hypertension.

Causes

1) Ulcerative/Erosive

a) Peptic ulcer disease

- ❏ Idiopathic

- ❏ Drugs (nonsteroidal anti-inflammatory drugs (NSAIDs), corticosteroids, immunosuppression)

- ❏ Infectious (*Helicobacter pylori*, cytomegalovirus (CMV), herpes simplex)

- ❏ Stress ulcer (postoperative, post-trauma, intensive care patients)

b) Oesophagitis

- ❏ Peptic

- ❏ Infectious

- ❏ Pill-induced, e.g. potassium chloride

2) Portal hypertension

3) Trauma / Severe vomiting (Mallory-Weiss syndrome)

4) Vascular malformations (angiomas, hereditary haemorrhagic telangiectasia (Osler disease))

5) Tumours (benign, malignant)

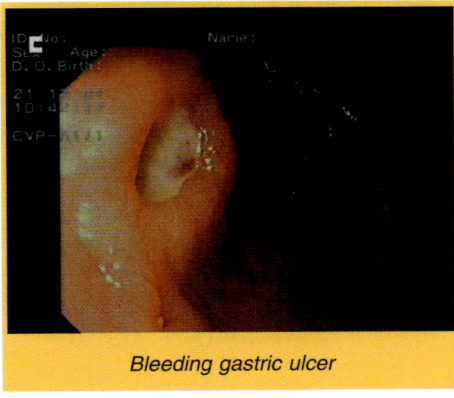

Bleeding gastric ulcer

Key Objectives

- Determine the haemodynamic stability of the patient and the resuscitation measures required.

- Select patients requiring admission to intensive care units.

- Select diagnostic studies after adequate resuscitation and stabilisation (to prevent complications of endoscopy) and deliver associated treatment if required.

General/Specific Objectives

- Through efficient, focused data gathering:

  - Diagnose the likely cause of haematemesis.

- Interpret critical clinical and laboratory findings which were key in the processes of exclusion, differentiation, and diagnosis:

  - Select appropriate investigations for the causes of haematemesis, and determine whether bleeding disorders are present.

  - List the indications for diagnostic endoscopy and diagnostic imaging.

  - List findings suggesting that likelihood of re-bleeding is high.

- Conduct an effective plan of management for a patient with haematemesis:

  - Outline the mechanism of action of various medical treatments.

  - List indications for pharmacological, endoscopic or surgical treatment.

  - Outline subsequent treatment to decrease recurrence.

  - Select patients in need of specialised care.

Overview

Haematuria is bleeding via the urinary tract and may be a dramatic presentation of renal or urinary tract pathology (frank haematuria) or a condition that is only detected on dipstick testing and/or microscopic examination. Phase contrast microscopy, except in frank haematuria, can indicate whether the bleeding is more likely to be of kidney origin (glomerular) or not.

Causes

1) Transient

  a) **Urinary tract infections (UTIs)**

  b) **Exercise-induced**

  c) **Glomerulonephritis**

  d) **Stones/Crystals**

  e) **Trauma**

  f) **Endometriosis**

  g) **Thromboembolism**

  h) **Anticoagulants**

2) Persistent

  a) **Extraglomerular**

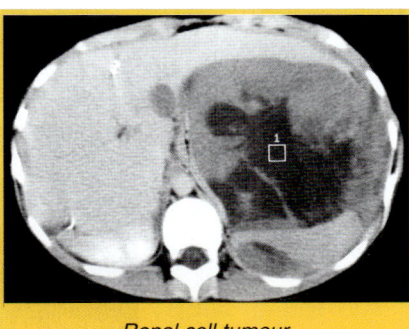

Renal cell tumour

    ❏ Renal
- Tumours
- Tubulointerstitial diseases (e.g. polycystic kidney disease, pyelonephritis)
- Vascular (e.g. papillary necrosis, sickle cell disease)

    ❏ Collecting system
- Tumours
- Stones

  b) **Glomerular**

    ❏ Isolated (e.g. immunoglobulin A (IgA) nephropathy, thin membrane disease)

    ❏ Post-infections (e.g. post-streptococcal)

    ❏ Systemic involvement (e.g. vasculitis, systemic lupus erythematosus (SLE))

Key Objective

- Differentiate red urine from haematuria, frank from microscopic haematuria, transient from persistent haematuria, and glomerular from extraglomerular haematuria.

General/Specific Objectives

- Through efficient, focused data gathering:

    - Determine whether the patient has true haematuria.

    - Diagnose the presence of UTIs.

    - Differentiate between glomerular and extraglomerular haematuria.

- Interpret critical clinical and laboratory findings which were key in the processes of exclusion, differentiation, and diagnosis:

    - Interpret reported urinalysis findings.

    - Outline significance of patient's age, gender, and lifestyle on diagnostic possibilities.

    - Formulate a diagnostic plan for a patient with frank haematuria.

- Conduct an effective plan of management for a patient with haematuria:

    - Select treatment for patients with UTIs appropriate for gender, and for lower and upper urinary tract.

    - Outline a plan for investigation of patients with recurrent nephrolithiasis.

    - Formulate a management plan for prevention of recurrent nephrolithiasis.

    - Discuss possible strategies for the detection and prevention of urinary tract tumours.

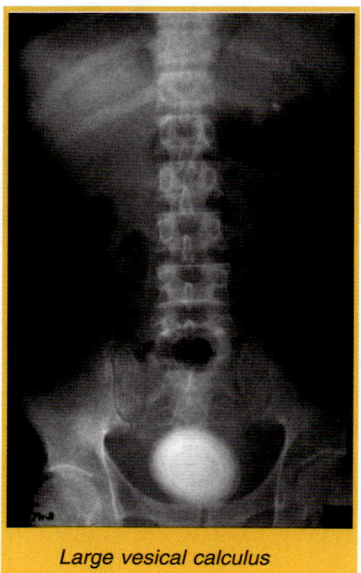

Large vesical calculus

Overview

Stroke is a focal neurologic deficit lasting longer than 24 hours, of presumed vascular origin. If the deficit lasts less than 24 hours, it is termed transient ischaemia. These arbitrary definitions are conventional but it is now recognised that a significant proportion of patients with transient ischaemic attacks will have pathological lesions on cerebral imaging (computed tomography (CT) and magnetic resonance imaging (MRI)). Vascular causes of neurological deficit usually have a sudden onset. Hemiplegia and hemianaesthesia arise from a lesion above the mid-cervical region, and aphasia indicates the involvement of the dominant cerebral hemisphere. The occurrence of a stroke or transient ischaemia indicates significant vascular, cardiac or haematological disease demanding investigation and appropriate medical or surgical treatment.

Causes

1) Stroke or transient ischaemia

  a) **Ischaemic**

    ❑ Embolism, thrombosis, hypoperfusion

  b) **Cerebral haemorrhage**

    ❑ 'Spontaneous'

    ❑ Vascular malformation

    ❑ Clotting disorder

  c) **Subarachnoid haemorrhage**

    ❑ Usually indicating intracerebral bleeding or vascular spasm

2) Postepileptic (Todd palsy)

3) Head trauma

  a) **Cerebral contusion with haemorrhage and oedema**

  b) **Extradural haematoma**

  c) **Subdural haematoma**

4) Intracranial space-occupying lesions

  a) **Primary and secondary malignancy**

  b) **Benign tumours**

  c) **Cerebral abscess**

5) Hemiplegic migraine

a) Encephalomyelitis

b) Multiple sclerosis

7) **Infections**

a) Encephalitis

b) Toxoplasmosis (in AIDS)

Key Objectives

• Recognise the risk factors for stroke within the community, and recommend appropriate preventive measures.

• Diagnose the cause of hemiplegia, on the basis of history, clinical findings and neuro-imaging studies.

• Diagnose the cause of transient ischaemia and minor stroke and recommend appropriate medical or surgical treatment to prevent further stroke.

General/Specific Objectives

• Through efficient history-taking:

- Differentiate between the causes of hemiplegia based on history, time course, clinical findings and risk factors.

- Identify transient ischaemic syndromes including transient monocular blindness (amaurosis fugax), transient hemispheric syndromes and vertebrobasilar syndromes including visual, brainstem and cerebellar symptoms.

• Interpret critical clinical findings, laboratory data and CT and MRI scan images necessary to arrive at a presumptive diagnosis.

- Recognise the CT scan appearance of large vessel and lacunar cerebral infarction, cerebral haemorrhage, subarachnoid haemorrhage, extradural haematoma, subdural haematoma, cerebral contusion and intracranial space occupying lesion.

- Recommend other appropriate laboratory and imaging studies (including contrast CT and MRI) if required to arrive at a definitive diagnosis.

• Recommend an immediate plan of investigation and treatment for all patients presenting with transient ischaemia.

- Describe an effective plan of management for a patient with hemiplegia:
  - Outline the acute medical management of patients with ischaemic and haemorrhagic strokes.
  - Discuss the primary and secondary preventive measures used in the prevention of ischaemic stroke, including medications (anti-platelet and anticoagulant) and carotid endarterectomy.
  - Outline the management in the prevention of stroke of a patient with atrial fibrillation.
  - Select patients in need of specialised care.
  - Understand the effective and timely use of rehabilitation.

050A Paraplegia/Paraparesis

Overview

Acute paraplegia should be identified as a medical emergency which may require urgent surgery. Spinal cord lesions cause lower motor neuron signs at the level of the lesion and upper motor neuron signs below that level. High cervical lesions will cause tetraplegia (quadriplegia). Lesions at lower cervical level or below cause paraplegia or paraparesis, with sensory loss affecting trunk and lower limbs. Cord compression also causes neurogenic bladder involvement with bladder distension and overflow incontinence.

Causes

1) With cord compression

    a) Spinal fractures/dislocations

    b) Intervertebral disc prolapse

    c) Metastatic or primary neoplasms

    d) Vascular malformations

2) Without cord compression

    a) Vascular thrombosis

    b) Syringomyelia

    c) Demyelinating disease

    d) Nutritional deficiency (vitamin B_{12})

Key Objective

* Recognise acute paraplegia as a medical emergency and identify causes associated with cord compression.

General/Specific Objectives

- Through efficient, focused data gathering, diagnose level and cause of paraplegia/paraparesis.

    - Define the upper limit of sensory loss to help determine level of injury.

    - Describe and explain the dissociated sensory loss and other findings in hemi-section of the spinal cord (Brown-Séquard syndrome) and outline other causes of paraplegia with dissociated sensory loss.

    - Describe the role of investigation by plain X-ray, computed tomography (CT) scanning, magnetic resonance imaging (MRI) and isotope bone scan in making the diagnosis of causative lesions.

Overview

Expectoration of blood can range from blood streaking of sputum to massive haemoptysis (greater than 1,000 ml/day) that may be acutely life-threatening. Bleeding usually starts and stops unpredictably, but under certain circumstances may require immediate establishment of an airway and control of the bleeding.

Causes

1) Airway disease

a) **Neoplasms**

- ❏ Bronchogenic carcinoma
- ❏ Endobronchial metastatic carcinoma (melanoma, breast, renal, colon)
- ❏ Bronchial carcinoid
- ❏ Kaposi sarcoma (in patients with AIDS)

b) **Inflammatory**

- ❏ Bronchitis (acute, chronic)
- ❏ Bronchiectasis

c) **Other (foreign body, trauma, arteriovenous fistula)**

2) Pulmonary parenchymal disease

a) **Infectious (tuberculosis (TB), pneumonia, abscess, aspergilloma)**

b) **Inflammatory/Immune (Goodpasture syndrome, pulmonary haemosiderosis, Wegener granulomatosis, lupus pneumonitis)**

3) Vascular

a) **Elevated capillary pressure (left ventricular failure, mitral stenosis)**

b) **Pulmonary embolus**

c) **Arteriovenous malformation**

4) Bleeding disorders

5) Anticoagulant therapy

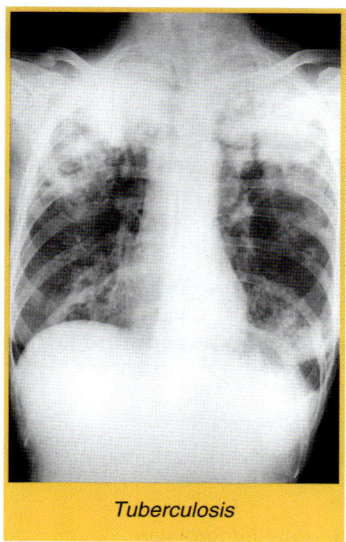

Tuberculosis

Key Objectives
- Determine whether the blood in sputum is true haemoptysis (originates below the vocal cords) rather than upper respiratory tract or upper gastrointestinal bleeding (haematemesis).
- Understand management principles for life-threatening haemoptysis.

General/Specific Objectives
- Through efficient, focused data gathering:

  - Differentiate between the causes of haemoptysis: contrast the disproportionate amount of blood flow in the pulmonary arteries (virtually the entire cardiac output) to the bronchial arteries (usually two branches off the aorta) to the origin of haemoptysis (more than 90% of the time from the bronchial arteries).

- Interpret critical clinical and laboratory findings which are key in the processes of exclusion, differentiation, and diagnosis:

  - Select investigations to determine the cause of haemoptysis (X-ray, computed tomography (CT) scan); if arteriogram is eventually selected, select imaging of the bronchial arteries first.

  - List indications for bronchoscopy.

- Conduct an effective plan of management for a patient with haemoptysis:

  - In the presence of massive haemoptysis (greater than 1,000 ml/day), establish airway first and consult a specialist capable of controlling the bleeding.

  - Outline the management of causes of haemoptysis which are not life-threatening and do not require immediate referral to a specialist.

  - Select patients in need of specialised care and/or consultation.

Overview

Hirsutism is a common problem, particularly in dark-haired, darkly pigmented, white women. However, if accompanied by virilisation, then a full diagnostic evaluation is essential.

Causes

1)   Androgen excess (may be associated with virilisation)

    a) Ovarian source
- Polycystic ovary syndrome
- Ovarian tumour (arrhenoblastoma)

    b) Adrenal Source
- Congenital adrenal hyperplasia
- Cushing syndrome
- Adrenal tumour (adenoma, carcinoma)

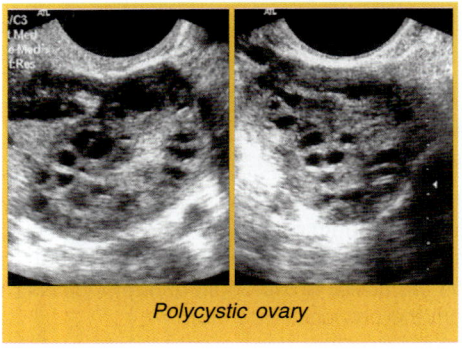

Polycystic ovary

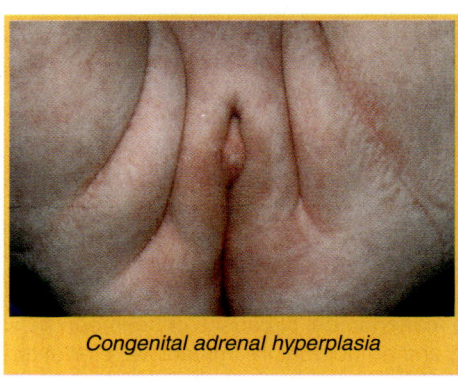

Congenital adrenal hyperplasia

2) Drugs (usually not associated with virilisation)

a) Phenytoin

b) Antihypertensives (minoxidil)

c) Cyclosporine

3) Familial (usually not associated with virilisation)

4) Idiopathic (usually not associated with virilisation)

Key Objective

- Outline the laboratory investigation for patients with signs of androgen excess.

General/Specific Objectives

- Through efficient, focused data gathering:

  - Determine which patients with recent onset of hirsutism require investigation.

  - Determine which patients with clinical symptoms and signs of defeminisation (i.e. amenorrhoea) and virilisation require investigation.

- Interpret critical clinical and laboratory findings which were key in the processes of exclusion, differentiation and diagnosis:

  - Select appropriate laboratory and imaging studies.

- Conduct an effective plan of management for a patient with hirsutism and virilisation:

  - Outline the medical management of patients with idiopathic hirsutism.

  - Outline the medical management of patients with polycystic ovary syndrome.

  - Counsel and educate patients with hirsutism on conservative methods of managing excess hair.

  - Select patients in need of specialised care.

Overview

Diabetes mellitus is a very common disorder. The morbidity and mortality associated with diabetic complications may be reduced by preventive measures. Intensive glycaemic control will reduce congenital malformations and neonatal complications in pregnancy-associated diabetes as well as complications associated with all other forms of diabetes.

Causes

1) Type I (beta-cell destruction insulin deficiency)

    a) Immune-mediated

    b) Idiopathic

2) Type II (insulin resistance)

3) Other specific types

    a) Genetic defects (*beta*-cell function or insulin action)

    b) Diseases of the pancreas (pancreatitis)

    c) Endocrinopathies (acromegaly, Cushing syndrome)

    d) Drugs (glucocorticoids, thiazides)

4) Gestational diabetes mellitus

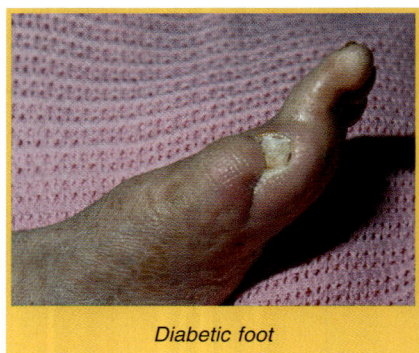

Diabetic foot

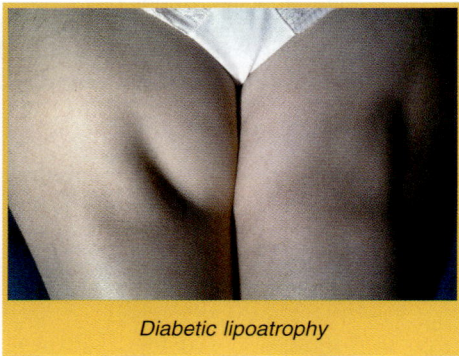

Diabetic lipoatrophy

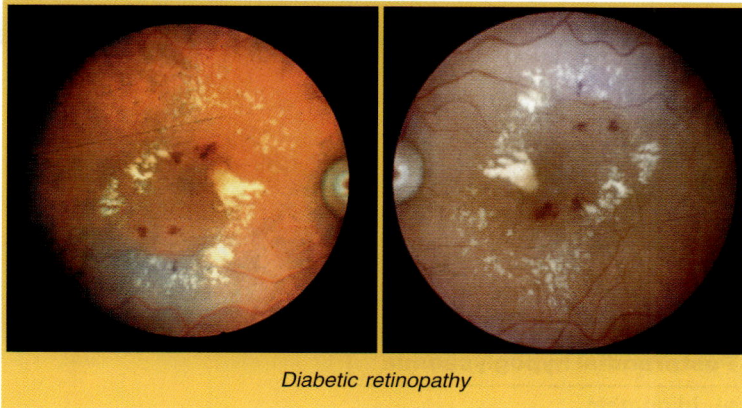

Diabetic retinopathy

053A Hypoglycaemia

Overview

Maintenance of the blood sugar within normal limits is essential for health. In the short term, significant hypoglycaemia is more dangerous than hyperglycaemia.

Causes

1) Postprandial hypoglycaemia

a) **Idiopathic**

b) **Alimentary hyperinsulinism (previous gastrectomy, gastrojejunostomy)**

2) Fasting hypoglycaemia

a) **Secondary to overutilisation of glucose**
- ❏ Associated with hyperinsulinism
  - Exogenous insulin, sulfonylureas (including factitious hypoglycaemia)
  - Insulinoma
  - Miscellaneous drugs (pentamidine, quinine)
- ❏ Associated with normal insulin levels
  - Large extrapancreatic tumours

b) **Secondary to impaired glucose production**
- ❏ Hormone deficiencies
  - Adrenal insufficiency
  - Hypopituitarism
- ❏ Substrate deficiency (severe malnutrition, muscle wasting)
- ❏ Drugs (alcohol, salicylate intoxication)
- ❏ Enzyme defects (glucose-6-phosphatase deficiency)
- ❏ Critical illnesses (severe hepatic failure, cardiac disease, sepsis)
- ❏ Autoimmune hypoglycaemia

Key Objectives
- Differentiate the causes of hypoglycaemia based on whether it occurs in the postprandial or fasting state.

- Determine the level of awareness of hypoglycaemia in patients prone to this condition.

General/Specific Objectives
- Through efficient, focused data gathering:

  - Identify those patients with true hypoglycaemia.

  - Differentiate the cause for hypoglycaemia.

- Interpret critical clinical and laboratory findings which were key in the processes of exclusion, differentiation and diagnosis; and important in formulating a differential diagnosis:

  - Evaluate the blood sugar in patients with symptoms suggestive of postprandial hypoglycaemia.

  - Outline the optimal laboratory work-up for a patient with fasting hypoglycaemia, which will include investigation at the time of the hypoglycaemia.

- Conduct an effective plan of management for a patient with hypoglycaemia:

  - Outline the management of an acute hypoglycaemic episode.

  - Counsel and educate patients with diabetes in relation to the symptoms and management (as well as prevention) of hypoglycaemia.

  - Select patients in need of specialised care.

Overview

Hypertension is a common condition affecting, in most countries, an increasing proportion of the population with increasing age and is a major contributor to the global burden of disease. A diagnosis of hypertension may require ambulatory blood pressure (BP) monitoring or self-monitoring. Appropriate management of hypertension can improve health outcomes. Central to an understanding of the impact of hypertension, through its effects on the cardiovascular system, is an appreciation of the family of cardiovascular risk factors and their interactions.

Causes

1) **Primary (essential hypertension)**

2) **Secondary**

   a) **Renal parenchymal disease (e.g. glomerulonephritis, reflux nephropathy, polycystic kidney disease, renal failure)**

   b) **Syndrome X**

   c) **Diabetes mellitus**

   d) **Sleep-apnoea syndrome**

   e) **Mineralocorticoid excess (e.g. adrenal adenoma or hyperplasia, glucocorticoid-suppressible hyperaldosteronism)**

   f) **Angiotensin II excess (e.g. unilateral renal artery stenosis)**

   g) **Catecholamine excess (e.g. phaeochromocytoma, drugs)**

   h) **Coarctation of the aorta**

   i) **Endocrine disorders (hypothyroidism, hyperthyroidism, hyperparathyroidism (HPT), Cushing syndrome)**

   j) **Genetic disorders (e.g. glucocorticoid-suppressible hyperaldosteronism, polycystic kidney disease, Liddle syndrome, multiple endocrine neoplasia)**

   k) **Drugs (sympathomimetics, cocaine, nonsteroidal anti-inflammatory drugs (NSAIDs), carbenoxalone, liquorice)**

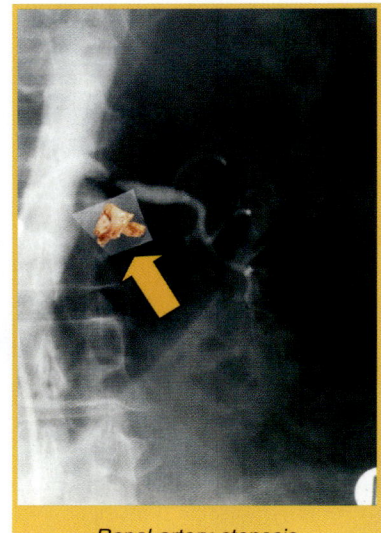

Renal artery stenosis

Key Objective

- Avoid mislabelling patients, select patients suitable for investigation for secondary causes, identify other cardiovascular risk factors and select the most appropriate management for each individual with hypertension.

General/Specific Objectives

- Through efficient, focused data gathering:

  - Diagnose hypertension and 'white coat' ('isolated clinic') hypertension.

  - Select patients suitable for investigation of secondary causes.

  - Identify end organ damage.

  - Characterise the patient's cardiovascular risk factor profile.

  - Identify hypertensive emergencies (e.g. hypertensive encephalopathy, dissecting thoracic aortic aneurysm, malignant hypertension).

- Interpret critical clinical and laboratory findings which were key in the processes of exclusion, differentiation, and diagnosis:

  - Diagnose renal parenchymal disease.

  - Select patients in need of specialised diagnostic care.

  - Discuss cost-effectiveness of investigation of hypertension.

- Conduct an effective plan of management for a patient with hypertension:

  - Risk stratification.

  - Define associated clinical conditions and comorbidities.

  - Set target BP levels and consider self-monitoring.

  - Outline non-pharmacological management strategies for patients, prior to pharmacological ones.

  - Select antihypertensive medication which will not adversely affect concomitant conditions such as diabetes mellitus, asthma, gout, and congestive heart failure.

  - Select appropriate agents for hypertensive emergencies (e.g. encephalopathy, dissection).

  - Communicate to patients the importance of consultation with other healthcare professionals (e.g. dieticians).

  - Determine factors contributing to non-compliance and discuss possible management strategies.

  - Discuss cost-effectiveness of management of hypertension.

054A Hypertension in Childhood

Overview
The prevalence of hypertension in children is less than one percent, but often results from identifiable causes (usually renal or vascular). Consequently, vigorous clinical investigation is warranted.

Causes

1) **Neonates and young infants (ischaemic or congenital renal disease, coarctation of the aorta, hypercalcaemia, neurogenic tumours, umbilical vessel catheterisation)**

2) **Children (1 to 10 years) (renal disease, both vascular and parenchymal, coarctation, or less commonly as above)**

3) **Children and adolescents (11 to adolescence) (renal disease, primary hypertension, or less commonly as above)**

Key Objectives
- Perform blood pressure (BP) measurements in infants and very young children with automated devices, and check BP tables for normal values.
- State that hypertension is a systolic or diastolic value greater than 95th percentile, appropriately measured.

General/Specific Objectives
- Through efficient, focused data gathering:
    - Diagnose hypertension and pseudohypertension; discuss 'white coat' hypertension.
    - Elicit or rule out signs of secondary hypertension.

- Interpret critical clinical and laboratory findings which were key in the processes of exclusion, differentiation, and diagnosis:

  - Outline value and use of ambulatory BP monitoring.

  - Diagnose renal parenchymal disease.

  - Select patients in need of diagnostic imaging and other laboratory investigation.

  - Discuss cost-effectiveness of investigation of hypertension.

- Conduct an effective plan of management for a paediatric age group patient with hypertension:

  - Outline for patients dietary treatment only if obese.

  - Select antihypertensive medication and dose.

  - Select appropriate agents for hypertensive emergencies (e.g. encephalopathy, cardiac failure).

  - Select patients in need of specialised care.

054B Pregnancy-Associated Hypertension

Overview
Preeclampsia is generally a self-limited disease with rapid resolution of hypertension and a low recurrence rate in future pregnancies (less than 7%). However, when severe, and especially when it occurs in the second trimester, preeclampsia is not so benign. Such patients are at high risk for recurrence in subsequent pregnancies (as high as 65% when the preeclampsia is in the second trimester) and also at high risk for hypertension later in life. The incidence of fetal growth retardation is about 10%.

Causes

1) Pregnancy-induced hypertension

   a) Preeclampsia

   b) Eclampsia

2) Chronic (pre-existing) hypertension / Chronic renal disease

   a) Preeclampsia superimposed on chronic hypertension

Key Objectives
- Describe the normal changes of blood pressure (BP) in pregnancy and define hypertension in pregnancy with these changes in mind.

- Outline the treatment of preeclampsia including consideration for early diagnosis, medical supervision, and timely delivery. This should include:

  - Control BP.

  - Assess maternal condition – urine, blood tests required.

  - Look for underlying medical condition.

  - Assess fetal condition.

  - Prevent eclampsia.

  - Delivery – timing and mode.

- Through efficient, focused data gathering:

  - Differentiate preeclampsia from chronic hypertension and transient hypertension.

  - Elicit symptoms and signs indicative of risk for eclampsia (e.g. headache, epigastric pain, visual abnormalities, proteinuria).

- Interpret critical clinical and laboratory findings which were key in the processes of exclusion, differentiation, and diagnosis:

  - Select and interpret laboratory investigation useful to the diagnosis of preeclampsia and 'HELLP' syndrome (*H*aemolysis, *E*levated *L*iver enzymes, *L*ow *P*latelets).

- Conduct an effective plan of management for a patient with hypertension in pregnancy:

  - Discuss the goals of management of hypertension in pregnancy (first, with respect to the safety of the mother, and second, the delivery of a live infant not requiring intensive, prolonged neonatal care) as listed in *Key Objectives* above.

  - Discuss strategies for the prevention of pregnancy-induced hypertension.

  - List drugs indicated and contraindicated in the management of hypertension in pregnancy.

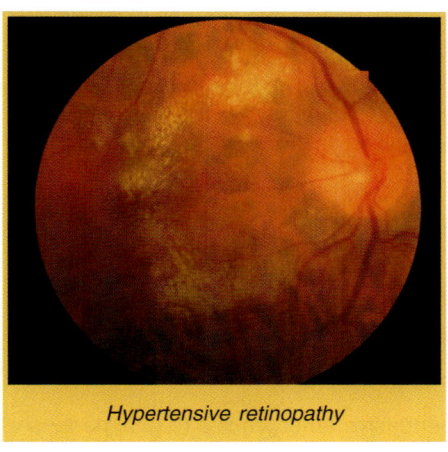

Hypertensive retinopathy

054C Hypertension in the Elderly

Overview

Elderly patients (older than 60–65 years) have hypertension much more commonly than younger patients do, especially systolic hypertension. The prevalence of hypertension among the elderly may reach 60%–80%.

Causes

Causes are the same as for hypertension in younger patients, but if age more than 50 years, secondary hypertension becomes more likely.

1) Primary hypertension

(see #054 Hypertension)

2) Secondary hypertension

(see #054 Hypertension)

Key Objectives

- Define hypertension in the elderly in a manner similar to younger patients; define pseudohypertension.

- Conduct antihypertensive pharmacologic treatment for systolic hypertension in elderly patients when systolic blood pressure (BP) is consistently greater than 160 mm Hg (use standing BPs as a guide to therapy), since evidence of benefit exists.

- State that the benefit of treating hypertension in the elderly is two to four times greater than that achieved in the treatment of younger patients with primary hypertension.

General/Specific Objectives

- Through efficient, focused data gathering:

    - Diagnose hypertension and pseudohypertension.

    - Select patients suitable for investigation of secondary causes.

    - Identify end organ damage.

    - Identify hypertensive emergencies (e.g. hypertensive encephalopathy, dissecting aortic aneurysm, malignant hypertension, transient ischaemic attacks).

- Interpret critical clinical and laboratory findings which were key in the processes of exclusion, differentiation, and diagnosis:

    - Diagnose renal parenchymal disease.

    - Select patients in need of specialised diagnostic care.

    - Discuss cost-effectiveness of investigation of hypertension.

- Conduct an effective plan of management for an elderly patient with hypertension:

    - Outline for patients non-pharmacological management strategies prior to pharmacological ones.

    - Select antihypertensive medication which will not adversely affect concomitant conditions such as diabetes mellitus, asthma, and congestive heart failure.

    - Select appropriate agents for hypertensive emergencies (e.g. encephalopathy, dissection).

    - Communicate to patients the importance of consultation with other healthcare professionals (e.g. dieticians).

    - Determine factors contributing to non-compliance and discuss possible management strategies.

    - Discuss cost-effectiveness of management of hypertension in the elderly.

    - Select patients in need of specialised care.

    - Define the goals of treatment in elderly hypertensive patients and contrast these with the goals for younger patients.

054D Malignant Hypertension

Overview
Malignant hypertension and hypertensive encephalopathy are two life-threatening syndromes caused by marked elevation in blood pressure (BP).

Causes

| 1) | **Primary hypertension (longstanding, uncontrolled, drug withdrawal)** |

| 2) | **Secondary hypertension** |

    a) Increased cardiac output (secondary increase in vascular resistance)

- ❏ Chronic renal failure, uraemia with volume overload
- ❏ Acute renal disease (glomerulonephritis, scleroderma crisis)
- ❏ Primary hyperaldosteronism (Conn syndrome)

    b) Increased vascular resistance

- ❏ Renovascular hypertension (renal artery stenosis)
- ❏ Phaeochromocytoma
- ❏ Drugs (cocaine, food or drug interactions with monoamineoxidase inhibitors, nonsteroidal anti-inflammatory drugs (NSAIDs))

Key Objectives
- Differentiate primary malignant hypertension (marked hypertension with diastolic BP usually greater than 140 mm Hg, associated with grade three to four retinopathy, proteinuria and renal impairment) from secondary conditions such as uraemia with fluid overload, subarachnoid or cerebral haemorrhages, brain tumours, head injury, seizure, etc.

- Conduct initial hypertension lowering treatment in a manner which lowers the BP gradually over hours, not precipitously.

General/Specific Objectives
- Through efficient, focused data gathering:

  - Determine quickly whether other hypertensive emergencies are present (e.g. aortic dissection, acute pulmonary oedema, acute or impending myocardial infarction (MI), cerebrovascular events) and make BP lowering the first concern.

  - Once BP control is in place, diagnose the cause of the BP elevation.

- Interpret critical clinical and laboratory findings which are key in the processes of exclusion, differentiation, and diagnosis:
  - Have an appropriate investigation strategy, since certain medications can interfere with some biochemical tests.
- Conduct an effective plan of management for a patient with malignant hypertension:
  - Recognise that the control of BP in a patient with malignant hypertension usually requires admission to an intensive care unit (ICU).
  - Outline the immediate management of malignant hypertension with parenteral drugs with intra-arterial BP monitoring in an ICU setting and with other medications if an ICU is not available.
  - Discuss advantages and disadvantages of various BP-lowering drugs used in malignant hypertension and other hypertensive emergencies.
  - Describe and explain the potential hazards of too rapidly lowering BP levels below 100–105 mm Hg diastolic or greater than 25% of baseline.
  - Outline a long term management strategy.

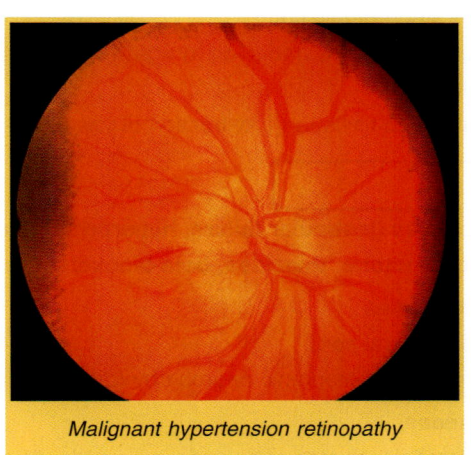

Malignant hypertension retinopathy

055 Infertility / Impotence / Sexual Dysfunction

Overview

Infertility affects about 10–15% of couples. Both partners should be investigated simultaneously since male-associated factors account for at least one-third of infertility problems, and problems are often identified in both male and female partners.

Causes

1) Infertility

a) **Female**
   (see #063 Menstrual Cycle Abnormal)

   ❏ Disorders of ovulation – causes at level of hypothalamus, pituitary, or ovary

   ❏ Disorders of tubal function

   ❏ Other causes – fibroids, endometriosis

b) **Male – disordered semen specimen**

   ❏ Endocrine causes – hypothalamic/pituitary causes (panhypopituitarism, haemochromatosis) – may have associated decreased androgenisation.

   ❏ Testicular (viral orchitis, radiation, drugs, liver disease, renal failure)

   ❏ Varicocele

   ❏ Abnormal sperm transport (obstruction of vas deferens)

2) Impotence

a) **Endocrine causes (testicular failure, hyperprolactinaemia)**

b) **Drugs (spironolactone, thiazides, *beta*-blockers, tricyclics, alcohol)**

c) **Neurologic diseases**

   ❏ Diseases of spinal cord

   ❏ Polyneuropathy / Autonomic neuropathy (diabetes)

d) **Vascular disease**

   ❏ Atherosclerotic occlusion of cavernous or pudenda arteries

   ❏ Venous leak

e) **Psychogenic**

Key Objectives

- Outline the investigation for couples with infertility.

- Outline the therapeutic options for couples with infertility.

General/Specific Objectives

- Through efficient, focused data gathering:

  - Diagnose the most likely cause of infertility.

  - Determine which patients are likely to have an organic cause for their impotence.

- Interpret critical clinical and laboratory findings which were key in the processes of exclusion, differentiation, and diagnosis:

  - Order and interpret a semen analysis.

  - Outline the laboratory investigation of a female with infertility.

- Conduct an effective plan of management for a patient with infertility or impotence:

  - Outline the medical and surgical management of a female/couple with infertility, considering the various causes of infertility and the treatment modalities for each (including the use of modern reproductive techniques of invitro-fertilisation (IVF) / intra-cytoplasmic sperm injection (ICSI) and gamete donor use).

  - Determine the therapy for impotence based on the underlying cause.

  - Describe the role of specific injectable and oral medications and the potential for surgical correction in patients with erectile dysfunction.

  - Select patients in need of specialised care.

  - Counsel and educate couples with infertility including the option of adoption.

Overview

Insomnia is a symptom that affects one-third of the population at some time, and is a persistent problem in 10% of the population. Affected patients complain of difficulty in initiating and maintaining sleep, and this inability to obtain adequate quantity and quality of sleep results in impaired daytime functioning.

Causes

1) Transient and short term insomnia

a) **Change in sleeping environment / Excessive noise / High or low ambient temperature**

b) **Jet-lag**

c) **Change in work shift**

d) **Stressful life events / Acute illness**

e) **Stimulant medication (theophylline, steroids, *beta*-agonists, thyroxine)**

2) Chronic insomnia

a) **Psychiatric disorders (depression, anxiety disorders, schizophrenia)**

b) **General medical disorders**
   - Cardiac (heart failure, coronary artery disease (CAD))
   - Respiratory (chronic obstructive pulmonary disease (COPD), asthma)
   - Gastro-intestinal (reflux, peptic ulcer disease)
   - Arthropathies / 'Fibromyalgia' / Lyme disease
   - AIDS
   - Chronic fatigue syndrome

c) **Neurologic**
   - Strokes (central hemispheric and brain stem)
   - Neuro-degenerative (Alzheimer disease, Parkinson disease)
   - Brain tumours
   - Neuromuscular (painful neuropathies)
   - Headaches (see #046 Headache)
   - Fatal familial insomnia

d) **Drug/Alcohol insomnia**

e) Primary sleep disorders

- ❏ Primary or idiopathic
- ❏ Psycho-physiologic
- ❏ Sleep state misperception
- ❏ Circadian rhythm disorders
  - • Delayed sleep phase syndrome
  - • Advanced sleep phase syndrome
  - • Hypernychthemeral syndrome
- ❏ Restless legs syndrome / Periodic limb movement disorder
- ❏ Altitude insomnia
- ❏ Insufficient sleep syndrome
- ❏ Central sleep-apnoea syndrome

Key Objective
- • Elicit a history of sleep habits involving the entire 24-hour cycle, including history from bed partner or caregiver (sleep habits, drug/alcohol consumption, medical or psycho-neurologic disease, psycho-social stressors, etc.).

General/Specific Objectives
- • Through efficient, focused data gathering:
  - - Conduct an examination of the patient to detect concomitant medical conditions which can adversely affect sleep.
  - - Describe to the patient a 'sleep log' and request one.
- • Interpret critical clinical and laboratory findings which were key in the processes of exclusion, differentiation, and diagnosis:
  - - State that laboratory investigation is not required in the routine evaluation of insomnia.
  - - List situations for which polysomnography may be indicated.
- • Conduct an effective plan of management for a patient with insomnia:
  - - State that management depends on the underlying cause.
  - - Outline some non-pharmacologic strategies for management of idiopathic chronic insomnia.
  - - State that pharmacologic therapy is generally not the treatment of first choice and should always be combined with non-pharmacologic therapies (e.g. sleep hygiene).

057 Involuntary Movement Disorders / Tic Disorders

Overview

Motor function may be impaired in a number of different ways, involving either a paucity or an excess of movements. Abnormal movements may be spontaneous (at rest), postural, or only with intention. They may involve dyskinesias, choreoathetosis, tremors, tics, myoclonic jerks or fasciculations.

Causes

1) **Akinesia (Parkinson disease: idiopathic or drug-induced)**

2) **Rigidity (Parkinson disease: idiopathic or drug-induced)**

3) **Akathisia (drug-induced, Parkinson disease, delirium)**

4) **Chorea (hereditary, basal ganglia disease, Huntington disease, rheumatic chorea, thyrotoxicosis, systemic lupus erythematosus (SLE), neuroleptics, pregnancy, polycythaemia)**

5) **Athetosis (cerebral palsy, Wilson disease, cerebral anoxia)**

6) **Hemiballismus (contralateral subthalamic pathology, hypertension, diabetes mellitus)**

7) **Dystonia**

   a) Primary (idiopathic, inherited)

   b) Secondary (kernicterus, Wilson disease, heavy metals, cerebral anoxia, drug-induced)

   c) Focal (spasmodic torticollis, cranial, occupational, drug-induced)

8) **Myoclonus**

   a) Physiological (sleep, anxiety, exercise, hiccough)

   b) Essential (familial, sporadic)

   c) Epileptic (benign, infantile, progressive, petit mal)

   d) Symptomatic (encephalopathy, basal ganglia disease, dementias, metabolic, toxic, physical, focal central nervous system (CNS) damage).

9) **Tremor**

   a) Familial/Essential

   b) Physiological (anxiety, fatigue, alcohol, caffeine)

   c) Orthostatic

   d) Symptomatic (Parkinson disease, cerebellar disease)

10) Restless legs syndrome

11) Asterixis (metabolic/hepatic)

12) Habit spasms and tics (Tourette syndrome)

Key Objectives
- Describe the abnormal movement accurately after careful observation both at rest and in action.
- Conduct appropriate testing to exclude treatable conditions:
    - Wilson disease, thyrotoxicosis, SLE, heavy metal poisoning, carbon monoxide poisoning and syphilis, etc.
- Be aware of common drug-induced causes of involuntary movements:
    - Neuroleptics, anticholinergics, antidepressants, antipsychotics, lithium, 1-dopa, haloperidol, thyroxine, caffeine, alcohol, bromocriptine.

General/Specific Objectives
- Through efficient, focused data gathering and neurological examination:
    - Differentiate between the various causes of movement disorders.
- Interpret critical clinical and laboratory findings which were crucial in the processes of exclusion, differentiation, and diagnosis:
    - Select patients in need of referral for investigation or specialised care.
    - Conduct testing for Wilson disease.
- Develop an effective management plan for a patient with an involuntary movement disorder / tic disorder.
- Contact family members and consider screening if either Wilson disease, Huntington disease or Tourette syndrome is diagnosed.

Overview

Jaundice is not usually detectable clinically until the serum bilirubin is greater than 30 mmol/L. Excess haemolysis causes mild acholuric jaundice (bilirubin attached to albumin does not appear in the urine) whereas cholestatic jaundice is associated with dark urine (conjugated bilirubin passes through the kidneys into the urine). Dark urine is usually the first symptom in cholestatic jaundice. Jaundice resulting from hepatobiliary disease may represent a benign heritable condition or severe life-threatening disease.

Causes

1) Unconjugated hyperbilirubinaemia

a) **Overproduction**
   - ❏ Haemolysis
   - ❏ Ineffective erythropoiesis

b) **Decreased hepatic uptake (sepsis)**

c) **Decreased bilirubin conjugation**
   - ❏ Hereditary transferase deficiency (Gilbert syndrome, Crigler-Najjar syndrome)
   - ❏ Neonatal jaundice
   - ❏ Acquired transferase deficiency (breast milk, hepatocellular disease)

2) Conjugated hyperbilirubinaemia

a) **Intrahepatic cholestasis**
   - ❏ Drugs (erythromycin, oral contraceptive pill (OCP))
   - ❏ Hepatocellular disease (hepatitis)
   - ❏ Cirrhosis
     - Infectious diseases including postviral
     - Hereditary diseases (alpha-1-antitrypsin deficiency, haemochromatosis, Wilson disease)
     - Primary biliary cirrhosis
     - Alcohol
   - ❏ Miscellaneous (fatty liver, sepsis)

b) **Extrahepatic cholestasis**
   - ❏ Intraductal obstruction
     - Gallstones
     - Sclerosing cholangitis
     - Biliary malformation (stricture)
     - Malignancy (cholangiocarcinoma)
   - ❏ Compression of biliary ducts (malignancy)

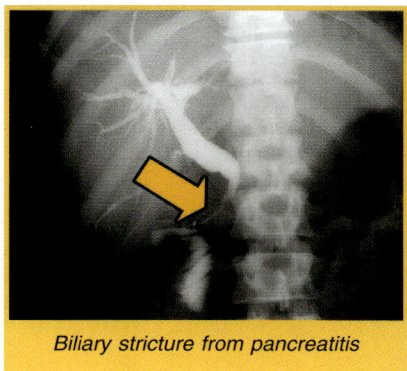

Biliary stricture from pancreatitis

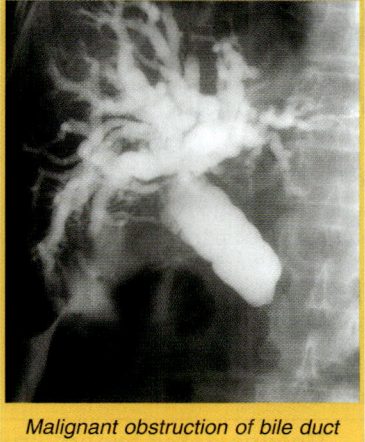

Malignant obstruction of bile duct

Key Objectives
- Determine which patients have significant liver dysfunction and evaluate the progression of the jaundice.

- Appreciate that alcohol is the commonest cause of cirrhosis.

General/Specific Objectives
- Through efficient, focused data gathering:

  - Differentiate between the various causes for jaundice and determine which are treatable.

  - Describe and demonstrate complications related to the presence of liver disease.

- Interpret critical clinical and laboratory findings which were key in the processes of exclusion, differentiation, and diagnosis:

  - Indicate changes in the sclera, skin, urine and faeces with the various causes.

  - Select and interpret appropriate investigations for patients with jaundice.

  - Order and interpret a blood smear in patients with unconjugated hyperbilirubinaemia.

  - List the indications for and interpret an abdominal ultrasound including the significance of dilated bile ducts.

- Conduct an effective plan of management for a patient with jaundice:

  - Outline a management plan for common causes of jaundice.

  - Outline a management plan for patients with acute hepatic failure.

  - Select patients in need of specialised care and/or in need of urgent hospitalisation.

058A Neonatal Jaundice

Overview
Jaundice is the most prevalent problem in the newborn period; up to 65% of full-term neonates develop transient jaundice. Although some causes are ominous, the majority are transient and without consequences. Physiologic jaundice comprises a transient decrease in the conjugation of bilirubin, appears on the second or third day of life and disappears within two weeks.

Causes

1) Unconjugated hyperbilirubinaemia

a) Increased bilirubin production

- ❏ Haemolytic causes – Coombs positive
  - • Isoimmune (Rh and ABO blood types, other blood antigens), autoimmune (systemic lupus erythematosus (SLE))
  - • Acquired red cells defects (e.g. drugs)
- ❏ Haemolytic causes – Coombs negative
  - • Red cell membrane defects (elliptocytosis, pyknocytosis, etc.)
  - • Red blood cell (RBC) enzyme deficiencies (pyruvate kinase, glucose-6-phosphate dehydrogenase)
  - • Haemoglobinopathy (with or without thalassaemia)
  - • Microangiopathy (haemolytic-uraemic syndrome)

b) Decreased bilirubin conjugation

- ❏ Metabolic/Genetic (Gilbert syndrome, Crigler-Najjar syndrome, hypothyroidism)
- ❏ Physiologic jaundice / Breast milk jaundice

c) Gastrointestinal absorption (pyloric stenosis, meconium ileus, sequestered blood)

2) Conjugated hyperbilirubinaemia

a) Decreased bilirubin uptake

- ❏ Infections (sepsis, neonatal hepatitis) / Toxic (parenteral nutrition)
- ❏ Metabolic/Genetic (galactosaemia, Gaucher disease, Niemann-Pick disease, decreased Y protein)

b) Decreased bilirubin excretion / Obstructive (biliary atresia, obstruction, choledochal cyst)

Key Objectives

- Determine whether jaundice presented at birth or within 24 hours, as in general such presentation is pathologic.

- State that hyperbilirubinaemia is most threatening when the onset is rapid, and the bilirubin is unconjugated. In the relatively immature central nervous system (CNS) of the neonate, especially in the premature, unconjugated bilirubin may be deposited and can result in severe brain damage.

General/Specific Objectives

- Through efficient, focused data gathering:

  - Elicit a history regarding family history of haematological disorders, previously affected children, maternal blood type, and antibody status, delivery history, how colouration was noticed, vital signs, and any medications.

  - Perform examination of scleral and mucous membranes, skin, liver and spleen, ascites, circulatory status, urine and stool.

  - Differentiate physiologic from organic causes of neonatal jaundice.

- Interpret critical clinical and laboratory findings which were key in the processes of exclusion, differentiation, and diagnosis:

  - Select investigations that will differentiate conjugated from unconjugated hyperbilirubinaemia.

  - Select investigations that will differentiate pathologic hyperbilirubinaemia from exaggerated physiologic jaundice.

  - State that conjugated hyperbilirubinaemia is never physiologic and select tests for immediate investigations.

- Conduct an effective plan of management for a neonatal patient with jaundice:

  - Outline initial monitoring and management in neonatal jaundice.

  - Explain advantages and disadvantages of phototherapy, exchange blood transfusions, and pharmacologic therapy.

  - Select appropriate consultants in the management of neonatal jaundice.

Overview

Pain involving a single joint, with painful limitation of movement, is a common presenting symptom. Conditions such as an infective arthritis are important to identify since failure to make the correct diagnosis could lead to permanent harm to the patient.

Causes

1)	Infection (bacterial, mycobacterial, fungal, viral, spirochaetes)

2)	Crystal (gout, pseudogout)

3)	Haemarthrosis (trauma/fracture, anticoagulants / bleeding disorders)

4)	Tumour (osteoma, sarcoma)

5)	Systemic rheumatic disease (rheumatoid arthritis (RA), systemic lupus erythematosus (SLE), sarcoid)

6)	Osteoarthritis (erosive variant)

Key Objectives

- Evaluate a patient with mono-articular arthritis first for the possibility of infection, since this relatively common cause of acute pain and swelling in a single joint can result in cartilage destruction within a few days if unrecognised.

- Recognise that the differential diagnosis of mono-articular arthritis overlaps with that of poly-articular arthritis, initially presenting as a single swollen joint.

General/Specific Objectives

- Through efficient, focused data gathering:

  - Differentiate articular from non-articular disorders.

  - After considering infection, diagnose other causes of mono-arthritis.

- Interpret critical clinical and laboratory findings which were key in the processes of exclusion, differentiation, and diagnosis:

  - Select appropriate investigations including diagnostic joint aspiration and synovial fluid analysis.

- Conduct an effective plan of management for a patient with mono-articular joint pain:

  - Outline appropriate treatment of septic arthritis.

  - Select appropriate treatment for other causes of arthritis.

  - List the indications, contraindications, and adverse effects of drugs commonly used in the treatment of arthritis (e.g. nonsteroidal anti-inflammatory agents).

  - Select patients in need of specialised care and/or referral.

Overview

Poly-articular joint pain ('polyarthralgia') is common in medical practice, and causes vary from some that are self-limiting to others which are potentially disabling and life-threatening. The term 'arthritis' includes inflammatory, infective, and degenerative joint disease. Arthritis is usually characterised by the spontaneous development of pain exacerbated by joint movement; and in superficial joints is often associated with swelling of the joints.

The most common types of arthritis seen in Australia are degenerative osteoarthritis and rheumatoid arthritis.

Causes

1) Degenerative osteoarthritis

2) Infectious (Lyme disease, bacterial endocarditis, gonococcus, viral)

3) Post-infectious (reactive)

a) Rheumatic fever

b) Reiter syndrome

c) Enteric infections

4) Seronegative spondyloarthritides

5) Systemic rheumatic diseases

a) Rheumatoid arthritis (RA)

b) Systemic lupus erythematosus (SLE)

c) Systemic vasculitis

d) Systemic sclerosis

e) Polymyositis /
     Dermatomyositis

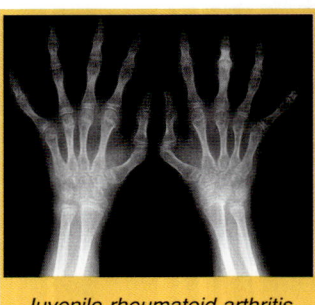

Juvenile rheumatoid arthritis

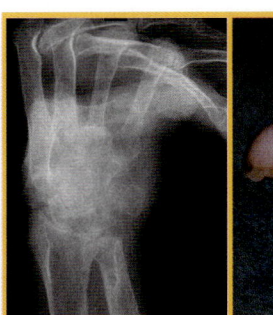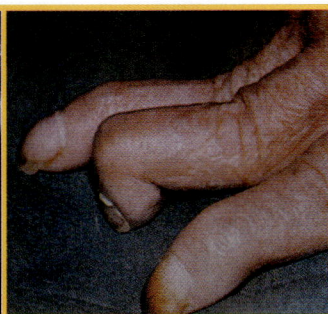

Rheumatoid arthritis – swan neck deformities

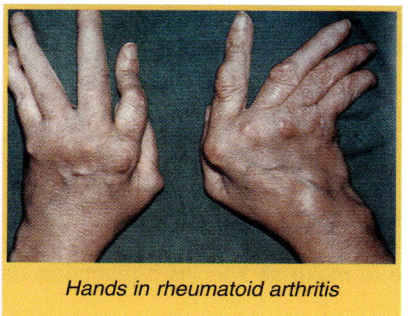

Hands in rheumatoid arthritis

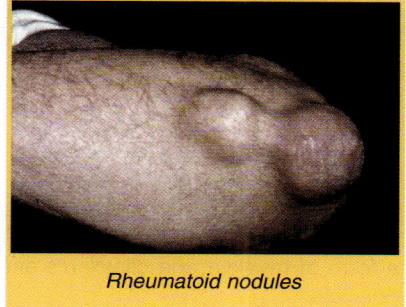

Rheumatoid nodules

6) Other (sarcoidosis, inflammatory osteoarthritis)

Key Objectives
- Differentiate articular from non-articular pain by clinical criteria; and between inflammatory and noninflammatory arthritis.

- Determine whether the patient has a musculoskeletal or neurologic emergency, compartment syndrome or acute myelopathy, versus radiculopathy or neuropathy.

- Differentiate neurologic causes by the burning quality associated with numbness, paraesthesia, constancy, worse at night, and unrelated to motion.

General/Specific Objectives
- Through efficient, focused data gathering:

  - Differentiate between inflammatory and non-inflammatory arthritis.

  - Describe articular and extra-articular manifestations and complications.

- Interpret critical clinical and laboratory findings which were key in the process of exclusion, differentiation, and diagnosis:

  - Select and interpret investigations including synovial fluid analysis.

- Conduct an effective plan of management for a patient with poly-articular joint pain:

  - Outline the principles of multidisciplinary management of RA and other inflammatory and non-inflammatory arthritides.

  - Outline a management plan for patients with inflammatory and non-inflammatory arthritis including drug therapy, physiotherapy, occupational therapy, and treatment of joint deformities.

  - Select patients in need of specialised care and/or referral.

  - Conduct counselling and education of patients.

(See also #089G Hip Pain, #089H Knee Pain)

Overview

Growing pains is a general diagnosis that is being made less frequently as clinicians become more expert in making specific diagnoses. Although *growing pains* do exist as a form of myalgia, the clinician's aim should be to make as specific a diagnosis as possible.

Causes

1) Trauma (stress fracture, traumatic epiphyseal injury)

(see #041 Fractures / Dislocations)

2) Infections (septic arthritis, osteomyelitis)

(see #071 Painful Limb)

3) Inflammatory (juvenile rheumatoid arthritis (RA), reactive arthritis, toxic synovitis of hip)

4) Other

a) **Hip**
   - ❏ Legg-Calvé-Perthes disease
   - ❏ Slipped capital femoral epiphysis

b) **Knee**
   - ❏ Osgood-Schlatter disease or epiphysitis
   - ❏ Chondromalacia patellae
   - ❏ Patella (tendon partial rupture, osteochondritis, subluxation, dislocation)
   - ❏ Meniscal injuries
   - ❏ Popliteal cyst

5) Growing pains

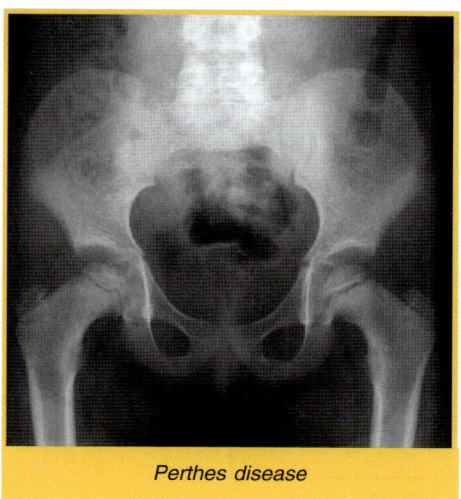

Perthes disease

Key Objectives
- Determine whether the pain originates in joints or soft tissue.

- Recognise that the most serious diseases causing leg pain in children are usually unilateral.

General/Specific Objectives
- Through efficient, focused, data gathering:
  - Communicate to child and parents that pain or limp lasting for longer than two to three weeks is unlikely to be the result of trauma even in the presence of trauma history.
  - Determine if the limp or pain are caused by serious entities.
  - Calculate leg length discrepancies (greater than 1 cm may cause pelvic tilt and limp), describe gait.
- Interpret critical clinical and laboratory findings which were key in the processes of exclusion, differentiation, and diagnosis:
  - Select patients in need of diagnostic imaging or specialised care for further investigation.
- Conduct an effective plan of management for a child with pain in the lower extremity and/or limp:
  - Select patients in need of specialised care.

Overview

Patients with focal lymphadenopathy at one site (groin, axilla, neck, abdomen) require careful assessment initially to identify neoplastic or inflammatory causes within regional fields. Generalised lymphadenopathy requires search for malignant or inflammatory disease. Finally, aspiration cytology is often diagnostic in the assessment of the lymph node swellings. Lymph nodes may be normally palpable in the groin, axilla or neck, but a lymph node swelling of 2 cm or greater which is persistent and firm, demands investigation.

Causes

1) Localised

a) **Infectious causes**
   - ❏ Bacterial (streptococci, staphylococci, cat scratch, tuberculous)
   - ❏ Viral (herpes simplex)

b) **Reactive (usually secondary to undiagnosed infection)**

c) **Malignant diseases**
   - ❏ Metastatic disease
   - ❏ Localised lymphoma

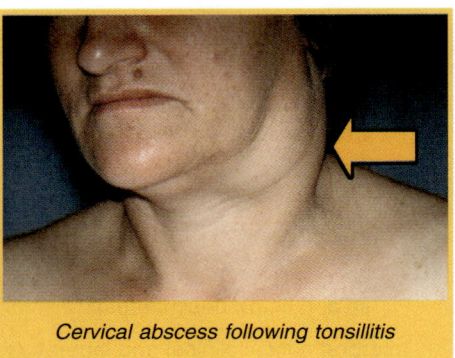

Cervical abscess following tonsillitis

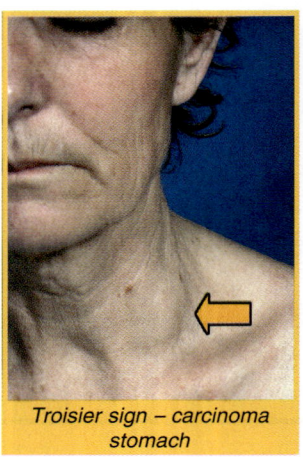

Troisier sign – carcinoma stomach

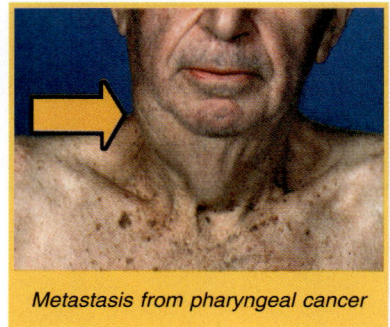

Metastasis from pharyngeal cancer

a) **Infectious causes**
   - ❏ Viral (Epstein-Barr virus (EBV), cytomegalovirus (CMV), infectious hepatitis, rubella, HIV)
   - ❏ Bacterial (brucellosis)
   - ❏ Fungal (histoplasmosis, coccidioidomycosis)

b) **Inflammatory diseases**
   - ❏ Collagen diseases (rheumatoid arthritis (RA), systemic lupus erythematosus (SLE), dermatomyositis, Sjögren syndrome)
   - ❏ Serum sickness
   - ❏ Drug hypersensitivity (allopurinol, phenytoin)
   - ❏ Sarcoidosis
   - ❏ Amyloidosis

c) **Malignant diseases**
   - ❏ Lymphoma
   - ❏ Acute or chronic lymphocytic leukaemia

Key Objective
- Differentiate the cause of lymphadenopathy based on its location and distribution.

General/Specific Objectives
- Through efficient, focused data gathering:

  - Differentiate benign from malignant causes for lymphadenopathy.

- Interpret critical clinical and laboratory findings which were key in the processes of exclusion, differentiation, and diagnosis:

  - Outline the laboratory investigation for a patient with generalised lymphadenopathy.

  - List the indications for a lymph node biopsy.

- Conduct an effective plan of management for a patient with lymphadenopathy:

  - Determine which patients require further investigation for their lymphadenopathy.

  - Select patients in need of specialised care.

063A Amenorrhoea (also Oligomenorrhoea)

Overview

The average age of menarche is less than 13 years (11–15 years). Most young women (phenotypic) failing to develop menses simply have delayed menarche, but rarely some (older than 16–17 years) fail to menstruate at all (primary amenorrhoea). Patients who have menstruated but have stopped (more than four to six months), have secondary amenorrhoea (commonest cause during reproductive years is pregnancy). Oligomenorrhoea investigation should include important issues such as nutrition and medications.

Causes

Primary amenorrhoea, secondary amenorrhoea and oligomenorrhoea. The causes which only apply to primary amenorrhoea are marked with an asterisk (*). The others can apply to all of these causes.

1) Pregnancy (also gestational trophoblastic tumours)

2) Endocrine causes:

   a) Hypothalamic – physiologic (exercise, stress, weight loss or gain, drugs) – pathologic – tumour

   b) Pituitary – tumour or hypopituitarism (including Sheehan syndrome)

   c) Thyroid – underactivity, overactivity

   d) Adrenal – congenital adrenal hyperplasia, tumour

   e) Ovarian – polycystic ovary syndrome, ovarian failure, ovarian agenesis*, streak gonads (45X)*, hormone-producing ovarian tumour

3) Uterine/Outflow tract anatomic defects

   a) Congenital absence of vagina* / Imperforate hymen*, transverse vaginal septum*

   b) Cervical stenosis

   c) Intra-uterine adhesions / Uterine absence* / Mal-development / Asherman syndrome

Key Objective

- First determine whether the woman is pregnant if aged 10–50 years; order a pregnancy test. If not pregnant, consider other diagnoses. Be aware of special causes of primary amenorrhoea.

General/Specific Objectives

- Through efficient, focused data gathering:

    - Determine degree of maturation of breasts, pubic and axillary hair, and external genitalia.

    - Determine current oestrogen status and presence or absence of outflow tract anatomic defect.

    - Determine patient's diet, drugs, and stress level; presence of galactorrhoea, hirsutism, acne.

- Interpret critical clinical and laboratory findings which were key in the processes of exclusion, differentiation, and diagnosis:

    - List indications for serum prolactin, gonadotropins, oestrogen and progesterone investigations.

    - List indications for obtaining a chromosomal karyotype.

    - List indications for assessing androgen status and what tests should be done.

    - List indications for a pelvic ultrasound examination.

- Conduct an effective plan of management for a patient with amenorrhoea:

    - Outline a management plan in a patient with functional hypothalamic amenorrhoea, including a rational basis for the agents used to induce ovulation if pregnancy is desired, and the place for hormone replacement therapy (HRT) if pregnancy is not desired.

    - Outline a management plan for a patient with ovarian failure, consider 'pros' and 'cons' of HRT.

    - Select patients in need of specialised care.

063B Pre-Menstrual Syndrome / Dysmenorrhoea

Overview
Approximately 30–50% of post-pubescent women experience painful menstruation and 10% of women are incapacitated by pain one to three days per month. Dysmenorrhoea is the single greatest cause of lost working hours and school days among young women.

Causes

1)	**Pre-menstrual syndrome**

2)	**Dysmenorrhoea**

    a) **Primary (no pelvic abnormality)**

    b) **Secondary (acquired)**

        ❏ Fibroids

        ❏ Endometriosis

        ❏ Infections / Foreign body

        ❏ Cervical occlusion

        ❏ Congenital abnormalities

Key Objective
- Differentiate primary (within the first two to three years of menarche, with regular ovulatory menstruation) from secondary dysmenorrhoea (usually many years after menarche).

General/Specific Objectives

- Through efficient, focused data gathering:

  - Differentiate between pre-menstrual syndrome (pain and other symptoms 2–12 days before, and improve with menses), and dysmenorrhoea.

  - Differentiate between primary and secondary dysmenorrhoea.

  - Perform pelvic examination to diagnose possible causes of secondary dysmenorrhoea.

- Interpret critical clinical and laboratory findings which were key in the processes of exclusion, differentiation, and diagnosis:

  - Order Papanicolaou (Pap) smear, wet smear, cultures.

  - Select patients in need of referral for additional investigation.

- Conduct an effective plan of management for a patient with pre-menstrual syndrome or dysmenorrhoea:

  - Outline initial management of pre-menstrual syndrome or dysmenorrhoea.

  - Select patients in need of specialised care.

Overview

Women live about one-third of their lives after ovarian function ceases. As the population ages, quality of life and disease prevention strategies are inherent in managing the post-menopausal symptoms in women.

Causes

1) Physiologic

    a) Oocytes responsive to gonadotropins progressively disappear from the ovaries

    b) Oocytes do not respond to gonadotropins – ovarian resistance

2) Pathologic or induced

    a) Infections or tumours of reproductive tract resulting in destruction or removal of a significant amount of ovarian tissue

    b) Ionising radiation

    c) Chemotherapy (cytotoxic agents)

    d) Surgery impairing ovarian blood supply

    e) Autoimmune or other processes disturbing ovarian function

Key Objectives

- Counsel women with menopause that nothing can prevent physiologic menopause (ovarian function cannot be prolonged indefinitely) and nothing can be done to postpone its onset or slow its progress. However, reassure patient that sudden ageing will not occur, sexual activity can continue, and hormone replacement therapy (HRT) can prevent many of the adverse effects seen.

- Explain the physiologic events being experienced by a woman in menopause in order to dispel fears and assess symptoms such as anxiety, depression, or sleep disturbance.

- State that osteoporosis is one of the most important health hazards associated with the menopause, along with an increase in coronary artery disease (CAD), Alzheimer disease, macular degeneration of the retina, urinary continence problems and bowel malignancy (all have a lesser incidence in women taking HRT).

General/Specific Objectives

- Through efficient, focused data gathering:

    - Differentiate from other causes of amenorrhoea (see #063 Menstrual Cycle Abnormal, #117 Vaginal Bleeding, Excessive in Amount or Irregular in Timing and #118 Vaginal Discharge / Urinary Symptoms, Vulvar Lesions, Sexually Transmitted Diseases (STDs)).

    - Determine whether there has been a decrease in amount and duration of menstrual flow, tapering to spotting, or cessation; determine length of time since onset of amenorrhoea.

    - Determine whether there are symptoms associated with vaginal changes to exclude other pathology (brownish discharge, bleeding with coitus, vaginal pruritus or leucorrhoea, excessive vaginal dryness, dyspareunia).

    - Elicit history of urinary tract symptoms, change in breasts, hot flush, cardiovascular symptoms, skin and hair changes, or any psychological complaints.

    - Perform a diagnostic pelvic examination.

    - Obtain a relevant family history regarding risks of cancer, osteoporosis and cardiovascular disease.

- Interpret critical clinical and laboratory findings which were key in the processes of exclusion, differentiation, and diagnosis:

    - Select patients requiring cytologic smears, hormone measurements, or bone density studies.

- Conduct an effective initial plan of management for a patient with menopause:

    - Counsel patients regarding prevention of osteoporosis, advantages and disadvantages of oestrogen replacement (e.g. endometrial cancer, breast cancer, hepatic function, hypertension, thromboembolic disease, lipid metabolism).

    - List contraindications to HRT.

    - Outline guidelines for hormonal (or oestrogen and progestin) replacement therapy.

    - List alternatives to oestrogen therapy for some of the symptoms of menopause.

Overview

Depressive illness is one of the commonest illnesses in medicine and is often confused with other illnesses. Depressed and anxious patients often present to doctors with somatic symptoms used as 'tickets-of-entry', when their primary disorders are psychological.

Although the return to the pre-depressive state, either spontaneously or with treatment, is the rule, untreated depressive episodes may last six months, they are usually recurrent, and chronic outcomes are not rare.

Bipolar disorders are episodic recurrent illnesses which have an onset at an early age and with a great deal of variation in cycling patterns.

Causes

1) Major depression

    a) With melancholic features

    b) With psychotic features

    c) Postpartum

    d) Seasonal

    e) Atypical

    f) Recurrent

2) Dysthymia

3) Cyclothymic disorder

4) Bipolar I disorder

    a) Hypomanic

    b) Manic

    c) With psychotic features

    d) Postpartum

    e) Seasonal

    f) Rapid cycling

    g) Mixed

5) Bipolar II disorder

    a) Hypomanic

    b) Depressed

    c) Melancholic

    d) Atypical

    e) Postpartum

Key Objectives

• Differentiate between the presence of one of the mood disorders (illness) and normal (non-illness) conditions such as bereavement and periods of sadness.

• Recognise the depressed patient at risk of suicide.

General/Specific Objectives

• Through efficient, focused data gathering:

    - Determine the intensity, duration (weeks, years) of depression and its effect on function (loss of interest in all activities, change in sleep, appetite, libido, energy).

    - Determine whether a general medical condition is present, use or abuse of drugs (or withdrawal).

    - Elicit history of sense of worthlessness, excessive guilt, inability to concentrate, suicidal thoughts.

    - Examine for slowness of thought, speech, motor activity or signs of agitation such as fidgeting, moving about, hand-wringing, nail-biting, hair-pulling, lip-biting; examine vital signs, pupils, and skin for previous suicide attempts, stigmata of drug and/or alcohol use, thyroid gland.

    - Elicit history of elevated mood, expansive or irritable mood (for at least one week) with impairment in function or without impairment and lasting only four days.

- Interpret critical clinical and laboratory findings which were key in the processes of exclusion, differentiation, and diagnosis:

  - Select patients only when high index of suspicion requires further investigation for medical condition or drugs that affect mood (e.g. thyroid function, toxicology screen, serum electrolytes, liver function tests).

- Conduct an effective plan of management for a patient with mood disorders:

  - Outline and describe treatments available for mood disorders under categories of medications, physical treatment, and psychologic treatment.

  - Select patients in need of specialised care.

Overview

Although many disease states can affect the mouth, the three most common and most important ones are: **dental caries**, **gingivitis**, and **oral carcinoma**.

Causes

1) Sore mouth problems in children

a) **Abnormalities in teeth (caries from pacifiers, eruptions, number, form, size)**

b) **Trauma (accidents, child abuse)**

c) **Gingival overgrowth (idiopathic, genetic, drugs)**

2) Mouth problems in adults

a) **Dental caries / Periapical dental abscess / Cellulitis (emergency)**

b) **Gingivitis / Periodontal / General mouth diseases**
- ❏ Oral hygiene
- ❏ Systemic factors (haematological disorders, HIV)
- ❏ Sexually transmitted / blood-borne infections

c) **Mouth ulcers / Lip lesions**
- ❏ Acute, painful (aphthous), herpetic
- ❏ Chronic persisting
  - • Malignant (squamous cell, muco-epidermoid, basal cell)
  - • Pre-malignant (leukoplakia, erythroplakia)

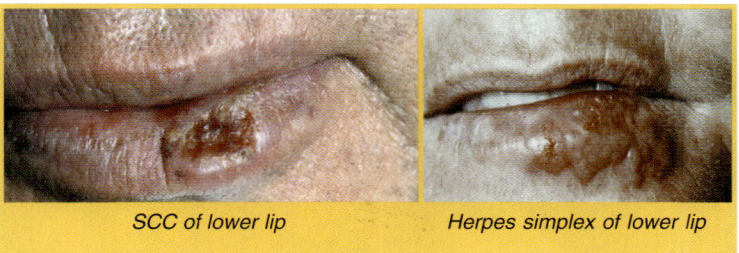

SCC of lower lip   *Herpes simplex of lower lip*

d) Pigmented lesions in the mouth
   - ❏ Tobacco, Betel nut
   - ❏ Lead, bismuth, iron
   - ❏ Drugs (antimalarials, oral contraceptive pill (OCP))
   - ❏ Addison disease
   - ❏ Peutz-Jeghers syndrome
   - ❏ Melanoma

e) Other (cellulitis, trauma, *Candida*)

f) Salivary glands (mumps, bacterial infections, sialolithiasis, tumour, mucuos cyst)

3) Mouth problems in the elderly

a) Receding gingivae/gums

b) Edentulism

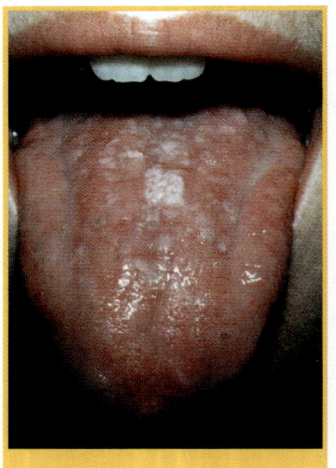

Leukoplakia tongue

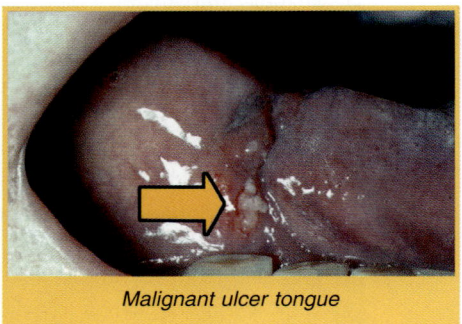

Malignant ulcer tongue

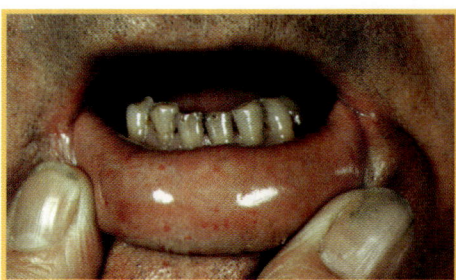

Peutz-Jeghers syndrome

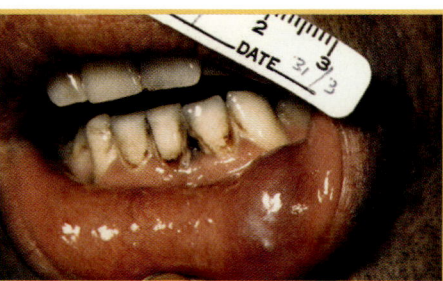

Mucous cyst

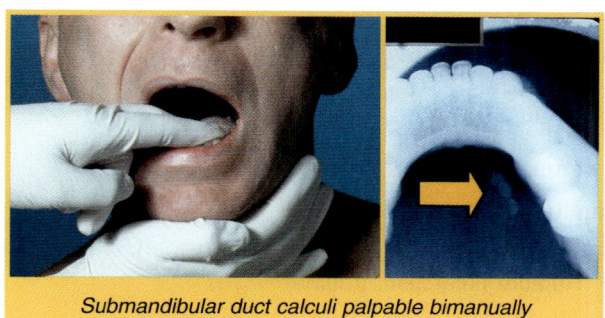

Submandibular duct calculi palpable bimanually

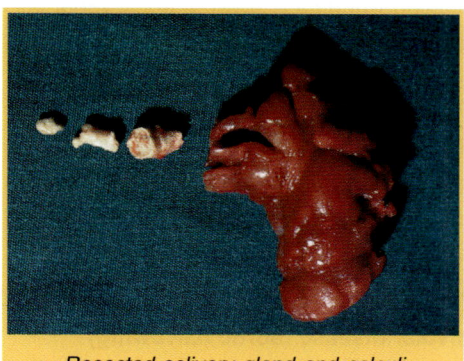

Resected salivary gland and calculi

067A   Systolic Murmur

Overview

Systolic murmurs are quite common, frequently 'innocent' flow murmurs. Good clinical examination techniques are required to differentiate the different cardiac lesions which give rise to systolic murmurs. The most common pathological lesions are **mitral regurgitation**, **aortic stenosis** and **tricuspid regurgitation**.

Causes

1)   Mitral regurgitation

a) **Leaflet**
- ❏ Rheumatic fever
- ❏ Collagen diseases (systemic lupus erythematosus (SLE), scleroderma)
- ❏ Connective tissue diseases (Marfan syndrome / congenital / mitral valve prolapse)
- ❏ Endocarditis
- ❏ Hypertrophic cardiomyopathy

b) **Chordae tendinae**
- ❏ Rupture (myocardial infarction (MI))
- ❏ Mitral valve prolapse
- ❏ Endocarditis
- ❏ Rheumatic fever
- ❏ Trauma

c) **Papillary muscle**
- ❏ Dysfunction (ischaemia/infarct, aneurysm, dilated cardiomyopathy)
- ❏ Rupture (infarction, trauma)

d) **Mitral annulus**
- ❏ Calcification (rheumatic fever, chronic renal failure)
- ❏ Dilatation (dilated cardiomyopathy)

2)   Aortic stenosis

a) **Leaflet disease**
- ❏ Unicuspid, bicuspid (congenital), tricuspid
- ❏ Rheumatic fever
- ❏ Degenerative

b) **Sub-valvular disease (hypertrophic cardiomyopathy)**

c) **Supra-valvular disease (aortic narrowing)**

Tricuspid regurgitation

a) **Dilatation of right ventricle / tricuspid annulus**

- ❑ Right ventricular myocardium (infarction, dilated cardiomyopathy)
- ❑ Pulmonary hypertension / right ventricular dilatation
  - Congestive heart failure
  - Mitral stenosis/regurgitation
  - Primary pulmonary disease (secondary pulmonary hypertension)
  - Primary pulmonary hypertension
  - Left to right shunt / Eisenmenger syndrome
  - Pulmonary valve stenosis

b) **Valve abnormality (rheumatic fever, endocarditis especially secondary to intravenous drug abuse, Ebstein anomaly, carcinoid syndrome)**

4) **Pulmonary stenosis**

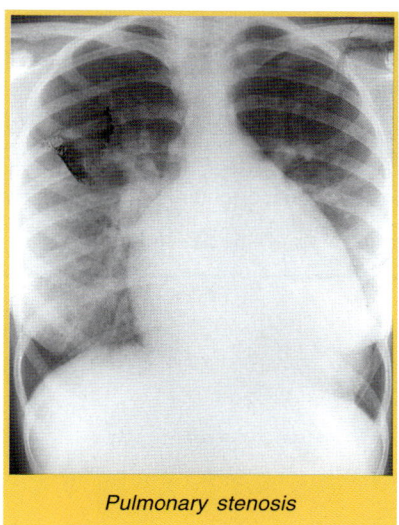

Pulmonary stenosis

5) **Ventricular septal defect (VSD)**

Key Objectives
- Determine whether the systolic murmur is innocent or pathologic.
- Determine aetiology of the murmur in the setting of clinical presentation, the patient's cardiovascular reserve, the clinical examination findings and evidence obtained from the electrocardiogram (ECG), chest X-ray and echocardiogram.
- Determine the need for specialist referral and intervention.
- Select patients in need of prophylaxis for bacterial endocarditis.

General/Specific Objectives

- Through efficient, focused data gathering:

  - Determine the origin of the murmur.

  - Define associated murmurs and evidence of structural cardiac disorders.

  - Determine whether heart failure is present, and whether left-sided, right-sided, or both.

  - Determine whether the heart rhythm is abnormal.

- Interpret critical clinical and laboratory findings which were key in the processes of exclusion, differentiation, and diagnosis:

  - Diagnose abnormal heart rhythm by means of clinical findings and ECG.

  - Select diagnostic imaging for further investigation of the systolic murmur.

- Conduct an effective plan of management for a patient with a systolic murmur:

  - Counsel and educate the patient concerning possible need for endocarditis prophylaxis.

  - Outline management of heart failure, including side-effects of prescribed medications.

  - Discuss the need for anticoagulants in patients with atrial fibrillation.

  - Select patients in need of specialised care.

067B Diastolic Murmur

Overview
A cardiac diastolic murmur is almost always indicative of cardiac pathology. The most common causes are **aortic regurgitation** and **mitral stenosis**. These can usually be differentiated using good clinical examination skills.

Causal Conditions

1) Aortic regurgitation

a) **Leaflet abnormality**
   - ❏ Bicuspid aortic valve (congenital: usually associated with aortic stenosis)
   - ❏ Endocarditis
   - ❏ Rheumatic fever
   - ❏ Rheumatoid arthritis (RA), ankylosing spondylitis
   - ❏ Trauma

b) **Aortic root and ascending aorta**
   - ❏ Hypertension
   - ❏ Marfan syndrome
   - ❏ Aortic valve replacement (artificial valve, allograft, xenograft)
   - ❏ Dissecting aneurysm
   - ❏ Reiter syndrome
   - ❏ Ankylosing spondylitis
   - ❏ Aortitis (syphilis)

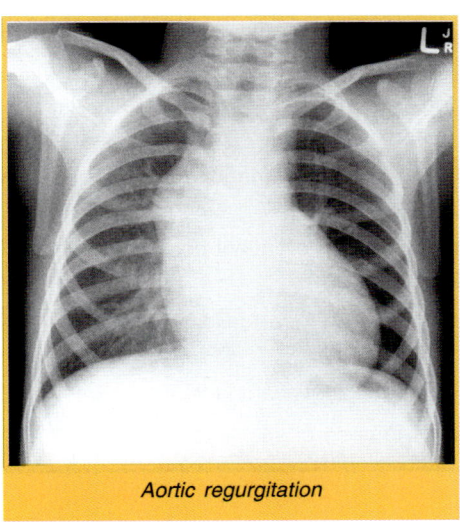

Aortic regurgitation

2) Pulmonary regurgitation

3) Mitral stenosis

❏ Rheumatic fever

❏ Congenital

❏ Collagen vascular disease (systemic lupus erythematosus (SLE), RA)

❏ Carcinoid syndrome

4) Tricuspid stenosis

Key Objectives

- Determine the aetiology of the murmur in the setting of the clinical presentation, the patient's cardiovascular reserve, the clinical examination findings and evidence obtained from the electrocardiogram (ECG), chest X-ray and echocardiogram.

- Determine the need for specialist referral and intervention.

- Select patients in need of prophylaxis for bacterial endocarditis.

General/Specific Objectives

- Through efficient, focused data gathering:

  - Determine the origin of the murmur.

  - Define associated murmurs and evidence of structural cardiac disorders.

  - Determine whether heart failure is present, and whether left-sided, right-sided, or both.

  - Determine whether the heart rhythm is abnormal.

- Interpret critical clinical and laboratory findings which were key in the processes of exclusion, differentiation, and diagnosis:

  - Diagnose abnormal heart rhythm by means of clinical findings and ECG.

  - Select diagnostic imaging for further investigation of the diastolic murmur.

- Conduct an effective plan of management for a patient with a diastolic murmur:

  - Counsel and educate the patient concerning possible need for endocarditis prophylaxis.

  - Outline management of heart failure, including side-effects of prescribed medications.

  - Discuss the need for anticoagulants in patients with atrial fibrillation.

  - Select patients in need of specialised care.

067C Heart Sounds, Pathological

Overview

Pathological heart sounds are clues to underlying heart disease.

Causes

1) Heart sound 1 (HS1) – mitral valve

  a) Loud (mitral stenosis, hyperthyroidism, short PR interval)

  b) Soft (mitral regurgitation, long PR interval, chronic obstructive lung disease, pericardial effusion)

2) Heart sound 2 (HS2) – aortic and pulmonary components

  a) Loud (systemic hypertension, pulmonary hypertension, increased pulmonary flow)

  b) Soft (hypotension, left heart failure, aortic valve stenosis, pericardial effusion)

  c) No split (Eisenmenger syndrome, severe pulmonary embolus, pulmonary valve stenosis)

3) Altered splitting of heart sounds

  a) Increased splitting of HS2

  ❏ Delayed pulmonary valve closure (pulmonary embolus, pulmonary hypertension, left-right shunt, right bundle branch block (RBBB)

  ❏ Early aortic closure (mitral regurgitation, ventricular septal defect (VSD))

  b) Fixed split (atrial septal defect (ASD))

  c) Paradoxical split (left bundle branch block (LBBB), hypertension, left ventricular outflow obstruction)

4) Heart sounds 3 and 4

  a) Physiological (young subjects)

  b) Third heart sound (dilated ventricle with volume overload, left or right heart failure, mitral/tricuspid regurgitation)

  c) Fourth heart sound (hypertension, heart failure, hypertrophic cardiomyopathy, aortic stenosis)

5) Extra heart sound and clicks

a) Ejection sounds (early systolic) – hypertension, aortic and pulmonary stenosis

b) Opening sounds (early diastolic) – mitral stenosis, tricuspid stenosis

c) Clicks (midsystolic) – mitral valve prolapse

d) Pericardial knock (pericardial effusion)

e) Prosthetic valve sounds

Key Objective
- Interpret the origin of heart sounds.

General/Specific Objectives
- Through efficient, focused, data gathering:

  - Determine whether underlying heart disease is present and how the heart sounds help to define this.

- Interpret critical clinical and laboratory findings which are key in the processes of exclusion, differentiation, and diagnosis:

  - Select common investigative tools such as chest X-ray, electrocardiogram (ECG), and echocardiography to assist with diagnosis and understand principles of interpretations of these tests.

- Conduct an effective plan of management for a patient with pathological heart sounds:

  - Select patients in need of specialised care.

Overview

Neck masses may come to clinical attention when noted by the patient as a presenting symptom, or as an incidental finding during routine physical examination or during a diagnostic imaging procedure. The most common causes of neck swelling are **lymph node** and **thyroid gland** swellings. Aspiration cytology of focal neck masses is often helpful in diagnosis of the cause.

Causes

1) Cervical lymph node swellings

    a) Associated with overt or occult neoplastic or inflammatory primary lesions of head and neck

    b) Associated with extracervical primary lesions (lung, abdomen, testis)

    c) Associated with general lymphadenopathy

2) Thyroid swellings (goitre)

    a) Uniform smooth diffuse enlargement (physiologic goitre, Graves disease)

    b) Multinodular enlargement (multinodular goitre)

    c) Uninodular (dominant nodule in multinodular goitre, or true solitary nodule)

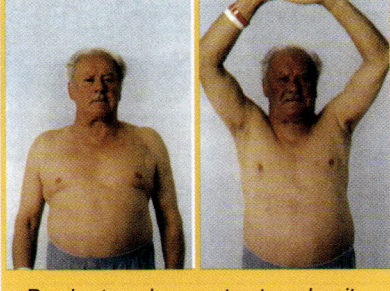

Pemberton sign – retrosternal goitre

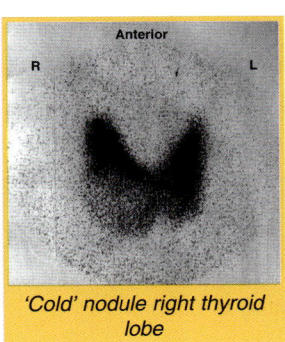

'Cold' nodule right thyroid lobe

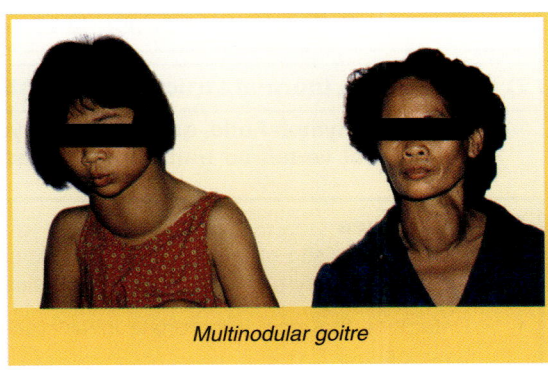

Multinodular goitre

3) Salivary gland swelling

    a) Neoplasm (pleomorphic adenoma, adenolymphoma, etc.)

    b) Obstructions (stone)

    c) Inflammations (acute or chronic)

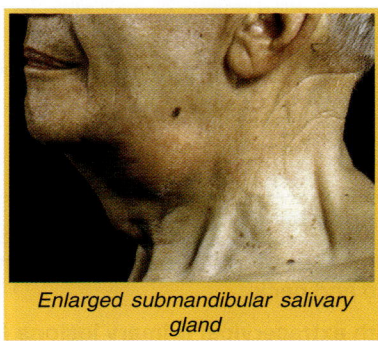

Enlarged submandibular salivary gland

4) Embryologic remnants

    a) Branchial cyst or fistula

    b) Thyroglossal cyst

    c) Lymphoepithelial cyst

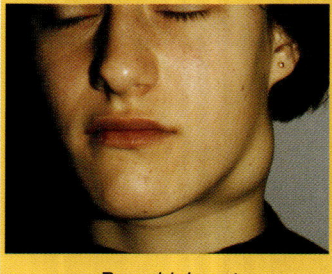

Branchial cyst

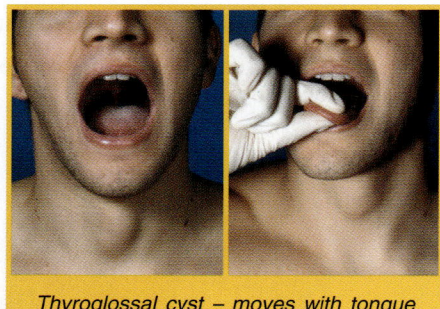

Thyroglossal cyst – moves with tongue

5) Vascular / Neuroendocrine

    a) Carotid body tumour (chemodectoma)

6) Musculoskeletal (sternomastoid tumour, cervical rib)

7) Subjective (normal structure presenting as lump)

    a) Normal lymph node, greater cornu hyoid, laryngeal structures, cervical vertebrae transverse processes

---

Key Objectives

- Identify likely site of origin and diagnostic significance of neck or facial lumps by history-taking and careful physical examination.

- Determine the most appropriate investigations required to confirm diagnosis.

General/Specific Objectives

- Through efficient, focused data gathering:

    - Determine whether the lesion is of rapid onset or insidious.

    - Determine the presence of hyperthyroidism (including findings typical of Graves disease) or hypothyroidism.

    - Perform examination of the thyroid gland, cervical lymph nodes, salivary glands and other neck and facial structures.

- Interpret the critical clinical and laboratory findings which were key in the processes of exclusion, differentiation, and diagnosis:

    - Discuss the utility of thyroid stimulating hormone (TSH) determination for screening patients suspected of thyroid abnormalities.

    - Select other thyroid function studies if TSH is abnormal, and outline their utility.

    - In a patient with a thyroid nodule, discuss the use of fine needle aspiration cytology (FNAC) and high-resolution thyroid ultrasonography.

- Conduct an effective plan of management for a patient with a neck mass due to goitre/thyroid disease:

    - Outline a management plan for hyperthyroidism, hypothyroidism, thyroiditis, and thyroid nodule.

    - Discuss control of symptoms of hyperthyroidism; discuss advantages and disadvantages of anti-thyroid drugs and radioactive iodine.

    - Discuss types of thyroid cancer and their various presentations.

- Discuss diagnosis and management of a patient presenting with clinical abnormalities of thyroid function without a neck swelling.

- Develop an algorithm for a patient presenting with a neck lump believed clinically to be a focal cervical node swelling.

- Develop diagnostic and management plans for a patient with generalised enlargement of cervical lymph nodes.

- Develop diagnostic and management plans for a patient presenting with a swelling involving left supraclavicular lymph nodes.

- Develop diagnostic and management plans for a patient presenting with a focal lymph node swelling in whom FNAC has revealed:

    - Metastatic adenocarcinoma.

    - Metastatic squamous cell carcinoma (SCC).

    - Hodgkin lymphoma.

- Develop diagnostic and management plans for a patient presenting with a salivary gland swelling.

- Select patients in need of specialised care.

Overview

Disordered sensation may be alarming and highly intrusive. The clinician requires a framework of knowledge in order to assess abnormal sensation, consider the likely site of origin, and recognise the implications.

Causes

1) Mononeuropathy

   a) Compression from nerve entrapment syndromes, e.g. carpal tunnel syndrome, ulnar neuropathy

   b) Radiculopathy (intervertebral disc lesion, foraminal encroachment)

2) Polyneuropathy (diabetes mellitus, alcoholism, renal failure, polyarteritis nodosa, systemic lupus erythematosus (SLE), systemic sclerosis, sarcoidosis, rheumatoid arthritis (RA), AIDS, leprosy)

3) Spinal cord lesion (cord tumour, infarction, multiple sclerosis, syringomyelia, vitamin B$_{12}$ deficiency)

4) Brain stem lesion (neoplasm, vascular lesion, demyelinating lesion)

5) Cerebral hemisphere lesion (tumour, demyelinating lesion, stroke)

6) Hyperventilation

Key Objective
- Determine whether the sensory complaint is positive, also called paraesthesia or dysaesthesia (tingling, pins and needles, pricking, burning, knifelike), or negative, termed hypoaesthesia or anaesthesia (numbness, diminution or absence of feeling).

General/Specific Objectives
- Through efficient, focused data gathering:

   - Determine the portion of the neural axis likely to be causing the symptoms.

   - Contrast peripheral neuropathies, spinal cord or brain stem dysaesthesia from cortical sensory dysfunction.

   - Recognise that only negative symptoms or hypoaesthesia may be detectable on physical examination.

   - Differentiate between possible causes of the lesion.

- Interpret critical clinical and laboratory findings which were key in the processes of exclusion, differentiation, and diagnosis:

  - Select initial laboratory investigations including such tests as nerve conduction / electromyelography (EMG) and serum vitamin B_{12} levels.

  - Select patients in need of specialised care for further investigation.

- Conduct an effective plan of management for a patient with numbness and tingling:

  - Outline initial management for mononeuropathy.

(See also #089 Regional Pain)

Overview

Because pain is understood to be a signal of disease, it is the most common symptom that brings a patient to a clinician's attention. Pain is an unpleasant somatic sensation, but it is also an emotion. Although control of pain and discomfort is a crucial endpoint of medical care, the degree of analgesia provided is often inadequate. All clinicians should be competent to recognise the development and progression of pain, and to develop strategies for its control.

Causes

1)	**Face pain (trigeminal neuralgia)**
2)	**Back pain**
3)	**Pain in the cancer patient**
4)	**Pain in the postoperative patient**
5)	**Somatic pain (burn, arthritis, bone metastasis)**
6)	**Visceral pain (intestinal colic, renal 'colic', cancer of pancreas)**
7)	**Neurologic pain (herniated intervertebral disc)**

Key Objectives

• State that the ideal treatment for any pain is to remove the cause.

• Because some conditions are so painful that rapid and effective analgesia is essential (e.g. in first aid, after injury, and after surgery), and in some conditions it is not possible to remove the cause (e.g. metastatic cancer), demonstrate familiarity with the use of analgesic medications as a first line of treatment in these cases.

• Discuss that depression, uncontrolled pain, the adverse effects of opioids, and fear of pain may precipitate suicidal thoughts or requests for aid in dying.

General/Specific Objectives

• Through efficient, focused, data gathering:

  - Determine the most likely cause of the pain (clinical features and use of provocative manoeuvres are key).

  - Because depression is the most common emotional disturbance in patients with chronic pain, elicit evidence of depression.

- Interpret critical clinical and laboratory findings which were key in the processes of exclusion, differentiation, and diagnosis:
  - Select laboratory investigations to identify cause of pain if required.
  - Select patients in need of specialised care for further investigation.
- Conduct an effective plan of management for a patient with acute or chronic pain:
  - Categorise and contrast drugs for relief of pain (non-narcotic analgesics, narcotic analgesics, anticonvulsants and anti-arrhythmics, tricyclic antidepressants, antispasmodics and steroids).
  - Discuss the use of combinations of medications.
  - Outline a multidisciplinary approach which utilises medications, counselling, physical therapy, nerve block, surgery, etc.
  - Since pain also adds to the discomfort of those caring for the patient with chronic pain, counsel caregivers.
  - Select patients in need of referral to a pain clinic or pain specialist.

070A Somatic Complaints / Somatoform Disorders

Overview

Non-specific somatic symptoms with no immediate organic explanation frequently present in primary care. Most are brief but some are persistent and result in repeated consultations. Somatisation implies the presentation of emotional distress as physical or bodily symptoms, which mask the underlying anxiety or mood disorder. These medically unexplained symptoms reflect patients' cognitive concerns and attributions about illness in general or about specific conditions, at either a conscious or unconscious level. Patients' interpretation of bodily sensations may be influenced by their medical experience and beliefs, their social circumstances and their personality. **Somatoform disorder** is the general term to cover all of the different categories of medically unexplained symptoms.

Causes

1) Acute transient somatic symptoms in response to stress

2) Subacute somatic symptoms in patients with depression or panic disorder

3) Chronic or recurrent somatic symptoms

    a) **Somatisation disorder**

    b) **Hypochondriasis**

    c) **Conversion disorder / Dissociative disorder**

    d) **Body dysmorphic disorder**

    e) **Somatoform pain disorder**

    f) **Factitious disorder**

    g) **Malingering**

Key Objective

- Differentiate various symptoms such as chest pain, palpitations, dyspnoea, abdominal pain, etc. which are due to an affective disorder or panic/anxiety, from similar symptoms due to organic causes.

General/Specific Objectives

- Through efficient, focused, data gathering:

  - Elicit history about current life stresses (separation, death, substance abuse), avoidance patterns or panic attacks, evidence of somatisation since adolescence, family history of somatisation.

  - Determine whether there was sexual abuse, physical abuse, emotional neglect.

- Interpret critical clinical and laboratory findings which were key in the processes of exclusion, differentiation, and diagnosis:

  - Select patients for limited laboratory testing, to exclude organic causes.

- Conduct an effective plan of management for a patient with somatic complaints:

  - Outline initial management including education about anxiety, supportive psychotherapy for life stressors, instruction in relaxation techniques.

  - Discuss medications available for treatment of somatic complaints / panic disorder.

  - Select patients in need of specialised care.

071A   Pain in the Upper Extremities

(See also #089E Shoulder Pain and #089F Hand/Wrist/Elbow Pain)

Overview
After backache, upper extremity pain is the next most common type of musculoskeletal pain.

Causes

1)   Trauma / Inflammation

- a) Torsion, contusion, fracture, dislocation
- b) Tendinitis, bursitis, arthritis
- c) Frozen shoulder / Traumatised joints

2)   Nerve impingement

- a) Carpal tunnel
- b) Cervical spondylosis / Disc herniation
- c) Neuritis
- d) Tumours

3)   Degenerative / Rheumatic

- a) Arthritis
- b) 'Fibromyalgia'
- c) Renal osteodystrophy (pseudogout)

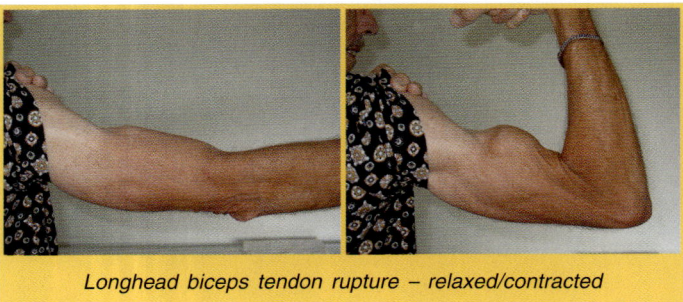

Longhead biceps tendon rupture – relaxed/contracted

4)   Vascular

- a) Arterial thromboembolism
- b) Raynaud phenomenon

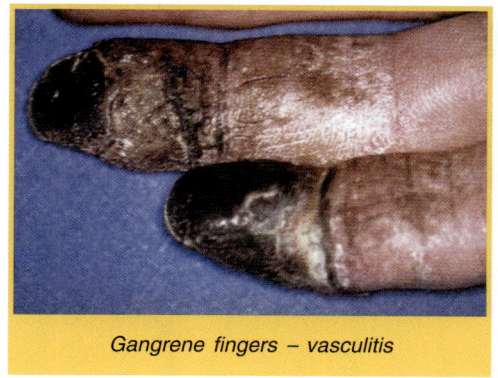

Gangrene fingers – vasculitis

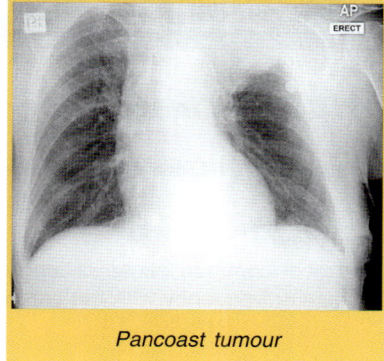

Pancoast tumour

   c) **Venous thrombosis**

   d) **Lymphoedema**

   e) **Thoracic outlet syndrome**

5)   Musculoligamentous (e.g. rotator cuff and other tendon tears and ruptures, myositis ossificans)

6)   Referred

   a) **Myocardial ischaemia**

   b) **Gallbladder disorders / Subphrenic abscess**

   c) **Apical lung tumour (Pancoast syndrome)**

Key Objective
- Demonstrate a careful physical examination with implementation of specific manoeuvres for diagnosis, since most cases can be diagnosed without imaging.

General/Specific Objectives
- Through efficient, focused, data gathering:
  - Differentiate between various causes of upper extremity pain.
- Interpret critical clinical and laboratory findings which were key in the processes of exclusion, differentiation, and diagnosis:
  - If necessary, select diagnostic imaging and laboratory investigation.
- Conduct an effective plan of management for a patient with pain in the upper extremities:
  - Outline a plan of management for various types of upper extremity pain.
  - Select patients in need of specialised care.

071B   Pain in the Lower Extremities

(See also #061 Limp / Pain in Lower Extremity in Children)

Overview

The most common cause of leg pain is muscular or ligamentous strain, seen with increasing frequency with the current interest in physical activity.

Causes

1)   Articular (degenerative joint disease)

  a) Hip (degenerative joint disease)

  b) Knee (degenerative joint disease, gout)

  c) Ankle

  d) Foot/Toes (gout)

2)   Non-articular

  a) Musculoligamentous (exercise, trauma)

  b) Vascular (thrombo-phlebitis, arterial insufficiency, varicose veins)

  c) Neurologic (lumbar disc disease, spinal stenosis)

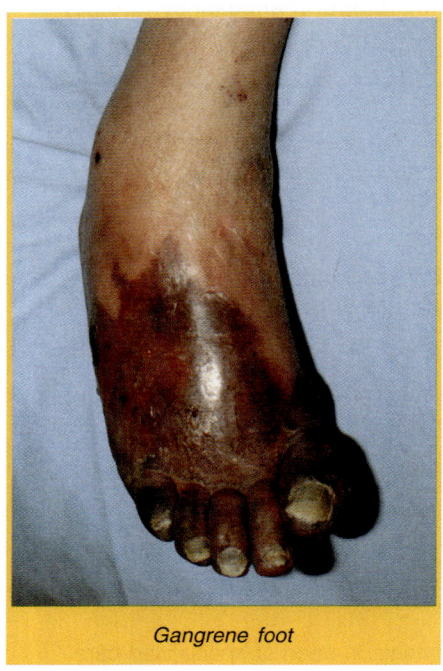

Gangrene foot

Key Objectives

- Determine whether the pain is articular (hip, knee, ankle) or non-articular (muscular, vascular, neurologic) and whether related to exertion or not.

- Recognise that degenerative joint disease and arterial insufficiency frequently co-exist.

General/Specific Objectives

- Through efficient, focused, data gathering:

  - Differentiate between different causes of lower extremity pain by eliciting essential information (e.g. precipitating events) and manoeuvres which reproduce the pain.

  - Perform examination of lower limb including observation of gait and posture, examination and determination of range of motion of joints, measurement of calves and thighs, and palpation of peripheral arteries.

- Interpret critical clinical and laboratory findings which were key in the processes of exclusion, differentiation, and diagnosis:

  - List indications for radiographic, magnetic resonance imaging (MRI), and arthroscopic examination.

- Conduct an effective plan of management for a patient with pain in the lower extremities:

  - Outline a multidisciplinary plan of management for lower extremity pain caused by degenerative joint disease.

  - Outline a multidisciplinary plan for prevention of peripheral vascular disease.

  - Outline a plan of management for exercise-induced injuries which makes possible the return to physical activity.

  - Select patients in need of specialised care.

071C Painful Lower Limb – Varicose Veins

Overview

Varicose veins are dilated, tortuous, elongated veins in the lower limb. They may present as concern with the cosmetic appearance of the visible venous swellings, or as a source of local chronic discomfort worse on standing and eased by recumbency. Acute symptoms result from localised acute thrombosis in superficial veins (superficial thrombophlebitis) causing a painful palpable subcutaneous cord. Deep venous thrombosis (DVT) may complicate superficial varices or arise independently (see #034B Unilateral Limb Oedema (Swollen Limb)). In the post-thrombotic syndrome, leg ulceration follows chronic deep venous insufficiency. Significant risk factors associated with 'primary' vascular veins are the female sex, pregnancy and multiparity, and a family history.

Causes

> **1)   'Primary' varicose veins of lower limb – cause unknown**

Often associated with female gender, systemic hormonal effects, pregnancies, familial influences, iliac (left) vein compression; or to primary valvular incompetence in superficial veins and in the communications between deep and superficial venous system.

> **2)   'Secondary' varicose veins of lower limb**

Superficial varices secondary to deep venous obstruction or incompetence, arteriovenous fistulae, or compression from pelvic mass.

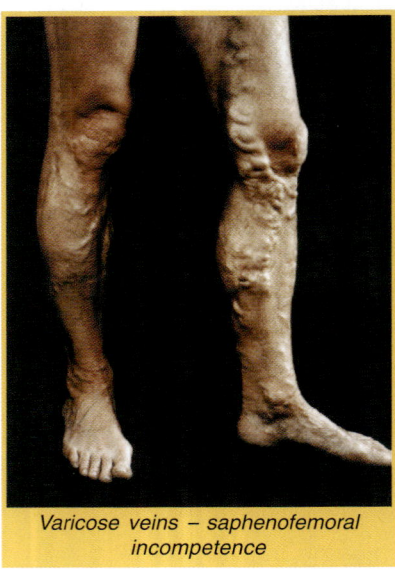

Varicose veins – saphenofemoral incompetence

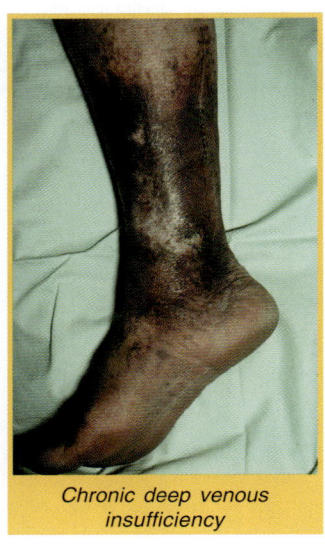

Chronic deep venous insufficiency

3) Miscellaneous causes of dilated superficial veins

a) Distal venous obstruction (e.g. retrosternal goitre)

b) Diversionary anastomotic channels (e.g. obstructed superior or inferior vena cava, effects of portal hypertension)

c) Arteriovenous malformations

Key Objectives

- Differentiate between uncomplicated, primary superficial varices and those associated with chronic deep venous insufficiency.

- Understand the principles of assessment of a patient presenting with symptomatic varicose veins.

General/Specific Objectives

- Through efficient, focused data gathering:

  - Appreciate the general anatomy and physiopathology of the superficial and deep venous systems of the leg, and their interrelationships during standing and activity.

- Interpret critical clinical and laboratory findings which were key in the processes of exclusion, differentiation, and diagnosis:

  - Recognise the common sites of communication between superficial and deep venous systems; and the principles and practice of tests for valvular incompetence.

  - Ability to answer the diagnostic questions:

    * Are definite superficial varices present, and do they involve the long or short saphenous system or both?

    * Are signs of vascular incompetence, particularly saphenofemoral incompetence, present; and are there signs of incompetent communicating or perforating veins below groin level?

    * Are the deep veins normal or is there evidence of deep venous circulatory insufficiency?

- Conduct an effective plan of management for a patient presenting with symptomatic varicose veins:

  - Outline noninterventional methods of management.

  - Outline indications and principles of sclerotherapy.

  - Outline indications for surgery and select patients for onward referral and further investigation.

Overview

The symptom of palpitations describes an abnormal subjective awareness of the heart beat. Patients can usually distinguish between occasional, intermittent or continuous bouts of palpitations and whether they are regular or irregular. In this regard, asking the patient to tap out the beats on a table can often clarify the important features. Palpitations are commonly associated with anxiety and vasodilatational states but may indicate a more serious cardiac arrhythmia where there are usually associated symptoms (sweating, breathlessness, dizziness, fainting, chest pain) which can give important clues to the diagnosis. The definitive diagnosis requires a clinical assessment and/or electrocardiogram (ECG) during a bout of palpitations.

Causes

1) Sinus rhythm

    a) **Vasodilatation / Sinus tachycardia (exercise, stress, fever, pregnancy, menopausal state, drugs)**

    b) **Anxiety**

    c) **Ectopic beats**

2) Atrial tachyarrhythmias

    a) **Atrial premature complexes**

    b) **Atrial flutter and fibrillation**
- Idiopathic (lone fibrillator)
- Ischaemic heart disease
- Hypertensive heart disease
- Valvular heart disease
- Thyrotoxicosis
- Cardiomyopathy (alcoholic, idiopathic, viral)
- Electrolyte disorders
- Drugs

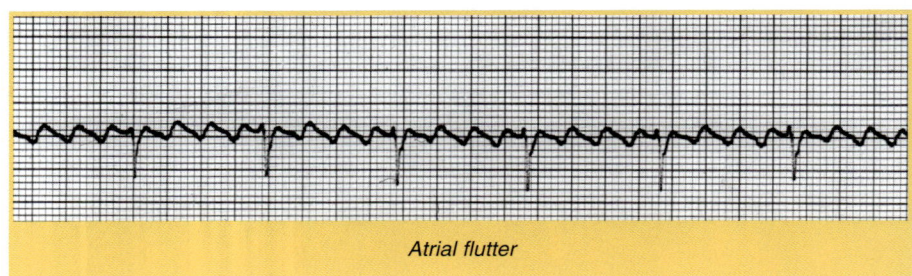

Atrial flutter

3) Supraventricular tachycardia

a) Paroxysmal supraventricular tachycardia

b) Wolff-Parkinson-White syndrome (WPW) / Concealed bypass tract

c) Multifocal atrial tachycardia

4) Ventricular tachyarrhythmias

a) Premature ventricular ectopics

b) Ventricular tachycardia
- ❏ Sustained
- ❏ Non-sustained

Key Objectives

- Select patients in need of urgent treatment.

- Differentiate palpitations due to intrinsic heart disease from those that are a manifestation of anxiety, exercise, or other systemic disease (differentiate from sinus tachycardia).

- Understand the indications for the use of drugs and when there are contraindications to particular drugs because of their pro-arrhythmic potential.

- Know when and how to use anticoagulant drugs in the patient with atrial fibrillation.

General/Specific Objectives

- Through efficient, focused data gathering:

  - Contrast benign palpitations to those associated with serious disease.

  - Diagnose major cardiac arrhythmias.

- Interpret critical clinical and laboratory findings which were key in the processes of exclusion, differentiation, and diagnosis:

  - Differentiate between causes of palpitations.

  - Elicit and interpret signs and symptoms which indicate that a cardiac arrhythmia requires immediate treatment.

  - Select and interpret appropriate investigations for patients presenting with palpitations, including cardiography and Holter monitoring.

- Conduct an effective plan of management for a patient with palpitations:

  - Outline initial management for the patient with an abnormal heart rhythm.

  - Select the patients in need of specialised care and/or consultation, including those with a benign or unknown aetiology.

  - Describe the indications for anticoagulant and/or anti-platelet therapy for patients with arrhythmias and perform initial and long term management.

Overview

The **anxiety disorders** are characterised by excessive and persistent worry, anxiety or fear, and avoidant or controlling behaviours and phenomena, accompanied by physical symptoms of hyperarousal and autonomic hyper-reactivity. They occur commonly, and may present acutely (for example panic attacks) or with chronic impairment (for example, generalised anxiety disorder). Presentation with predominantly somatic symptoms, either a single complaint (e.g. chest pain, neurological deficit) or a large number of multisystem symptoms, through the process of somatisation, is frequent. The anxiety disorders are:

❏ **Generalised anxiety disorder**: enduring six months or more of excessive worry and anxiety, with muscle tension and physical indicators of hyperarousal, such as sleep and concentration disturbance, fatigue.

❏ **Panic disorder, with or without agoraphobia**: sudden anxiety attacks; fear of collapse, loss of control, or death; and hyperarousal, especially hyperventilation and its sequelae; with situational avoidance.

❏ **Phobias (specific, agoraphobia, and social)**: excessive, unreasonable fear of specific situation, with avoidance, or extreme sensitivity and anxiety if endured.

❏ **Post–traumatic stress disorder**: exposure to extreme, threatening event and subsequent persistent hyperarousal, intrusive re-experiences, and avoidance of the trigger and allied events.

❏ **Obsessive–compulsive disorder**: recurrent and irrepressible thoughts, images or impulses, accompanied by anxiety symptoms, and repetitive driven habits or rituals to reduce distress or some anticipated dread.

Causes

1) Physical causes of anxiety

   a) **Cardiovascular (angina, arrhythmias)**

   b) **Drugs (caffeine, amphetamines, cocaine)**

   c) **Metabolic / Endocrine (thyroid, phaeochromocytoma)**

   d) **Neurological (encephalopathy, temporal lobe seizure, dementia)**

   e) **Respiratory (asthma, emboli, oedema)**

2) Non-physical conditions causing anxiety

   a) **Primary anxiety disorders (see *Overview*)**

   b) **Other psychiatric conditions – depression, substance abuse disorders, schizophrenia**

Key Objectives

- Identify the presence of a primary anxiety disorder and its type.

- Differentiate from secondary anxiety arising from other psychiatric conditions, physical causes or drugs, and from realistic anxiety arising from an environmental threat.

General/Specific Objectives

- Through efficient, focused data gathering:

  - Elicit a history of excessive anxiety, fear or worry along with other symptoms specific to the particular anxiety disorder.

  - Determine the level of social, occupational and general functional disability.

- Interpret those clinical and laboratory findings key to the diagnostic process.

- Implement an appropriate management plan for the particular anxiety disorder and level of disability:

  - Education about the condition, causes and symptom manifestations.

  - General anxiety management including relaxation methods, hyperventilation control, and graduated exposure to trigger situations.

  - Specific intervention with problem-solving techniques and cognitive behavioural therapy, or specialist referral.

  - Selected drug therapy such as antidepressants.

Overview
Any female patient who visits a clinician's office should have current screening guidelines applied and if appropriate, a Papanicolaou (Pap) smear should be recommended.

Causes

1) Normal

2) Abnormal

a) **Benign atypia**
  - ❏ Atypical glandular cells of uncertain significance (AGUS)
  - ❏ Atypical squamous cells of uncertain significance (ASCUS)
  - ❏ Infection

b) **Human papilloma virus (HPV)**

c) **Mild/Severe dysplasia – cervical intra-epithelial neoplasia (CIN)**
  - ❏ CIN 1 – also called mild dysplasia
  - ❏ CIN 2 – also called moderate dysplasia
  - ❏ CIN 3 – also called carcinoma-*in-situ*

d) **Invasive carcinoma (micro)**

3) False positive or negative smears

Key Objective
- Select patients in need of referral for further investigation including colposcopy and target biopsy after the report of a Pap smear becomes available.

General/Specific Objectives
- Through efficient, focused data gathering:
  - Determine whether the patient is at high risk for developing cervical dysplasia or invasive disease.
  - List situations which increase the index of suspicion for cervical dysplasia.
  - Describe how to obtain a Pap smear.
- Interpret critical clinical and laboratory findings which were key in the processes of exclusion, differentiation, and diagnosis:
  - Select additional investigation if appropriate.

- Conduct an effective plan of management for a patient with abnormal Pap smear:

  - List recommendations for prevention of cervical dysplasia / cervical cancer and identify health promotion strategies for young sexually active women.

  - Discuss the role of regular cervical cytology in the prevention of invasive disease.

  - Outline methods of treatment for pre-invasive disease of the cervix and list possible complications.

  - Discuss the association of HPV infection with CIN neoplasia and invasive cancer (including the most common HPV sub-types associated with progression to invasive cancer).

  - Discuss the specificity and sensitivity of Pap smear test, and factors leading to a false positive or negative test.

Overview

Pelvic masses are common in clinical practice and need to be investigated to find the cause.

Causes

1) Gynaecologic

a) **Ovary**
  - ❑ Functional cysts (follicular, corpus lutein cysts, theca lutein cysts)
  - ❑ Hyperplastic (polycystic ovary, endometriotic cyst)
  - ❑ Neoplastic
    - Serous cystadenoma / Carcinoma
    - Mucinous cystadenoma / Carcinoma
    - Thecomas / Granulosa cell tumours
    - Fibromas
    - Germ cell tumours (cystic teratoma, teratoma, gonadoblastoma, dysgerminoma)

b) **Tube (salpinx)**
  - ❑ Ectopic pregnancy
  - ❑ Inflammation (including hydrosalpinx/pyosalpinx), cysts (mesonephric, paramesonephric)

c) **Uterus**
  - ❑ Pregnancy
  - ❑ Haematometra / Pyometra
  - ❑ Leiomyoma/Adenomyoma
  - ❑ Sarcoma

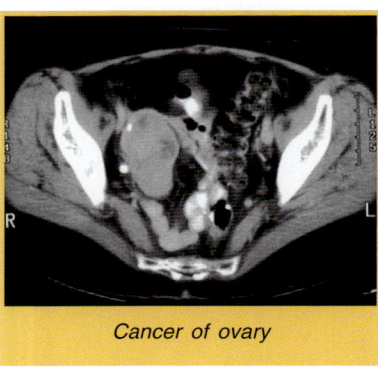

Cancer of ovary

2) Non-gynaecologic (bowel, bladder, other)

Key Objectives

- Determine whether the patient may be pregnant.

- Determine whether the mass is gynaecologic, and whether the origin is the ovary, tube, or uterus.

General/Specific Objectives

- Through efficient, focused data gathering:

   - Elicit a history including menstrual, fertility, and obstetrical history, sexual activity, and associated symptoms.

   - Perform abdominal and pelvic examination including speculum examination.

   - Describe features suggestive of androgenisation in the reproductive age and oestrogenisation in prepubertal age group.

- Interpret critical clinical and laboratory findings which were key in the processes of exclusion, differentiation, and diagnosis:

   - List blood tumour markers if malignancy is suspected; pregnancy test and/or cultures if indicated.

   - Select diagnostic imaging appropriate for mass, or endometrial biopsy if indicated.

- Conduct an effective plan of management for a patient with a pelvic mass:

   - Outline management of functional cysts.

   - Outline management of tubo-ovarian abscess.

   - Counsel patients with leiomyoma and outline medical management.

   - Select patients in need of specialised care.

Overview

Many hours each year are lost from school and work due to pelvic pain. Successful treatment requires a correct diagnosis. Once the diagnosis is established, specific and usually successful treatment may be instituted.

Causes

1) Pregnancy-related

a) Ectopic pregnancy

b) Aborting pregnancy

c) Gynaecological conditions in pregnancy – complicated ovarian cysts, red degeneration of a leiomyoma

d) Molar pregnancy

2) Gynaecological

a) Mittelschmerz

b) Torsion (e.g. ovarian)

c) Endometriosis

d) Bleeding into a pelvic mass / Ruptured pelvic mass

e) Infection (e.g. salpingitis)

f) Dyspareunia

3) Non-gynaecological (gastrointestinal, renal, musculoskeletal)

Key Objective

• Determine whether the pain is acute or chronic, whether pregnancy is likely, and stabilise the patient whose pain is acute and life-threatening.

General/Specific Objectives

• Through efficient, focused data gathering:

- Elicit a history including menstrual, fertility, and obstetrical history, sexual activity, and associated symptoms.

- Determine whether the patient's condition is haemodynamically stable and whether a candidate for possible emergency surgery.

- Perform abdominal and pelvic examinations including speculum examination.

- Interpret critical clinical and laboratory findings which were key in the processes of exclusion, differentiation, and diagnosis:

  - List guidelines for ultrasound in pregnancy; obtain pregnancy test.

  - Select appropriate diagnostic imaging; list indications for laparoscopy.

- Conduct an effective plan of management for a patient with pelvic pain:

  - List indications for dilatation and curettage, laparoscopy, and laparotomy for aborting pregnancy or ectopic pregnancy including impact on future fertility.

  - Outline initial management of endometriosis.

  - Outline management of acute salpingitis.

  - Counsel for the purpose of preventing sexually transmitted diseases (STDs).

  - Counsel and outline management of patients with chronic pelvic pain associated with psycho-emotional factors.

  - Outline management of dyspareunia.

  - Select patients in need of specialised care.

Overview

Periodically, patients visit clinicians' offices not because they are unwell, but because they want a 'check-up'. The periodic health examination is considered an opportunity to relate to an asymptomatic patient for the purpose of case finding and screening for undetected disease and risky behaviour. It is also an opportunity for health promotion and disease prevention, particularly in regard to immunisation, tobacco and alcohol abuse, and monitoring growth and weight.

Causal Conditions to be Considered

1)   Infant and toddler less than 3 years (e.g. delayed growth, development, abuse/neglect)

2)   Child 3–12 years (visual/hearing deficit, accidents, development, abuse/neglect)

3)   Youth 13–24 years (motor vehicle accident (MVA), substance abuse, sexually transmitted diseases (STDs), sedentary)

    a) Female (rubella immunisation, contraception)

    b) Male (contraception)

4)   Adult 25–44 years (substance abuse, eating disorders, family violence)

    a) Female (cervical cancer, hypertension)

    b) Male (hypertension, elevated cholesterol, MVA)

5)   Middle age 45–64 years (lung cancer, colon cancer, skin cancer, obesity)

    a) Female (osteoporosis, breast cancer)

    b) Male (prostate cancer, ischaemic heart disease)

    c) Hypercalcaemia – both sexes

6)   Seniors older than 64 years (elder abuse, falls, drug-related morbidity, nutrition, cancer)

Key Objectives

- Determine patient's risks for common gender/age specific conditions.

- Elicit information about ethnic, family, socio-economic, occupational, lifestyle characteristics that are known to be at high-risk for a particular condition.

General/Specific Objectives

- Through efficient, focused data gathering:

  - In an infant, toddler, or child, elicit information about risk factors at conception, pregnancy, and birth, familial factors, and existing signs of illness or environmental risk factors (missed immunisation, diet, passive smoke inhalation, skin protection).

  - Determine height, weight, head circumference, medical status, and developmental milestones.

  - For a youth, elicit information about nutrition, physical activity, drug use, sexual/social/peer activities, emotional concerns, communication with parents.

  - In adults, elicit information about lifestyle patterns, psychological, social, and physical functioning, symptoms of any illness, and situational factors affecting mood.

  - In seniors, elicit information about past illness, lifestyle factors, mental function, drug use, physical and social activity, emotional concerns, social relations and support systems.

- Interpret critical clinical and laboratory findings which were key in the processes of exclusion, differentiation, and diagnosis:

  - Select investigation specific to age and gender concerns.

- Conduct an effective plan of management for a patient who is well and without disease, well and with disease, not well and with disease, not well and without disease:

  - Communicate regarding disease and accident prevention; encourage patient control over health.

  - Outline interventions that would reduce risk for an existing condition detected.

  - For a frequently encountered risk factor (e.g. colon cancer), outline interventions that would reduce the risk for the condition.

  - Remember when considering major interventions that it is difficult to make an asymptomatic patient feel better.

077A   Newborn Assessment/Nutrition

Overview
Primary care clinicians, paediatricians and obstetricians play vital roles in identifying children at risk for developmental disabilities. Parents require direction and reassurance regarding the health status of their newborn infant. In most cases, parental concerns regarding the child's language development, articulation, fine motor skills, and global development are likely to be associated with true developmental delays. Parental concerns with personal-social skills are associated with developmental delays in some cases.

Causes

1)	Developmental surveillance

2)	Nutrition (breastfeeding, bottlefeeding, solid foods)

3)	Well-newborn care

Key Objectives
- Determine development through ongoing monitoring because new circumstances may interfere (e.g. medical illness, family disruption) or because, as children develop, new categories of skills are gained (e.g. language delays cannot be detected before 18–24 months).

- Provide anticipatory guidance to parents in order to prevent unnecessary demands from healthcare providers.

General/Specific Objectives
- Through efficient, focused, data gathering:

  - Elicit history of parental concerns regarding the child's development, risk factors for developmental delays, and attainment of developmental milestones.

  - Perform examination of head circumference, congenital anomalies or dysmorphic features, skin lesions (e.g. *café-au-lait* spots, ash leaf macules, 'port-wine' naevi), muscle tone, hearing, vision, and developmental screening tests.

- Conduct an effective plan of management for the newborn:

  - Counsel parents regarding breastfeeding (maternal drug use during lactation, maternal nutrition and rest, breastfeeding technique, feeding frequency and intake), bottlefeeding technique, frequency and intake, formula types, and introduction of solid food, vitamin requirements and the indications for dietary supplements; discuss contraindications to breastfeeding.

  - Determine the measurements appropriate for normal infant growth and development.

  - Counsel parents about skin care, fontanelles, eye colour, strabismus, teeth, umbilicus, genitalia, urination and defaecation.

077B Infant and Child Immunisation

Overview
Immunisation has reduced or eradicated many infectious diseases and has improved overall world health. Recommended immunisation schedules are constantly updated as new vaccines become available.

Causes to be Prevented

1) **Poliomyelitis**

2) **Diphtheria-Tetanus-Pertussis**

3) **Measles-Mumps-Rubella**

4) **Hepatitis B**

5) **Chicken pox**

6) **Pneumococcal pneumonia**

7) **Meningococcal meningitis**

8) **Influenza**

Key Objectives
- Discuss the population health benefits of immunisation programmes.
- State that a lapse in immunisation schedule does not require re-instituting the initial series, merely correcting the lapse at the next visit.
- Communicate to patients and parents about vaccine benefits and risks.

General/Specific Objectives
- Through efficient, focused data gathering:
  - Obtain an immunisation history on all children and determine whether the child (or family member) is immunosuppressed or is receiving immunosuppressive drugs.
  - Determine whether the child has had splenectomy (also congenital or functional in sickle cell disease).

- Interpret critical clinical and laboratory findings which were key in the processes of exclusion, differentiation, and diagnosis:

  - Test immune status of susceptible children.

- Conduct an effective plan of management which will:

  - Discuss misconceptions about immunisation contraindications and actual contraindications.

  - List possible complications of immunisation.

  - Discuss immunisation of immuno-compromised children (e.g. with asplenia, chronic diseases or seizures).

077C Preoperative Assessment

Overview

Accurate and thorough evaluation of patients prior to surgery will maximise the chance of successful outcome. The objectives of such an evaluation include the determination of risk of the intended procedure to the patient and what measures may be required to minimise such risks. Pivotal in the process is counselling of the patient (and where appropriate, family members) with appropriate explanation of the procedure, its benefits and its risks.

Considerations in Preoperative Assessment

1) Understanding of the procedures – potential risks, complications and side-effects

2) Preoperative assessment of risk factors and comorbidities

    a) Optimal care of recognised diseases / risk factors

    b) Identification of unrecognised diseases / risk factors

    c) Identification/Management of potential complications

- ❏ Anaesthetic/Postoperative risk
  - Myocardial dysfunction
  - Autonomic neuropathy (e.g. diabetes mellitus)
  - Pulmonary risk (upper abdominal/thoracic surgery, duration greater than three hours, smoking and/or chronic obstructive lung disease, P_aCO_2 greater than 45 mm Hg, obesity, etc.)
  - Drugs (e.g. anticoagulants, analgesics, psychotropics)
- ❏ Exercise capacity
- ❏ Other

Key Objectives

- Identify factors likely to influence peri-operative and postoperative morbidity and mortality.
- Identify measures required to reduce morbidity and mortality of surgery.
- Communicate to the patient and the preoperative team the level of risk for the proposed surgery compared to average risk for the procedure rather than 'clearing' or 'not clearing' patients for surgery.

General/Specific Objectives
- Through efficient, focused data gathering; identify potential risks from history-taking, examination and preoperative investigations:

  - Elicit evidence of feeling unwell, serious past illnesses and any medications in previous three months.

  - Elicit evidence of dyspnoea, cough, wheeze, chest pain on exertion, ankle oedema.

  - Obtain history of allergies, previous anaesthetics, problems with anaesthetics (including in family); and in women, their last menstrual period.

  - Note history of previous surgery, bleeding tendency, aspirin, nonsteroidal anti-inflammatory drugs (NSAIDs) or anticoagulant medication, or previous transfusions.

- Interpret critical clinical and laboratory findings which were key in the processes of exclusion, differentiation, and diagnosis:

  - Select and interpret preoperative laboratory investigations based on known or clinically suspected diseases or risk factors (e.g. cardiac or pulmonary disease, diuretic use, diabetes, hypertension) or the age and sex of the patient.

  - Identify patient-related and procedure-related risk factors.

  - Grade surgical and anaesthetic risk according to the American Society of Anaesthiologists (ASA) classification.

- Conduct an effective plan of management for a patient with illnesses or risk factors:

  - Recommend smoking cessation eight weeks preoperatively in smokers.

  - Explain why 'routine' preoperative investigations are not indicated.

  - Discuss postoperative pain control including various analgesics, epidural analgesia, and intercostal nerve block in patients at risk for pulmonary complications.

077D Postoperative Patient Evaluation and Care

Overview

Wound care is required after any surgical procedure and any complications of the healing process need early diagnosis and management. General observational and nursing care of the surgical patient is equally important. Optimal patient care and regular systems review can avert potential complications or detect and reverse them at an early stage.

Causes of Potential Postoperative General Complications

1) Wound – delayed wound healing associated with haematoma/ seroma, infection, dehiscence; incisional hernia

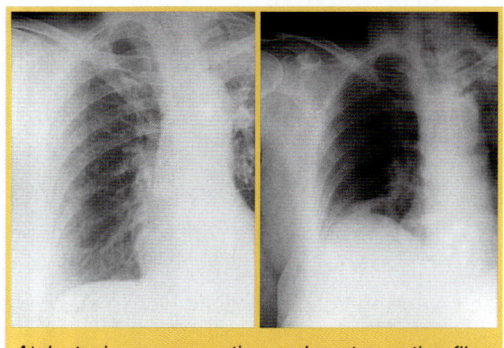

Atelectasis – preoperative and postoperative films

2) Airway/Breathing/Chest – atelectasis, aspiration, pneumonia, postoperative respiratory failure, pulmonary embolism

3) Circulation

    a) **Haemorrhage**

        ❏ Wound – primary, reactionary, secondary; overt or concealed

        ❏ Gastrointestinal haemorrhage – stress ulcer syndrome

    b) **Shock – haemorrhagic, cardiogenic, obstructive/embolic, septic**

    c) **Cardiac – arrhythmias/arrest, myocardial infarction (MI), cardiac failure**

4) Gastrointestinal – postanaesthetic nausea/vomiting, disturbed bowel function, bowel obstruction, gastrointestinal haemorrhage, jaundice, parotitis

5) Urinary – retention, infection, acute renal failure (ARF)

6) **Integument and vascular access** – thrombophlebitis, extravasation of intravenous solutions, pneumothorax (central cannulation), incompatible blood transfusion, diathermy burn, pressure sore

7) **Cerebral** – delirium: hypoxia; drugs/intoxication/withdrawal; sleep loss / disorientation; metabolic disturbance; sepsis

8) **Fever** – atelectasis; focal or systemic sepsis; thrombophlebitis; deep venous thrombosis (DVT) and thromboembolism; tissue necrosis / gout / MI; incompatible blood transfusion; drug allergy

Key Objectives

- Optimally monitor postoperative course by regular wound assay, observation of vital signs, focused systems review and followup.

- Encourage early return of preoperative functions.

- Achieve early detection and treatment of complications.

General/Specific Objectives

- Through efficient, focused data collection, including investigations where appropriate:

  - Monitor early postoperative progress, supervise and maintain uncomplicated postoperative progress.

  - Check for adequate pain relief; and that vital signs are normal from nursing observations. Check wound status and fluid balance; intravenous drip sites and urethral catheter care if present; assess chest, abdomen, legs for DVT, circulation and temperature at regular intervals.

  - Anticipate postoperative pharmaceutical requirements, followup by surgeon, and by patient's own family doctor to co-ordinate overall patient care.

  - Liaise with other health workers including ward and district nursing staff, paramedical care including: physiotherapy, occupational therapy, speech pathology, social worker and community service workers as required.

  - Communicate with family members, other relatives and friends as appropriate.

  - Communicate with patient's doctor verbally and arrange early transmission of summary of admission, operative and postoperative details.

  - Communicate accurately, empathically and at an appropriate level with patient during early convalescence and prior to discharge and answer any continuing concerns.

077E Work-Related Health Issues

Overview

Doctors will encounter health hazards in their own work place, as well as in the work place of their patients. These hazards need to be recognised and addressed.

Causes

1) **Disability management and work fitness**

2) **Public health and surveillance**

   a) Hazard recognition, evaluation, and control

   b) Occupational and environmental injury/illness

   c) Underlying medical condition and environment

3) **Clinical preventive services**

Key Objective

- Determine whether the work place or environmental conditions are potentially hazardous, the impact on the health of the workers, and recommend preventive strategies.

General/Specific Objectives

- Through efficient, focused data gathering:

   - Elicit history of patient's occupation and possible exposure to toxic or hazardous environments and identify potential relationship to patient presentation.

- Interpret critical clinical and laboratory findings which were key in the processes of exclusion, differentiation, and diagnosis.

- Conduct an effective plan of management for a patient with work-related health issues:

   - Select patients in need of specialised care and provide followup care.

   - Counsel patients about safety issues and report findings to affected patients as well as employers (considering medical confidentiality issues).

- Gain an understanding of Australian WorkCover law:
  - Legal obligations of employers:
    - To provide a safe workplace.
    - To indemnify employees against work-related injury.
  - The process of completing and submitting an Australian WorkCover form when treating patients with work-related injury or illness.
  - The limits of the indemnity cover provided by WorkCover law in Australia.

077F Health of Special Populations

Overview

The health of groups frequently reflects the influences of health determinants such as the ones considered in #077G Population and #077H Environment. The conditions resulting from these adverse factors do not differ from those considered under the numbered clinical presentations indicated, but are here re-considered in order to alert learners to the most common conditions to be considered in these respective groups.

Causal Conditions to be Considered in Individual Population Groups

1) The health of indigenous aboriginal peoples

a) Trauma / Poisoning / Sudden infant death syndrome (SIDS) / Acute life-threatening event (ALTE)

(see #079 Poisoning, #099 Sudden Infant Death Syndrome (SIDS), (Acute Life-Threatening Event (ALTE)), #107 Substance Abuse/Addiction, #108 Suicidal Behaviour/Prevention, #113 Trauma/Accidents/Prevention)

b) Circulatory diseases (including rheumatic fever)

(see #020 Chest Discomfort, #032 Dyspnoea and/or Cough / Prevention of Cancers and Chronic Respiratory Diseases, #054 Hypertension, #067 Murmur / Extra Heart Sounds)

c) Neoplasms

(see #016 Bleeding with Defaecation / Acute Lower Gastrointestinal Bleeding / Melaena / Occult Blood in Stool / Prevention of Cancer, #048 Haematemesis / Melaena, #049 Haematuria, #051 Haemoptysis, #070 Pain, #125 Weight Loss / Eating Disorders / Anorexia / Nutritional Disorders)

d) Diseases of respiratory system

(see #032 Dyspnoea and/or Cough / Prevention of Cancers and Chronic Respiratory Diseases, #126 Wheezing / Respiratory Difficulty / Stridor)

e) Infection (gastroenteritis, otitis media, infectious hepatitis)

(see #027 Diarrhoea/Constipation, #033 Ear Pain, #040 Fever and Chills (Adult and Paediatric), #058 Jaundice)

f) Diabetes

(see #053 Hyperglycaemia / Diabetes Mellitus)

g) Skin disorder

(see #101 Skin Blisters – Boils – Comedones – Ulcers, #101A Chronic Leg Ulcer)

2

The health of seniors

a) Musculoskeletal (including falls and injuries)

(see #037 Falls, #059 Joint Pain, Mon-Articular (Acute, Chronic), #060 Joint Pain, Poly-Articular (Acute, Chronic), #089 Regional Pain)

b) Hypertension/Heart diseases

(see #020 Chest Discomfort, #032 Dyspnoea and/or Cough / Prevention of Cancers and Chronic Respiratory Diseases, #054 Hypertension, #067 Murmur / Extra Heart Sounds)

c) Respiratory diseases

(see #032 Dyspnoea and/or Cough / Prevention of Cancers and Chronic Respiratory Diseases, #126 Wheezing / Respiratory Difficulty / Stridor)

d) Dementia

(see #024 Dementia / Memory Disturbances)

3) The health of children in poverty (single mothers, immigrants)

a) Low birth weight

(see #123 Weight (Low) at Birth / Intra-uterine Growth Aberration)

b) Trauma / Poisoning

(see #079 Poisoning, #113 Trauma/Accidents/Prevention)

c) Mouth problems

(see #066 Mouth Problems)

d) Fever / Infectious diseases

(see #040 Fever and Chills (Adult and Paediatric), #058 Jaundice)

e) Psychiatric problems

(see #065 Mood Disorders, #073 Panic and Anxiety, #078 Personality Disorders, #107 Substance Abuse/Addiction, #108 Suicidal Behaviour/ Prevention, #119 Violence/Aggression and Mental Illness, #125 Weight Loss / Eating Disorders / Anorexia / Nutritional Disorders)

4) The health of people with disabilities

Key Objective
- When providing a periodic health examination to a person belonging to one of the above groups, evaluate conditions common to the group and determine whether evidence exists that the individual has such a condition.

077G Population

Overview

Some people are healthy while others are not, for reasons other than biology, genetic endowment, and the physical environment. The social environment exerts a profound influence on health, and social stimuli may exert a profound effect on physical responses.

Causal Determinants of Health

1) **Income and social status**

2) **Social support network**

3) **Education**

4) **Personal health practices and coping skills**

5) **Healthy child development**

6) **Health services (access and barriers to access)**

7) **Employment and working conditions**

   (see #077E Work-Related Health Issues)

8) **Physical environment**

   (see #077H Environment)

9) **Biology and genetic endowment**

Key Objectives

- Discuss the three levels of disease prevention (primary, secondary, and tertiary) and strategies for health promotion (e.g. education, communication/behaviour change, social marketing, healthy public policy, community development and organisation, community-wide prevention, and diffusion of innovations).

- Explain that factors such as geographic location, gender, and ethnic origin influence some of the determinants of health, but health status is in turn influenced by differential allocation and distribution of health service resources.

General/Specific Objectives

- Through efficient, focused, data gathering:

  - Identify needs of population with survey information and other sources in order to select interventions or management strategies for clinical presentations (e.g. education about seat belts, education about herbal medications since some weight reduction herbal medications can cause chronic renal failure).

  - Elicit history concerning occupation, education, level or absence of control, cultural issues, etc. that may have had an impact on presenting condition.

- Interpret critical clinical and laboratory findings which were key in the processes of exclusion, differentiation, and diagnosis.

- Conduct an effective plan of management for patients with conditions related to determinants of health:

  - Select population issues better managed by means of health promotion rather than traditional medical interventions.

077H   Environment

Overview

Environmental issues are important in medical practice because exposures may be causally linked to a patient's clinical presentation, or a patient's reported environmental exposure may necessitate interventions to prevent future illness. Clinician involvement is important in the promotion of global environmental health.

Exposures to Causal Environmental Pollutants

1)   Air pollutants

a) **Biological**
   - ❏ Pollen
   - ❏ Home exposures (dust mites, cockroaches, etc.)

b) **Chemicals**
   - ❏ Lead
   - ❏ Fossil fuel related (e.g. CO, SO_2)
   - ❏ Indoor air pollutants (e.g. formaldehyde)
   - ❏ Secondhand tobacco smoke

c) **Physical (energy transfer)**
   - ❏ Radiation (e.g. ultraviolet (UV) from ozone layer destruction by chlorofluorocarbons)
   - ❏ Electricity

2)   Water pollutants (drinking/recreational water)

a) **Bacterial**

b) **Chemical/Industrial**

3)   Soil pollutants (chemical/industrial)

4)   Food pollutants

a) **Biological (toxins/bacteria)**

b) **Chemical**
   - ❏ Drugs (antibiotics, hormones)
   - ❏ Food preservatives
   - ❏ Pesticides

Key Objectives

- Describe clinical presentations caused or aggravated by environmental exposures that are virtually indistinguishable from ones caused by other conditions (e.g. headache from carbon monoxide poisoning is similar to tension headache or migraine; asthma).

- In patients whose immediate (e.g. allergic reaction), subacute (e.g. asthma), or delayed (e.g. pneumoconiosis) presentation may be linked to environmental exposure, elicit an environmental history and identify potential sources of problems.

General/Specific Objectives

- Through efficient, focused, data gathering:

  - Determine whether symptoms are worse at home, work, or at leisure activities, on weekends or work days and are related to recent or past exposures (e.g. fumes, dusts, chemicals, radiation).

  - Determine whether an illness is occurring in an unexpected person (e.g. lung cancer in a non-smoker) or whether symptoms have developed without a clear aetiology.

  - Determine presence of nearby industrial plants, commercial businesses, or dump sites.

  - Determine home insulation, heating and cooling systems, cleaning agents, pesticide use, water supply, water leaks, recent renovations, air pollution, hobbies, hazardous waste contamination, spills, or other exposures.

- Interpret critical clinical and laboratory findings which were key in the processes of exclusion, differentiation, and diagnosis:

  - Select and consult labels or Material Safety Data Sheets (MSDS), poison control centres, consultants, agencies, and other references for information.

  - Select consultants (environmental medicine specialists, toxicologists, governmental agencies, industrial hygienists, etc.) for the purpose of documenting and quantifying exposure.

  - Select laboratory tests for the patient to establish exposure or select investigations to establish the presence of adverse health effects on target organs (e.g. blood lead levels to assess exposure to lead and serum creatinine to look for effects on kidney function).

- Conduct an effective plan of management for a patient with possible environmental exposure:

  - If evidence supports, or a strong suspicion exists, for a causal connection between exposure and the clinical presentation, notify the appropriate authorities to inspect the site and thereafter to decrease or eliminate exposure.

Overview

Personality disorders are deeply ingrained, inflexible and persistent maladaptive behaviours, which have been present since adolescence. These enduring patterns of behaviour exhibited over a wide variety of social, occupational and relationship contexts have adverse effects on the individual and on society. Abnormal personalities predispose to anxiety, mood disorders and alcohol and substance abuse, although they may co-exist with positive and favourable traits. Abnormal personalities occur in about five percent of the general population and thus need to be recognised by clinicians.

Causes

1)	'Odd' personality (paranoid, schizoid, schizotypal)

2)	'Dramatic' personalities (borderline, histrionic, narcissistic)

3)	'Anxious' personalities (dependent, avoidant, obsessive-compulsive)

4)	Antisocial personality disorder

5)	Others (passive-aggressive, explosive)

6)	Mixed patterns

Key Objective

- Determine whether the pattern of behaviour exhibited is enduring and exhibited over a wide variety of social and personality contexts leading to impairment in social and occupational functioning.

General/Specific Objectives

- Through efficient, focused data gathering:

  - Determine whether the patient is excessively suspicious or jealous, isolative, aloof or emotionally cool with little need for personal relationships, or has eccentric ideas or disturbances in thinking and communication.

  - Determine whether there is excessive sensitivity or depression, perfectionism and inflexibility, shyness and withdrawal, or excessive dependence on others.

  - Elicit history of lying, truancy, fights, thefts, cruelty, arson, substance or illegal activity before the age of 15 years; along with a pattern of manipulation and exploitation of others; impulsivity; a lack of empathy or remorse; and instability of mood or affect.

  - Determine whether there is excessively dramatic, flamboyant attention-seeking, excitable, grandiose and emotional behaviour.

- • Develop an effective management plan for a patient with a personality disorder:

  - - Outline differences between supportive therapy; insight-oriented therapy; cognitive and behavioural therapy; family or couple therapy and group therapy.

  - - Identify patients who will need drug and alcohol counselling.

  - - Identify patients who will benefit from treatment for anxiety or mood disorders.

  - - Select and refer patients who will benefit from specialised assessment and care.

079 Poisoning

Overview

Exposures to poisons or drug overdoses account for 5–10% of emergency department visits, and greater than 5% of admissions to intensive care units. More than 50% of these patients are children less than six years of age.

Causes

1) Common

a) Cleaning substances (detergents, soap, shampoo)

b) Cough and cold remedies

c) Cosmetics

2) Potentially lethal

a) Alcohol/Antifreeze

b) Analgesics (paracetamol, aspirin, nonsteroidal anti-inflammatory drugs (NSAIDs), opiates)

c) Psychotropics (neuroleptics, antidepressants, hypnotics, anxiolytics, lithium)

d) Carbon monoxide

e) Street drugs

f) Cardiovascular drugs

Key Objectives

- Perform supportive care, decontamination or prevention of further absorption, give antidote where indicated, and enhance elimination of the poison.

- Determine whether poisoning has occurred, the substance involved, how severe the exposure was, how toxic it is likely to become, and the causticity of substance.

- Discuss special considerations in the management of poisoning with aspirin, paracetamol, tricyclic antidepressants, and methanol.

General/Specific Objectives

- Through efficient and focused data gathering:

  - Determine the drug or poison causing the problem, using patient's vital signs, mental status, pupil size, appearance, smell, etc. as potential clues in addition to history from patient, paramedics, police, clinician, pharmacist, friends and relatives (if intentional, history is frequently unreliable).

- Interpret the critical clinical and laboratory findings which were crucial in the processes of exclusion, differentiation, and diagnosis:

  - Select and interpret drug screen based on clinical information.

  - Select laboratory and diagnostic imaging investigation for toxic effects in addition to diagnosis.

  - Calculate anion and osmolar gap; explain and interpret findings.

- Conduct an effective plan of management for a poisoned patient:

  - Perform supportive care before or at the same time as data gathering and investigation, such as ensuring airway adequacy, haemodynamic stability and intravenous access, cardiac monitoring and electrocardiogram (ECG), pulse oximetry, etc.

  - Outline initial management in a patient with poisoning with altered consciousness.

  - Discuss advantages and disadvantages of various strategies for prevention of poison absorption (also termed decontamination) in a patient who is less than one hour after intake of poison.

  - Discuss strategies for enhancing the elimination from the body of various poisons.

Overview

The reason for evaluating patients with elevated haemoglobin levels (male greater than 185 g/L, female greater than 165 g/L) is first to ascertain the presence or absence of polycythaemia vera, and subsequently to differentiate between the various causes of secondary erythrocytosis.

Causes

1) Polycythaemia vera – low or normal erythropoietin

2) Secondary erythrocytosis – elevated erythropoietin

   a) Hypoxaemia
- ❏ Pulmonary (sleep-apnoea, chronic obstructive pulmonary disease (COPD), pulmonary hypertension)
- ❏ Eisenmenger syndrome

   b) Abnormal haemoglobin function

   c) Erythropoietin – secreting tumour (hepatocellular, renal cell, ovarian)

   d) Other (polycystic kidney, post-transplant, hydronephrosis, androgens)

3) Relative polycythaemia (decreased plasma volume: e.g. burns, diarrhoea)

4) Inapparent polycythaemia (increased plasma volume: e.g. renal failure)

Key Objective
- Discuss whether the determination of red cell mass is necessary for the diagnosis of polycythaemia or whether measurements of haemoglobin levels convey the same information.

General/Specific Objectives
- Through efficient, focused data gathering:
  - Determine whether the patient has any other polycythaemia-related features.
  - Differentiate between causes of secondary erythrocytosis in patients without polycythaemia-related features.

- Interpret critical clinical and laboratory findings which were key in the processes of exclusion, differentiation, and diagnosis:

  - List indications for bone marrow biopsy.

  - Contrast the interpretation of low or normal erythropoietin levels to elevated levels in a patient with polycythaemia.

  - Contrast arterial oxygen saturation in primary and secondary polycythaemia.

- Conduct an effective plan of management for a patient with polycythaemia:

  - Select patients in need of further investigation and referral for specialised care.

081A Antepartum Care

Overview

The purpose of antepartum care is to help achieve as good a maternal and infant outcome as possible.

Aspects for Consideration in Antepartum Care

1)	**Pre-conception (counsel, if possible, about pregnancy and perform baseline investigations which may require action prior to pregnancy – rubella immunity, full blood examination (FBE), Papanicolaou (Pap) smear). Advise about folic acid ingestion**

2)	**Initial presentation**

3)	**First trimester / Second trimester / Third trimester**

4)	**Pre-labour (counsel for preparation of labour, and when to present to hospital)**

Key Objectives

- Determine whether the patient is pregnant and the most likely date of conception for the purpose of estimating the date of confinement; develop an appropriate relationship and rapport with prenatal patients.

- List physical findings associated with a normal first trimester pregnancy, including vital signs, skin changes, breast changes, and uterine changes.

General/Specific Objectives

- Through efficient, focused data gathering:

  - Elicit factors which might alter the expected date of conception, or might influence the course of the pregnancy (e.g. maternal age); determine uterine size in terms of weeks of gestation.

  - In the first trimester, determine whether pregnancy is progressing satisfactorily (normal pregnancy symptoms), or complications are present (hyperemesis, miscarriage, ectopic).

  - In the second trimester, determine whether pre-term labour may be present, any bleeding, or urinary symptoms, and determine maternal blood pressure (BP) and fetal heart rate.

  - In the third trimester, determine the presence of fetal movements or their decrease, and measure BP, maternal weight gain, and determine fetal lie and presentation.

  - Diagnose onset of labour.

- Interpret critical clinical and laboratory findings which were key in the processes of exclusion, differentiation, and diagnosis:

  - Discuss current recommendations for ultrasound screening in normal pregnancy, in second trimester, and list first trimester complications for which ultrasound is indicated.

  - Discuss recommendations for routine testing at the first antenatal visit (if not done pre-pregnancy) screening for Group B streptococcus, diabetes, bacterial vaginosis, and maternal serum screening in second trimester, proteinuria and glycosuria in third trimester.

  - List investigations for a patient with Rh-negative blood type and list indications for anti-D globulin; list indications for amniocentesis.

- Conduct an effective plan of management for a patient who is pregnant:

  - Outline nutrition management in normal pregnancy including recommendations for iron and folic acid.

  - List potential complications associated with smoking, alcohol in pregnancy (maternal and neonatal).

  - Counsel patient on medications which are safe and unsafe during pregnancy, physical and sexual activity, travel, vaccines and breastfeeding.

  - Outline management of urinary tract infections (UTIs) in pregnancy, nausea and vomiting, and constipation.

  - Outline initial management of a woman with symphyseal fundal height measurement significantly larger or smaller than expected.

  - Outline initial management of BP elevation, of bleeding in first, second, or third trimester.

  - Outline initial management if fetal movements decline.

  - Outline initial management of post-date pregnancy.

  - Outline initial management of diabetes in pregnancy.

  - Counsel patients regarding breastfeeding.

  - Counsel patients regarding maternal serum screening.

  - Outline the components of the Bishop score, and the relevance of the score in clinical practice.

  - Select patients in need of specialised care because of maternal or fetal problems.

081B Intrapartum/Postpartum Care

Overview

Intrapartum and postpartum care means the care of the mother and fetus during labour and the six-week period following birth during which the reproductive tract returns to its normal nonpregnant state. Of pregnant women, 85% will undergo spontaneous labour between 37 and 42 weeks of gestation. Labour is the process by which products of conception are delivered from the uterus by progressive cervical effacement and dilatation in the presence of regular uterine contractions.

Aspects for Consideration in Intrapartum/Postpartum Care

1) **Normal labour**

2) **Abnormal labour**

3) **Fetal surveillance**

4) **Postpartum care**

   a) **Normal puerperium**

   b) **Abnormal puerperium**
      - ❏ Fever
      - ❏ Pain
      - ❏ Haemorrhage

Key Objective

- Determine whether the patient is in labour, rupture of membranes is present, and determine her risk score.

General/Specific Objectives

- Through efficient, focused data gathering:

   - Determine the fetal presentation, lie, position, station, and presence of engagement.

   - Determine whether labour is in the latent or active phase, and state the approximate duration of each, as well as the duration of the second stage of labour, expected rate of cervical dilatation.

   - Determine whether physical findings are present which necessitate increased levels of maternal or fetal monitoring.

   - List maternal and fetal signs to be monitored; discuss indications and frequency for pelvic examination in the first and second stages of labour.

   - Diagnose prolonged, protracted, or arrested stages of labour, and factors in mother's history predisposing to them.

- Diagnose cause of abnormal labour in terms of uterine contraction, fetus, and passage.

- Determine whether the course of the puerperium is normal or abnormal physically and emotionally.

- Differentiate between causes of postpartum fever. Include genital tract infection, episiotomy or wound infection, urinary tract infection (UTI), breast infection, breast engorgement, intercurrent or viral infection, deep venous thrombosis (DVT) and/or pulmonary embolus.

- Determine cause of postpartum haemorrhage (uterine, cervical, vaginal, perineal, disseminated intra-vascular coagulation (DIC)).

- Interpret critical clinical and laboratory findings which were key in the processes of exclusion, differentiation, and diagnosis:

  - Order routine tests for a woman presenting to the labour and delivery ward.

  - List indications for fetal and uterine contractions monitoring and discuss significance of meconium in amniotic fluid.

  - Postpartum, in an Rh-negative woman, order maternal and neonatal blood to determine need for Rh immunoglobulin.

- Conduct an effective plan of management for a patient in labour and postpartum:

  - Counsel patient in labour about need for examination, reasons for examination, and permission to go ahead.

  - Describe mechanism of delivery for a fetus; define shoulder dystocia and list risk factors for this complication.

  - Describe signs of placental separation and normal duration of third stage of labour; describe the options for management of the third stage of labour; list components of Apgar score.

  - Discuss techniques for pain relief in labour; list indications for and complication of episiotomy; list the indications for and the complications of epidural analgesia/anaesthesia.

  - List risk factors for Group B streptococcal disease in the neonate and discuss use of prophylactic penicillin in labour.

  - List indications and contraindications of active management of third stage of labour with intravenous (IV) or intramuscular (IM) oxytocics.

  - Outline initial management of primary and secondary postpartum haemorrhage.

  - List methods to augment labour; list indications/complications of Caesarean section, forceps, or vacuum extraction.

  - Outline management of puerperal pain, dyspareunia, bladder and bowel dysfunction and depression.

  - Outline management of fever postpartum.

  - Select patients in need of specialised care.

081C Haemorrhage

(See #117 Vaginal Bleeding, Excessive in Amount or Irregular in Timing)

081D Obstetrical Complications

Overview

Virtually any maternal medical or surgical condition can complicate the course of a pregnancy and/or be affected by pregnancy. In addition, conditions arising in pregnancy can have adverse effects on the mother and/or the fetus (e.g. babies born prematurely account for greater than 50% of perinatal morbidity and mortality; an estimated 5% of women will describe bleeding of some extent during pregnancy, and in some patients, the bleeding will endanger the mother's survival).

Causes

1) Pre-existing maternal conditions

a) **Hypertension**

(see #054B Pregnancy-Associated Hypertension)

b) **Diabetes**

c) **Cardiac disease**

d) **Chronic renal disease**

e) **Thrombosis**

f) **Systemic lupus erythematosus (SLE)**

2) Maternal conditions arising in pregnancy

a) **Pregnancy-induced hypertension**

(see #054B Pregnancy-Associated Hypertension)

b) **Gestational diabetes**

c) **Gestational thrombocytopenia**

d) **Thrombosis**

e) **Viral infections ('TORCH' (_T_oxoplasmosis, _O_ther, _R_ubella, _C_ytomegalovirus, _H_erpes simplex virus), rubella, varicella, HIV)**

3) Fetal conditions arising in pregnancy

a) **Large for gestational age (twins)**

b) **Small for gestational age**

c) **Structural abnormality of fetus**

d) **Alloimmune disease (Rh isoimmunisation)**

a) **Antepartum haemorrhage**

(see #117 Vaginal Bleeding, Excessive in Amount or Irregular in Timing)

b) **Preterm labour**

c) **Preterm premature rupture of membranes**

d) **Polyhydramnios/Oligohydramnios**

Key Objective

- Determine the risk factors that increase chances of complication during the pregnancy at the initial visit for prenatal care.

General/Specific Objectives

- Through efficient, focused data gathering:

  - Elicit history of pre-existing maternal medical conditions, history of maternal or fetal problems in previous pregnancies, or any other complication inherent to pregnancy.

  - Elicit family history, history of nutrition, alcohol, smoking, obesity, drug use including recreational drugs, maternal age, viral infections, previous fetal structural or immune abnormalities, bleeding, leakage of fluid.

  - Perform physical examination of mother, uterine height, amount of amniotic fluid, and other fetal parameters.

- Interpret critical clinical and laboratory findings which were key in the processes of exclusion, differentiation, and diagnosis:

  - Select and order ultrasound and list ultrasound parameters of the biophysical profile (amniotic fluid, fetal movement, fetal tone, fetal breathing).

  - List indications for amniocentesis.

  - List investigations for specific maternal conditions including maternal blood type and antibody screen.

- Conduct an effective plan of management for a patient with obstetrical complications:

  - Outline preventive / 'improving outcome of pregnancy' programme (e.g. smoking cessation, folic acid, betamethasone to mother when preterm delivery imminent, screen for gestational diabetes, Rh immunoglobin to Rh-negative women).

  - Outline immediate management of preterm labour and premature rupture of membranes; diabetes.

  - Select patients in need of specialised care.

Overview

Ideally, the prevention of an unwanted pregnancy should be directed at education of patients, male and female, preferably before first sexual contact. Counselling patients about which method to use, how, and when is a must for anyone involved in healthcare. Counselling should also address prevention of sexually transmitted diseases (STDs).

Causes

1) Non-permanent

   a) Hormonal contraception (oral, injectable, morning after pill)

   b) Barrier methods (diaphragm, cap, condom)

   c) Intra-uterine devices

   d) Other (abstinence, breastfeeding, withdrawal, rhythm method, ovulation method)

2) Permanent contraception

   a) Sterilisation (male, female)

3) Termination

Key Objectives

- Determine whether there are any absolute or relative contraindications to the use of hormonal contraceptives.

- If permanent contraception is being contemplated, determine the level of determination and commitment to proceed, level of understanding of options, and surgical or medical risks.

- If faced with an unplanned pregnancy, discuss the alternatives for management.

General/Specific Objectives

- Through efficient, focused data gathering:

  - Elicit obstetric and gynaecologic history and determine risk factors for hormonal use.

  - Perform pelvic examination and exclude the presence of pregnancy if appropriate.

- Interpret critical clinical and laboratory findings which were key in the processes of exclusion, differentiation, and diagnosis:

  - Order appropriate cultures, Papanicolaou (Pap) smear, and pregnancy test if indicated.

- Order ultrasound to determine gestational age in a pregnant woman, and recognise the accuracy is best the earlier the ultrasound examination is done.

- Conduct an effective plan of management for a patient requesting contraception, pregnancy prevention or termination:

  - Outline methods of contraception, risks of failure, complications, and drug interactions.

  - Counsel patient about side-effects, adjustments if pill is missed, or need to add barrier techniques.

  - Counsel patient on benefit of barrier contraception in conjunction with hormonal contraception in reducing HIV transmission and STDs.

  - Counsel patient about failure rates of sterilisation, the importance of family being perceived complete, and complications of various approaches.

  - Counsel patient about the complications of pregnancy termination including potential guilt/emotional concerns, the effect of subsequent fertility and subsequent pregnancy outcome.

  - Select patients in need of specialised care.

  - Present contraceptive and termination alternatives while respecting the individual's own moral, ethical and religious beliefs.

  - Understand the legal position in regard to pregnancy termination, at varying gestations, in Australia.

Overview

The impact of premature birth is best summarised by the fact that although less than 10% of babies are born prematurely (less than 37 weeks gestation), these births account for greater than 50% of all perinatal morbidity and mortality. Most morbidity and mortality is due to delivery at less than 28 weeks gestation. Overall, the outcome, although guarded, can be rewarding given optimal circumstances and care.

Causes

Premature delivery can occur after spontaneous labour or when labour is induced prematurely because of maternal, placental or fetal problems. In many instances the cause of the spontaneous premature labour is unknown.

1) Fetal

   a) Multiple gestation

   b) Erythroblastosis and nonimmune hydrops

   c) Congenital anomalies

2) Placental

   a) Placenta praevia

   b) Placental abruption

3) Uterine

   a) Incompetent cervix

   b) Excessive enlargement (hydramnios)

   c) Distortion (leiomyomas, septate)

4) Maternal

   a) Preeclampsia

   b) Premature rupture of membranes

   c) Smoking, substance abuse

   d) Chronic medical illnesses

   e) Infections (urinary, cervical, amniotic) – Group B streptococcus, herpes, 'TORCH' (Toxoplasmosis, Other, Rubella, Cytomegalovirus, Herpes simplex virus), etc.

5) Iatrogenic (indicated induction of labour)

Key Objectives

- Contrast low birth weight (intra-uterine growth restriction) and prematurity.

- Identify risk factors for probable prematurity and initiate immediate and appropriate care of a premature baby.

General/Specific Objectives

- Through efficient, focused data gathering:

  - List the immediate and long term health problems faced by premature infants.

- Interpret critical clinical and laboratory findings which were key in the processes of exclusion, differentiation and diagnosis:

  - Investigate the maternal and fetal factors which may precipitate a premature birth.

- Conduct an effective plan of management for a premature baby:

  - Resuscitate and manage the health problems encountered by premature infants.

  - Outline the nutritional requirements of premature infants.

  - Select patients in need of referral and/or specialised care for premature infants.

  - Plan the care of a premature baby, born at 28 weeks of gestation, whilst awaiting transfer to a tertiary care facility 200 km away.

  - Care of a baby with respiratory distress syndrome in the newborn period.

  - Counsel parents about immediate and long term health problems encountered by premature infants.

  - Co-ordinate healthcare facilities for the short and long term care of premature infants.

- Conduct an effective plan of management for a patient in premature labour at varying gestations:

  - Use of drugs to inhibit uterine contractions.

  - Use of corticosteroid and other drugs to improve pulmonary maturity.

  - Mode of delivery.

(See also #115B Urinary Incontinence, Elderly)

Overview

Patients with pelvic relaxation present in many different and often subtle ways. In order to identify patients who would benefit from therapy, the clinician should be familiar with the types of pelvic relaxation and the approach to the patient with symptoms suggestive of this problem.

Causes

1)	**Uterine prolapse**
2)	**Vaginal vault prolapse**
3)	**Cystocele**
4)	**Rectocele**
5)	**Enterocele**

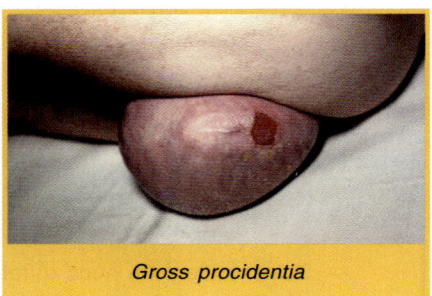

Gross procidentia

Key Objective

- Describe the progression of genital prolapse from grade one to procidentia, including the impact of chronic straining and hormone replacement therapy (HRT); explain to the patient the development and progression of urinary tract or gastrointestinal symptoms.

General/Specific Objectives

- Through efficient, focused data gathering:

    - Determine the severity of symptoms, effect on activity, predisposing factors (particularly after the menopause), and risk factors for surgery.

    - Differentiate between different types of pelvic relaxation according to associated difficulties (e.g. voiding, stress incontinence, defaecating).

    - Determine structure which is prolapsing on physical examination.

- Interpret critical clinical and laboratory findings which were key in the processes of exclusion, differentiation, and diagnosis:

    - State that there are no specific tests for the assessment of prolapse.

- Conduct an effective plan of management for a patient with pelvic relaxation or prolapse:

    - Counsel the patient on benefit and risks of no intervention, conservative measures including pelvic floor exercises and other physiotherapy, and surgery.

    - Select patients requiring referral for specialised care.

085 Proteinuria

Overview

Proteinuria is identified by positive dipstick on urinalysis during routine screening for insurance and other examinations, when examining patients with symptoms related to the urinary tract, or when following the progress of patients with secondary causes. Persistent proteinuria implies abnormal glomerular function and always requires further investigation.

Causes

1)	**Transient proteinuria**

2)	**Orthostatic proteinuria**

3)	**Persistent proteinuria**

    a) **Overflow**

    b) **Tubulointerstitial**

    c) **Glomerular (including nephrotic syndrome)**
- ❏ Primary
  - Minimal change disease
  - Focal segmental glomerulosclerosis (FSGS)
  - Membranous glomerulonephropathy
- ❏ Secondary
  - Diabetes mellitus
  - Secondary FSGS
  - Collagen diseases

Key Objective
- Differentiate between benign causes of proteinuria and proteinuria resulting from transient or permanent glomerular damage requiring specialist assessment.

General/Specific Objectives
- Through efficient, focused data gathering:
  - Exclude transient and orthostatic proteinuria; reassure patients about benign nature of conditions.
  - Differentiate between overflow and tubulointerstitial proteinuria, and glomerular proteinuria.
  - Diagnose common primary or secondary glomerular diseases.
- Interpret critical clinical and laboratory findings which were key in the processes of exclusion, differentiation, and diagnosis.

- Conduct an effective plan of management for a proteinuric patient:
  - State referral indications for a patient with proteinuria.
  - Formulate the most appropriate management to prevent or delay progression to chronic renal failure in patients with primary glomerular diseases.
  - Formulate the most appropriate management to prevent or delay diabetic nephropathy in patients with Type I or Type II diabetes mellitus.
  - Interpret and contrast the prognostic significance and possible clinical sequelae of light and heavy proteinuria.

Overview

Pruritus accompanies many skin disorders. In the allergic group pruritus is the predominant symptom. In the absence of a primary skin lesion pruritus can be indicative of systemic disease or psychological or emotional disorder.

Causes

1) Skin Lesions

a) **Primary skin disease**

- ❏ Skin blisters (papular/vesicular)
  - • Dermatitis herpetiformis
  - • Bullous pemphigoid
- ❏ Skin rash (papulosquamous)
  - • Mycosis fungoides
  - • Psoriasis
  - • Lichen planus

b) **Parasitosis (scabies, pediculosis)**

c) **Allergy (atopic dermatitis/eczema, urticaria, allergic dermatitis)**

d) **Arthropod bites**

e) **Factitious dermatitis**

2) No skin lesions

a) **Senile pruritus**

b) **Drugs/Foods**

c) **Obstructive biliary disease**

d) **Uraemia / Renal failure**

e) **Haematological**

- ❏ Polycythaemia vera / Microcytic anaemia
- ❏ Leukaemia
- ❏ Lymphoma

f) **Carcinoma / Carcinoid syndrome**

g) **Endocrine (diabetes, thyroid disease)**

3) Psychiatric, psychological and emotional disorders

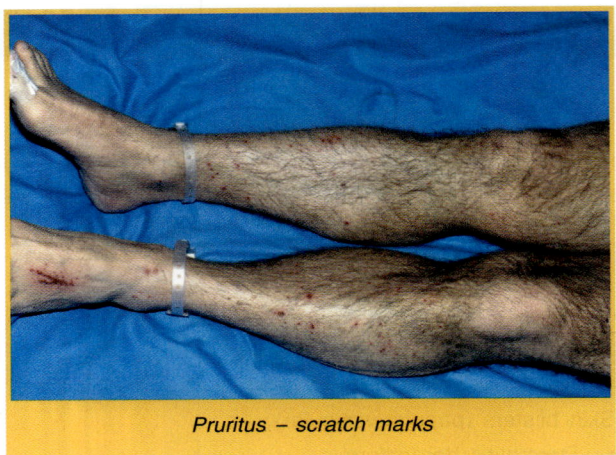

Pruritus – scratch marks

Key Objectives

- Identify the skin disorder causing pruritus.

- In the absence of primary skin lesions identify the underlying cause of the pruritus.

General/Specific Objectives

- Through efficient, focused data gathering:

  - Categorise primary skin lesions associated with pruritus.

  - In the absence of skin lesions, select investigations to diagnose systemic disorders.

- Conduct an effective plan of management for a patient with pruritus:

  - Outline local and other therapy for pruritus.

  - Treat underlying systemic disease if identified.

  - Select patients in need of specialised care.

086A   Pruritus Ani

Overview

Anal pruritus can be associated with defective local hygiene, generalised skin conditions, or local anal conditions. Pruritus vulvae may coexist.

Causes

1)	**Defaecatory habits, poor or excessive hygiene**

2)	**Localised anorectal conditions (skin tags, anal condylomas/ warts, fistulae, haemorrhoids, threadworms)**

3)	**Generalised skin or systemic disorders**

Key Objective

- Conduct a detailed history and local examination to identify likely causes.

General/Specific Objectives

- Through efficient, focused data gathering:

    - Identify likely general causal factors (diabetes mellitus, general skin disorders).

    - Perform full anorectal examination for local causes.

    - Detect yeasts, fungi, parasites from stool examination, skin scraping, microscopy.

- Outline a management plan based on appropriate local hygiene.

Overview

Psychosis refers to a group of severe mental disorders characterised by morbid, false beliefs (delusions), disturbances in sensory perception (hallucinations), disorganised speech patterns (thought disorder) and grossly disorganised or catatonic behaviour. There may be impaired or absent insight into the pathological nature of symptoms, affective flattening, apathy and lack of drive, and cognitive and conceptual impairments. Schizophrenia is both the most common and the classic psychotic disorder, but psychotic symptoms in isolation can occur in a range of other syndromes. There are about 200,000 people with schizophrenia in Australia. The illness typically begins in adolescence or early adult life and is associated with prolonged disability, stigma, under-employment and discrimination. Depending on the severity, schizophrenia may significantly affect the patient's social, occupational and interpersonal functioning.

Causes

1)	**Schizophrenia (and subtypes)**
2)	**Schizophreniform disorder (duration of illness less than six months)**
3)	**Schizoaffective disorders (concurrent mood disorder and psychosis)**
4)	**Delusional disorder (grandiose, persecutory, erotomanic, jealous, somatic)**
5)	**Brief psychotic disorder (duration less than four weeks)**
6)	**Psychotic disorder due to a general medical condition**
7)	**Substance-induced psychotic disorder – intoxication or withdrawal from**

   a) Alcohol

   b) Amphetamines

   c) Cannabis

   d) Cocaine

   e) Hallucinogens

   f) Inhalants

   g) Opioids

   h) Psychotropics

8)	**Shared psychotic disorder**

9) Other

Key Objective
- Differentiate patients with psychotic symptoms who have insight and are aware of their symptoms, from those who have no insight and are of concern to others.

General/Specific Objectives
- Through efficient, focused data gathering:

  - Establish a collaborative relationship with the patient.

  - Determine the extent of the psychotic symptoms, including the history of onset, progression and duration and any associated mood symptoms.

  - Determine any relationship between the psychotic symptoms and medical illness, alcohol and non-prescribed drugs or medication.

  - Assess personality and social strengths and current level of functioning.

  - Perform a mental status examination including risk of harm to self and others.

  - Perform baseline screening investigations and physical examination.

  - Refer for appropriate educational/social/vocational assessments.

- Interpret critical clinical and laboratory findings which were key in the processes of exclusion, differentiation, and diagnosis.

- Establish an effective plan of management for a patient with psychosis:

  - Outline modern management principles, including atypical antipsychotics, psychological and psychosocial therapies and the role of hospitalisation.

  - Tactfully counsel and educate patients and carers/family about the nature and natural history of the psychosis.

  - Provide ongoing support to carers and family and advocacy for patients and advise on support groups.

  - Select patients in need of specialised referral or rehabilitation.

Overview

Pupils should be black, round, equal and reactive to light and accommodation. The pupils dilate in dark surroundings and constrict in bright light, the size depending on a balance between parasympathetic and sympathetic innervation. Pupil size is influenced by local mydriatics or the effects of drugs. Any non-black area in the pupil implies media opacification in the anterior chamber, lens or vitreous. Abnormal pupillary reactivity and size after trauma may be important clues to intracranial pathology in the setting of head injuries; and pupillary abnormalities may be associated with a variety of neurological disorders.

Causes

1)   Local disorder of iris

2)   Inequality of pupil size (anisocoria)

    a) Impaired pupil constriction (third nerve palsy, tonic pupil, mydriatics)

    b) Impaired pupil dilatation (Horner syndrome)
- First order (hypothalamus, brain stem, spinal cord lesions)
- Second order / Preganglionic lesions
- Third order / Postganglionic lesions

3)   Impairment of pupil constriction (without anisocoria)

    a) Unilateral (optic nerve or retinal lesion)

    b) Bilateral (diabetes, syphilis, midbrain lesion, hydrocephalus, factitious)

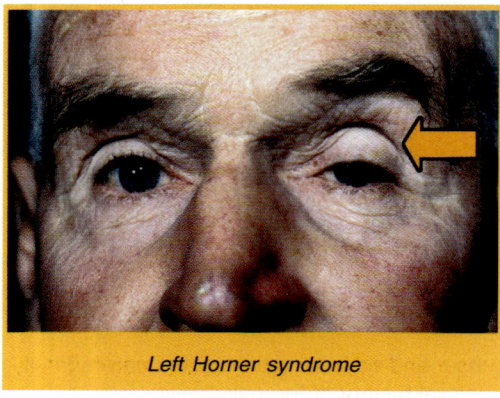

Left Horner syndrome

Key Objectives

- Determine whether there has been previous ocular inflammation, trauma, loss of vision, or eye pain in order to begin ruling out local disorders.

- Understand and interpret changes in pupillary appearance, size and reactivity.

- Select patients in need of urgent referral.

General/Specific Objectives

- Through efficient, focused data gathering:

  - Differentiate clinically between the various mechanisms of pupil abnormalities.

- Interpret critical clinical and laboratory findings which were key in the processes of exclusion, differentiation, and diagnosis:

  - Select patients in need of referral for further investigation.

- Conduct an effective plan of management for a patient with pupil abnormalities:

  - Select patients in need of referral for management.

089A Chronic Musculofascial Pain

Overview

'**Fibromyalgia**' (fibrositis, myofascial pain syndrome) is a very common but poorly defined condition of unknown aetiology associated with chronic pain affecting muscles and soft tissues such as tendons and ligaments. Symptoms include diffuse muscle pains and aches, stiffness, fatigue, sleep disturbance and focal points of tenderness without other abnormalities on physical examination, laboratory, or radiological studies. Concomitant anxiety and depression are common. The condition is more common in women.

Polymyalgia rheumatica is a rheumatic condition that is frequently linked to giant cell (temporal) arteritis. Polymyalgia rheumatica is a relatively common disorder, with a prevalence of about 700 out of 100,000 persons over 50 years of age. Synovitis is considered to be the cause of the discomfort. The erythrocyte sedimentation rate (ESR) is markedly raised in most patients.

Causes

1)	'**Fibromyalgia**'

2)	**Polymyalgia rheumatica**

3)	**Polymyositis/Dermatomyositis**

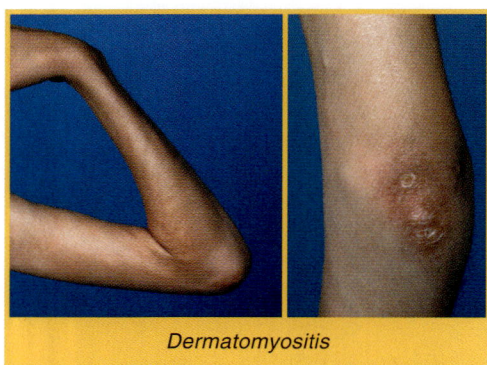

Dermatomyositis

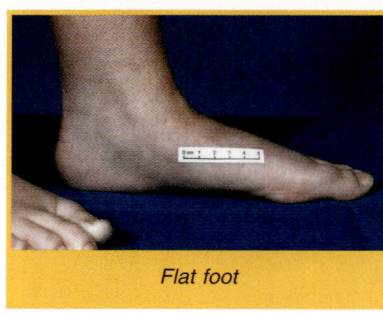

Flat foot

4)	Shoulder pain (rotator cuff injury, capsulitis, bursitis, tendinitis)

5)	Hand/Wrist pain (carpal tunnel, fracture/dislocation, tendinitis)

6)	Foot pain (flat feet, hallux valgus, metatarsalgia, neuroma, fasciitis, stress fracture, tendinitis, apophysitis)

7)	Knee pain (meniscal injury, cruciate/collateral ligament injury, patellofemoral disease)

8)	Nerve entrapments / Neuropathies

Key Objectives

- Differentiate between articular and non-articular pain.
- Differentiate between 'fibromyalgia' and polymyalgia rheumatica.

General/Specific Objectives

- Through efficient, focused data gathering:

  - Diagnose 'fibromyalgia', especially in women, from history and associated features, especially tender point examination of selected anatomic locations.

  - Diagnose polymyalgia rheumatica in patients 50 years or older with bilateral morning stiffness and aching (more than 30 minutes) for at least one month in neck or torso, shoulders or proximal arms and hips or proximal thighs, and an elevated ESR.

  - Differentiate local from referred pain, acute from chronic, muscle from nerve pain, etc.

- Interpret critical clinical and laboratory findings which were key in the processes of exclusion, differentiation, and diagnosis:

  - State that laboratory tests in patients with 'fibromyalgia' are normal, and in polymyalgia rheumatica only the sedimentation rate is usually elevated.

  - List indications for electromyelography (EMG).

- Conduct an effective plan of management for a patient with regional pain:

  - Outline management of 'fibromyalgia' including exercise, education, medication, and supportive psychosocial measures.

  - Describe complications of corticosteroids and nonsteroid anti-inflammatory agents.

  - List indication and contraindications in management of non-articular conditions of: rest, physiotherapy, anti-inflammatory medication, local corticosteroid injection, and surgery.

  - Select patients in need of specialised care.

089B Low Back Pain

Overview

Low back pain is an extremely common complaint. Most people experience at least one episode of acute low back strain at some period. Short-lived back pain of mechanical origin is not associated with a clearly definable aetiology. Most low back pain is of benign aetiology, with spontaneous recovery over the course of days or weeks. Imaging and other investigations are unnecessary and unlikely to be helpful. Concerning features, indicating the need for further investigation, include an insidious onset, a neurologic deficit, unremitting severe pain, evidence of systemic illness and a relevant medical history. Associated loss of bladder or bowel control indicates a potential surgical emergency. Low back pain remains a major cause of lost work time. In many patients with persisting and chronic back pain a precise pathological diagnosis is not possible. Chronic occupationally-related and litigation-linked low back pain may be associated with unconscious or conscious exaggeration of symptoms in the absence of demonstrative organic disease and with the presence of non-objective physical signs indicating abnormal illness behaviour.

Causes

1)	**Acute musculoligamentous lumbo-sacral strain – self resolving**

2)	**Chronic, persistent or recurrent low back pain**

a) **Mechanical**

   ❏ Age-related and degenerative spondylosis

      • Disc disease and prolapse, osteoarthritis of facet joints

      • Spondylolysis, spondylolisthesis, spinal canal stenosis

   ❏ Metabolic (osteoporosis)

   ❏ Neoplasms (myeloma, metastasis)

   ❏ Spinal infections (tuberculosis (TB), osteomyelitis)

   ❏ Inflammatory (seronegative spondyloarthropathy)

      • Ankylosing spondylitis

      • Reiter syndrome / Reactive arthritis

      • Enteropathic arthritis

      • Psoriatic arthritis

b) **Referred pain (renal, pancreatic, vascular aneurysm, retroperitoneal blood, gynaecologic, etc.)**

Key Objectives
- Perform an appropriately focused and accurate examination of back and spine.
- Recognise the rare serious causes of low back pain by being alert to warning flags in history and examination.

- Through efficient, focused data gathering:

    - Determine whether inciting event exists, pain location, radiation, and effect of back or leg motion.

    - Perform examination of the back and proximate anatomic areas that could lead to back pain.

    - Identify patients with neurologic defect.

    - Determine whether there is loss of sphincter tone or urinary retention, and state that the presence of such signs represent a surgical emergency.

- Interpret critical clinical and laboratory findings which were key in the processes of exclusion, differentiation, and diagnosis:

    - Outline management of acute back pain without neurologic or other abnormality on examination.

    - Outline clinical features and management plans in a patient with low back pain with nerve root impingement.

    - Select patients in need of specialised care.

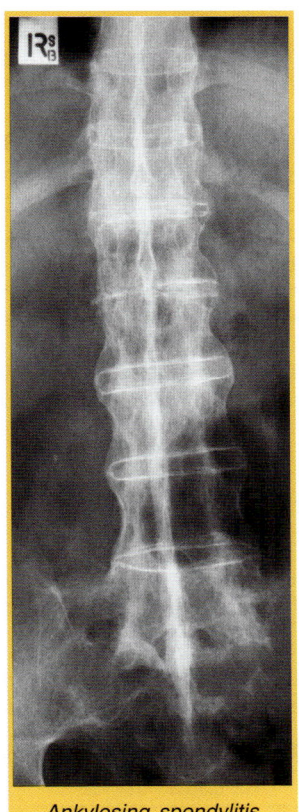

Ankylosing spondylitis

089C Neck Pain

Overview

Attacks of transient acute neck pain and stiffness are very common, the incidence increasing with age. Prolonged neck pain and stiffness are important sequelae to whiplash-associated motor vehicle collisions. Specific nerve root deficiencies are rarely found. Continuing chronic disabilities and impairments are often associated with compensation claims and secondary psychological problems.

Causes

1) Intrinsic disease

- a) Muscle spasm (awkward posture, certain occupations – assemblyline workers, violinists)

- b) Disc degeneration/herniation (with neural impingement, C6–C7 most commonly)

- c) Osteoarthritis / Cervical spondylosis

- d) Tumours

- e) Other (whiplash, myofascial pain syndromes, diffuse idiopathic skeletal hyperostosis, congenital spinal stenosis)

2) Systemic disease (rheumatoid arthritis (RA), ankylosing spondylitis, polymyalgia rheumatica, bone metastases)

3) Referred (from shoulder, angina pectoris, meningitis, diaphragm, or teeth and jaw pathology)

Key Objectives

- Determine whether the pain is caused by conditions that are intrinsic to the cervical spine or its musculature, by systemic conditions or by referred pain from elsewhere.

General/Specific Objectives

- Through efficient, focused data gathering:

  - Elicit a history including age, occupation, trauma, radiation of pain (if not correlated with neuro-anatomic pathways, consider myofascial pain or 'fibromyalgia').

  - Determine whether pain is nerve root, and which root, or whether the condition is central disc herniation with bilateral long tract signs.

  - Determine muscle and sensory function, tendon reflexes, neck mobility, trigger points.

- Interpret critical clinical and laboratory findings which were key in the processes of exclusion, differentiation, and diagnosis:

  - State that imaging (computed tomography (CT), magnetic resonance imaging (MRI)) may demonstrate significant lesions in asymptomatic patients.

  - Select diagnostic imaging when indicated.

  - List indications for electromyelography (EMG).

- Conduct an effective plan of management for a patient with cervical pain:

  - Outline conservative medical management for degenerative disc disease (posture modification, cervical collar, physical therapy, local pain relief, drugs, trigger point injections, etc.).

  - Select patients in need of specialised care.

089D Facial Pain

Overview
Facial pain can be separate from or can overlap with headache. Pain in the face itself has a miscellany of causes from local disorders. Referred pain from intracranial, cardiac and other causes needs to be excluded; the keys to accurate diagnosis are a careful history and physical examination aimed at recognising urgent causes and those requiring additional investigation.

Causes

1) **Dental pain (caries, third molar impaction, root abscess, etc.)**

2) **Sinuses (maxillary, frontal and ethmoid sinusitis)**

3) **Eye problems (glaucoma, iritis)**

4) **Temporomandibular joint (TMJ) dysfunction**

5) **Nasopharyngeal and oesophageal causes (inflammations, foreign body, neoplasms)**

6) **Migraine variants (facial migraine, cluster headaches)**

7) **Salivary gland disorders (sialitis, stone, neoplasm)**

8) **Trigeminal neuralgia ('tic douloureux')**

9) **Referred pain from extrafacial (intracranial, cardiac) causes**

Key Objectives
- Differentiate causes by careful history-taking and examination.
- Recognise referred pain from extrafacial causes.

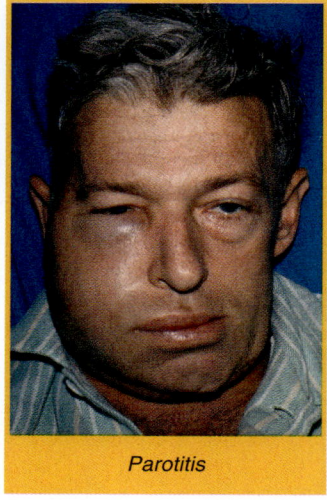

Parotitis

089E Shoulder Pain

(See also #071A Pain in the Upper Extremities)

Overview
Shoulder pain is commonly associated with painful limitation of arm movement, which aids identification of pain due to intrinsic shoulder disease from that referred from neck, diaphragm and mediastinum. Osteoarthritis of the glenohumeral joint is uncommon and in most instances the pain is due to rotator cuff problems, bursitis and acromioclavicular arthritis. The mobility of the joints associated with shoulder movements renders them liable to dislocation and recurrent dislocation, especially from sporting injuries.

Causes

1)	**Rotator cuff lesions / Subacromial bursitis**

2)	**Adhesive capsulitis ('frozen shoulder')**

3)	**Bicipital tendinitis/tear**

4)	**Acromioclavicular arthritis**

5)	**Referred pain**

  a) Ischaemic cardiac disease / Pericarditis

  b) Cervical spondylosis

  c) Gallbladder / Diaphragm

  d) Pancoast tumour

Key Objectives
* Diagnose most likely cause from history and examination.
* Exclude extrinsic causes of shoulder pain.
* Recognise requirements for investigation and specialised care.

089F Hand/Wrist/Elbow Pain

Overview

Pain in the upper limb involving hand, wrist or elbow is a common symptom, usually definable by careful history and examination into well-defined causes, and responding well to treatment. A smaller subgroup of predominantly functional illness linked with repetitive strain, of poorly defined aetiology and often associated with work-related compensation claims, is more difficult to treat.

Causes

1) Nerve entrapment/impingement syndromes

    a) Carpal tunnel (median nerve at wrist)

    b) Ulnar neuritis (cubitus valgus, Guyon canal, 'ulnar hammer' syndrome)

    c) Cervical spondylosis / Disc prolapse with nerve root radiculopathy

    d) Thoracic outlet syndrome with nerve root radiculopathy

2) Stenosing tenosynovitis

    a) de Quervain tenosynovitis

    b) Trigger finger

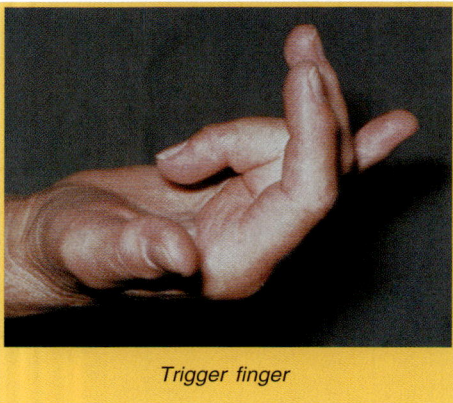

Trigger finger

3) Musculotendinous strain injuries

    a) Lateral and medical epicondylitis ('tennis elbow', 'golfer elbow')

4) Degenerative

   a) Rheumatoid arthritis (RA) (wrist/hands/fingers)

   b) Osteoarthritis (hands/thumb/fingers)

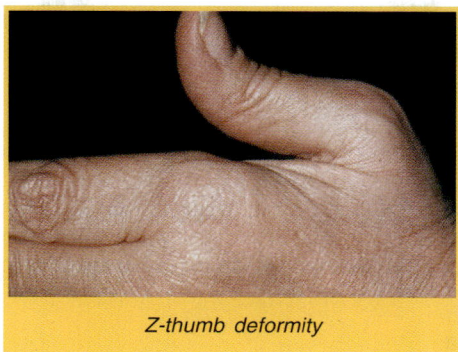

Z-thumb deformity

5) Vascular

   a) Raynaud syndrome, scleroderma

   b) Venous thrombosis (axillary vein thrombosis / effort thrombosis)

   c) Arterial thromboembolism (cervical rib, thoracic outlet syndrome, distal vascular effects)

   d) Lymphoedema

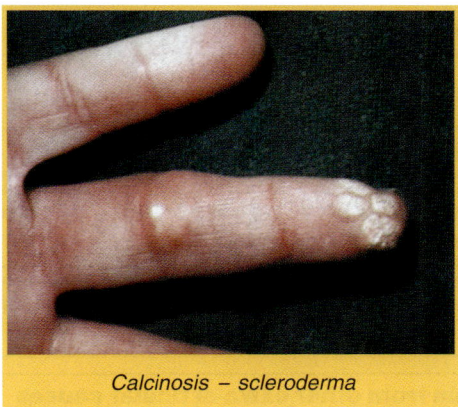

Calcinosis – scleroderma

6) Referred pain (cardiac, lung apex)

7) Reflex sympathetic dystrophy (chronic regional pain syndrome, Sudeck atrophy)

Key Objectives
- Diagnose most likely cause from history and examination.
- Recognise requirements for investigation and specialised care.

089G Hip Pain

(See also #059 Joint Pain, Mono-Articular (Acute, Chronic) and #061 Limp / Pain in Lower Extremity in Children)

Overview

Causes of pain in the hip tend to be age related. In childhood, a variety of potentially severe disorders can benefit from early diagnosis and treatment. In adults osteoarthritis is the most common cause of hip pain. Pain in the region of the hip can also be referred from the lumbar spine and sacro-iliac joints. Ischaemic claudicant muscle pain secondary to aorto-iliac occlusion can be confused with joint pain.

Causes in Children

1)	Developmental dysplasia of hip (DDH, CDH)

2)	Juvenile osteochondritis of femoral head (Legg-Calvé-Perthes disease)

3)	Septic arthritis

4)	Transient synovitis ('irritable hip')

5)	Slipped femoral head epiphysis

Causes in Adults

1)	Osteoarthritis of hip

2)	Osteonecrosis of femoral head (steroids, decompression sickness, previous dislocation)

3)	Musculofascial strain/bursitis ('snapping hip', trochanteric bursitis)

4)	Referred pain from other extra-articular causes

    a) Lumbar disc prolapse

    b) Cutaneous nerve entrapment (meralgia paraesthetica)

    c) Ischaemic aorto-iliac vascular disease

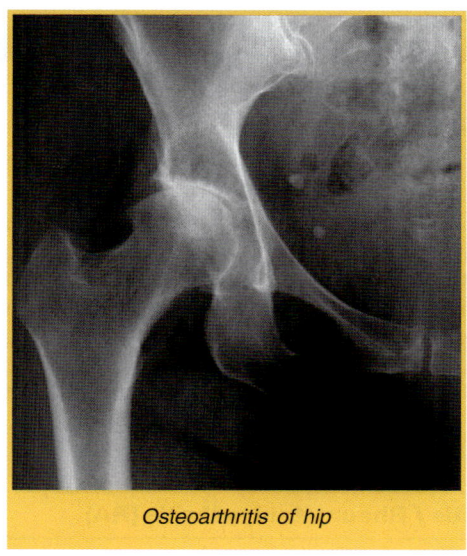

Osteoarthritis of hip

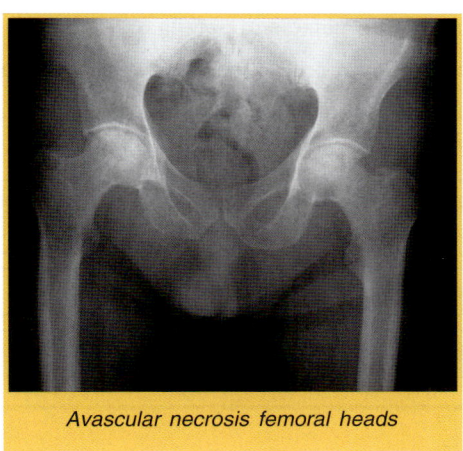

Avascular necrosis femoral heads

Key Objectives

- Diagnose most likely cause from history and examination.
- Recognise requirements for investigation and specialised care.

089H Knee Pain

Overview

The knee is the most complex and extensive of all body joints, and is the area of most active bone growth in childhood. The knee and adjacent long bones are the most common sites for osteomyelitis and primary bone tumours in childhood. The knee is particularly vulnerable to injuries in contact sports such as football; and depends for its stability on strong ligaments and the surrounding muscles, particularly quadriceps femoris. Surrounding bursae are prone to inflammatory complications. Osteoarthritis presents with painful stiffness, the incidence increasing with advancing age.

Causes

1)	**Osteoarthritis / Rheumatoid arthritis (RA)**

2)	**Traumatic derangements**

    a) **Meniscal, and crucial/collateral ligamentous damage**

    b) **Traumatic chondromalacia of patella or condyle**

    c) **Traumatic osteochondritis dissecans / osteonecrosis**

    d) **Traumatic musculoligamentous strains (extensor apparatus injuries, Osgood-Schlatter apophysitis)**

3)	**Bursitis (prepatellar, pretibial, anserine, semimembranosus, Baker cyst)**

4)	**Vascular disease – popliteal aneurysm**

5)	**Referred pain (hip)**

Key Objectives

- Diagnose most likely cause from history and examination.

- Recognise requirements for investigation and specialised care (including arthroscopy).

089I   Foot and Ankle Pain

Overview

Apart from ischaemic pain and proximal neuropathies, which are important to exclude, most causes of chronic foot pain are due to local abnormalities. Chronic foot strain is exacerbated by obesity and improper footware.

Footcare in diabetics to prevent ulcerative neuropathic, ischaemic, and infective complications has a high priority in preventive primary care practice.

Causes

1) Forefoot pain (metatarsalgia)

    a) Anterior flat foot, hallux valgus, bursitis ('bunion')

    b) Claw toe / Hammer toe / Over-riding toe

    c) Plantar digital neuritis/neuroma ('Morton metatarsalgia')

    d) Stress fracture ('march fracture'), metatarsal necks

    e) Plantar warts/callosities

    f) Ischaemic and neuropathic pain (diabetes, atheroma)

2) Heel and ankle pain

    a) Plantar fasciitis

    b) Achilles tendinitis/bursitis/tear

    c) Peroneal tendinitis/dislocation

    d) Tarsal tunnel syndrome

    e) Traumatic osteochondritis/osteonecrosis

        ❑ Calcaneum (Sever)

        ❑ Navicular (Köhler)

        ❑ Metatarsal (Freiberg)

Key Objectives
- Diagnose most likely causes from history and examination.
- Recognise cases needing investigation and specialised care.

089J Spinal Compression / Osteoporosis

Overview

Spinal compression is one manifestation of osteoporosis, the prevalence of which increases with age. As the proportion of our population in old-age rises, osteoporosis becomes an important cause of painful fractures, deformity, loss of mobility and independence, and even death.

Causes

1)	**Type I (oestrogen/testosterone deficiency or menopause – ratio male:female = one:six)**

2)	**Type II (age related – ratio male:female = one:two)**

3)	**Disuse**

a) Lack of weight-bearing activity (inactivity, prolonged bed rest)

b) Paralysis / Paresis / Weightlessness in space

4)	**Diet**

a) Malnutrition / Anorexia nervosa (inadequate calcium / vitamin C,D / protein)

b) Alcoholism / Smoking

5)	**Chronic disease**

a) Rheumatoid arthritis (RA)

b) Drugs (increased cortisol, heparin, methotrexate)

c) Genetic (peak bone mass, osteogenesis imperfecta)

d) Metabolic acidosis

e) Neoplasms (myeloma/lymphoma)

6)	**Endocrine causes**

a) Hyperparathyroidism (HPT) / Hyperthyroidism

b) Hypercortisolism

Key Objectives

- Define osteoporosis as a metabolic bone disease with decreased density (mass/unit volume; bone is abnormally porous and thin). The reduced bone mass weakens the mechanical strength of the bone, thus making it much more likely to break, often with little or no trauma.

- Outline how osteoporosis and its complications can be prevented or minimised.

General/Specific Objectives

- Through efficient, focused data gathering:

  - In a patient with spinal compression or other fractures, determine extent of trauma causing break or whether the fracture occurred at rest or routine activity.

  - Determine the presence of spinal deformity (kyphosis), loss of height, and abdominal protrusion.

  - Differentiate osteoporosis from osteomalacia (defective bone mineralisation)

  - Check for risk factors of osteoporosis.

- Interpret critical clinical and laboratory findings that were key in the processes of exclusion, differentiation, and diagnosis:

  - Select patients requiring investigation for less common causes of bone loss.

  - Select patients in need of bone density assessment to prevent or minimise osteoporosis.

- Conduct an effective plan of management for a patient with osteoporosis and/or spinal fracture:

  - Outline management of pain relief in vertebral compression fractures as well as supportive measures and mobilisation.

  - Outline prevention and treatment of osteoporosis including nutrition, calcium and vitamin D supplementation, drug (oestrogen, biphosphonates) therapy, and activity.

089K Cancer Pain

(See also #030 Dying Patient)

Overview

The most common cancers causing death in Australia are lung, bowel, breast, prostate, lymphoma and pancreas. Chronic pain is a major symptom in many or most patients with advanced cancer. Doctors dealing with such patients must appreciate the principles of global palliative care combined with adequate pain control and prevention. Broad-spectrum analgesic management using an 'analgesic ladder' approach to maximise analgesic effect is required.

Use of adjuvant analgesics, psychotropic medications, laxatives when using opioid analgesics, and anti-emetics form part of this approach. All cancer patients requiring analgesics need close and compassionate supervision to achieve maximum comfort with minimal adverse effects.

Causes

Pain can be associated with most cancers; the most common associations in Australia are with lung, bowel, breast, prostate, lymphoma and pancreas.

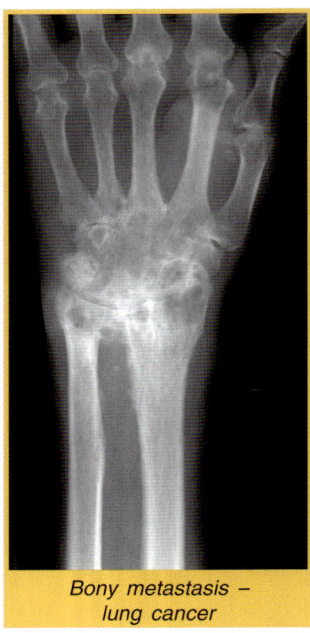

*Bony metastasis –
lung cancer*

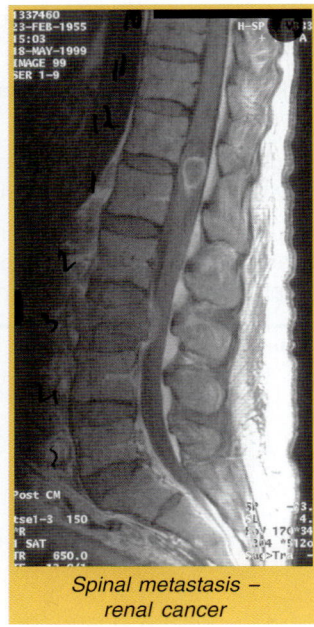

*Spinal metastasis –
renal cancer*

Agents used for pain relief in cancer patients

1) **Non-opioids (paracetamol, nonsteroidal anti-inflammatory drugs (NSAIDs))**

2) **Weak opioids (codeine, etc.)**

3) **Strong opioids (morphine)**

4) **Adjuvant (non-conventional) analgesics**
   a) Steroids
   b) Antidepressants
   c) Anticonvulsants
   d) Muscle relaxants
   e) Nerve transmission blockade (transcutaneous electrical nerve stimulation (TENS), acupuncture, epidural injection, implantable devices)

Key Objective
- Maintenance of maximum pain control with the lowest attainable adverse effects.

090 Renal Failure, Acute (Anuria/Oliguria / Acute Renal Failure (ARF))

Overview

A sudden and rapid rise in serum creatinine is a common finding. A competent clinician is required to have an organised approach to this problem. Prompt diagnosis and treatment of extrarenal causes can prevent progression to established acute renal failure (ARF).

Causes

1) Pre-renal causes of oliguria/azotaemia

    a) Hypovolaemia (haemorrhage, volume loss, third space loss)

    b) Distributional shock (sepsis)

    c) Cardiac causes of hypotension (myocardial infarction (MI))

    d) Obstructive causes of hypotension (pulmonary embolus)

2) Renal causes of oliguria/azotaemia

    a) Glomerular (crescentic glomerulonephritis, haemolytic uraemic syndrome (HUS), etc.)

    b) Tubular (acute tubular necrosis (ATN))

    c) Tubulo-interstitial

       ❑ Acute interstitial nephritis (drugs, toxins)

       ❑ Cast nephropathy

    d) Vascular (e.g. malignant hypertension, renovascular disease)

3) Post-renal causes of oliguria/azotaemia (prostate obstruction, cervical cancer, stone, etc.)

4) Drugs

Key Objectives

- Contrast the clinical findings of acute and of chronic renal failure, and determine whether the serum creatinine rise is primarily acute or chronic, or an acute problem superimposed on a chronic one.

- Identify treatable extrarenal causes and correct these.

General/Specific Objectives

- Through efficient, focused, data gathering:

  - After determining that the rise in serum creatinine is caused by an acute problem (or acute superimposed on chronic), differentiate pre-renal, from renal, and post-renal ARF.

- Interpret critical clinical and laboratory findings which were key in the processes of exclusion, differentiation, and diagnosis:

  - Select appropriate laboratory and diagnostic imaging investigations.

  - Compare results, and discuss which of the three types of ARF is most likely.

- Conduct an effective plan of management for a patient with ARF:

  - In patients suspected of having post-renal failure, select the insertion of a patent urethral catheter as an initial investigative as well as therapeutic measure; institute early ultrasound of upper urinary tract if anuria/oliguria confirmed.

  - Outline initial management of fluid and dietary restrictions in a patient with ARF.

  - Select initial intervention(s) in the management of complications of ARF.

  - Select patients in need of specialised care.

  - Outline indications for renal and peritoneal dialysis.

  - Outline principles of haemodialysis and haemofiltration.

Overview

Although specialists in nephrology will care for patients with chronic renal failure, generalist clinicians will care for other common medical problems that afflict these patients. Clinicians must realise that patients with chronic renal failure have unique risks and that common therapies may be harmful because kidneys are frequently the main routes for excretion of many drugs.

Causes

1)   Pre-renal causes

    a) Renal vascular disease (occlusion)

    b) Cholesterol emboli

2)   Renal causes

    a) Glomerular diseases, primary (focal segmental glomerulosclerosis (FSGS), immunoglobulin A (IgA) nephropathy)

    b) Glomerular diseases, secondary (diabetic nephropathy, hypertensive nephropathy, systemic lupus erythematosus (SLE))

    c) Chronic interstitial nephritis

    d) Polycystic kidney disease

3)   Post-renal causes (obstructive nephropathy)

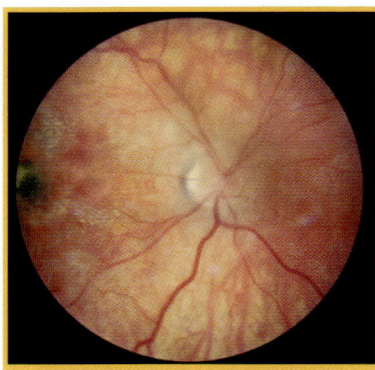

Papilloedema – chronic renal failure

Key Objective

- Determine which patients with elevated serum creatinine levels have chronic rather than acute renal failure (ARF), and communicate as early as possible to such patients that progression to chronic renal failure may be avoided or delayed with conservative management. Select such patients for referral.

General/Specific Objectives

- Through efficient, focused, data gathering:

    - Diagnose chronic renal failure, its underlying aetiology, and associated complications.

- Interpret critical clinical and laboratory findings which were key in the processes of exclusion, differentiation, and diagnosis.

- Conduct an effective plan of management for a patient with chronic renal failure:

    - Outline secondary prevention management for chronic renal failure.

    - List indications and contraindications for dialysis in chronic renal failure.

    - Counsel and educate patients about secondary and tertiary prevention strategies.

    - Counsel and educate patients about choosing to start chronic dialysis / preparation for renal transplantation.

    - Outline principles of management for patients with irreversible renal failure.

    - Select patients in need of specialised care.

Overview

Rhinorrhoea and sore throat occurring together indicate a viral upper respiratory tract infection (URTI) such as the 'common cold', transmitted by infected saliva or nasal secretions. Sore throat alone may be caused by bacterial pathogens particularly Group A streptococci, when specific therapy is indicated. Rhinorrhoea alone is not infective and may be seasonal (hay fever or allergic rhinitis) or chronic (vasomotor rhinitis).

Causes

1)	Infections (viral, bacterial, mycoplasma, *Chlamydia*, candidiasis)

2)	Noninfectious chronic rhinitis and allergic rhinitis

3)	Obstruction (foreign body in nasal passage, polyps, deviated septum)

4)	Neoplasm

Key Objectives

- Discuss that making a clinical diagnosis of streptococcal tonsillo-pharyngitis is difficult, but excluding the diagnosis is easier in the presence of rhinorrhoea, cough, hoarseness, and normal temperature. Such patients usually have a viral URTI and do not require diagnostic tests or treatment.

- Discuss the benefit of antibiotic treatment in Group A streptococcal pharyngitis with respect to prevention of acute rheumatic fever and acute glomerulonephritis.

General/Specific Objectives

- Through efficient, focused data gathering:

    - Determine whether testing for Group A streptococci is indicated.

    - Determine if an allergy or more unusual cause for rhinorrhoea is present.

- Interpret critical clinical and laboratory findings which were key in the processes of exclusion, differentiation, and diagnosis:

    - Select throat culture of the posterior pharynx in patients suspected of having streptococcal infection, or rapid antigen detection test.

- Conduct an effective plan of management for a patient with rhinorrhoea and/or sore throat:

  - Outline the management of contacts of patients with proven streptococcal infections.

  - Outline management in a patient with streptococcal, non-streptococcal URTI or other causes for symptoms.

  - Select patients in need of specialised care.

Overview

A swelling confined to the scrotum must be differentiated from an inguinoscrotal swelling in continuity (virtually diagnostic of an indirect inguinal hernia). Most true scrotal swellings are benign, often requiring only reassurance. Tumours of the testis are uncommon (only one to two percent of malignant tumours in men), but represent a very important tumour in young men (20–40 years). Advances in management have markedly improved survival rates.

Causes

1) Inguinoscrotal swelling (indirect inguinal hernia)

2) True scrotal swelling

   a) Cystic (transilluminable)
- ❏ Hydrocele (primary, secondary)
- ❏ Epididymal cyst (spermatocele)

   b) Venous (soft, compressible)
- ❏ Varicocele (almost invariably left-sided, lessens on recumbency)

   c) Solid (firm, non-transilluminable)
- ❏ Testicular malignancy
  - Seminoma
  - Teratoma
  - Mixed
  - Lymphoma
  - Other
- ❏ Epididymitis
- ❏ Chronic bacterial (tuberculosis (TB))
- ❏ Granulomatous orchitis / Testicular abscess

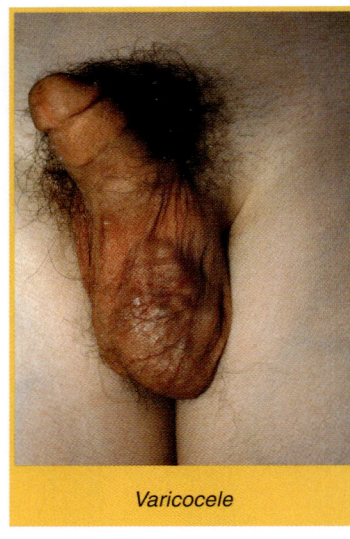

Varicocele

Key Objectives

- Differentiate true scrotal swellings from inguinoscrotal swellings (check for reducibility of inguinoscrotal indirect inguinal hernia).

- Differentiate benign scrotal masses from those suspicious of testicular tumour.

- Differentiate *solid* true scrotal swelling (testicular tumour until disproved) from:

  - Benign cystic swelling (trans-illuminates):

    * Hydrocele – surrounds testis.

    * Epididymal cyst – above and behind testis.

  - Varicocele (soft squishy 'bag of worms' feel, lessens on recumbency).

- Differentiate secondary hydrocele hiding tumour, from primary hydrocele (younger age, use of ultrasound and tumour markers as diagnostic aids) in suspicious presentations.

General/Specific Objectives

- Through efficient, focused data gathering:

- Distinguish between **suspicious** and **non-suspicious** lumps.

  - **Non-suspicious** – primary hydroceles in older patients, epididymal cysts also mainly in older patients.

  - **Suspicious** – all solid masses of testis and epididymis.

- Differentiate from primarily painful lesions (see #094 Scrotal Pain (Acute)).

- Recognise importance of avoiding scrotal needling/aspiration of suspicious lumps.

- Selection of suspicious lumps needing scrotal ultrasound; abdominal, pelvic and chest computed tomography (CT) scanning; and search for tumour markers.

- Elicit history of undescended testicle, infertility, previous testicular tumour, breast enlargement/tenderness.

  - Perform abdominal examination including inguinal areas, and an examination of the male genitalia (erect and supine), including rectal examination to assess the prostate and seminal vesicles in suspicious lumps.

- Interpret critical clinical and laboratory findings which were key in the processes of exclusion, differentiation, and diagnosis:

  - Select patients for CT scanning of chest, abdomen, and pelvis.

- Conduct an effective plan of management for a patient with a scrotal mass:

  - Outline management options for masses which are not testicular tumours.

  - Select patients in need of specialised care.

Overview

Most scrotal swellings are painless. Acutely painful swellings mandate early diagnosis and treatment. Occasionally pain precedes or is independent of a scrotal mass.

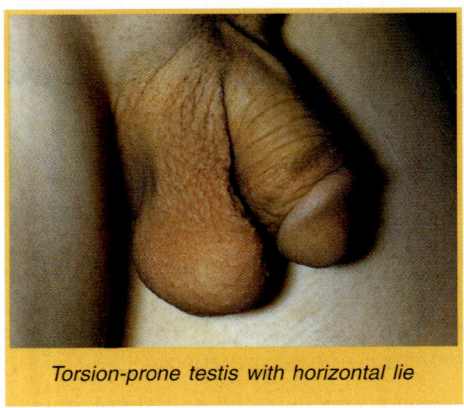

Torsion-prone testis with horizontal lie

Causes

1) Torsion

    a) Torsion of testis

    b) Torsion of testicular appendage

2) Inflammation

    a) Acute epididymitis, orchitis, trauma

3) Tumours

    a) Acute haemorrhage into testicular tumour

4) Conditions arising outside scrotum

    a) Acute strangulation of inguinoscrotal hernia

    b) Referred pain – renal 'colic'

Key Objective

- Acute scrotal pain accompanied by a tender testis is a surgical emergency caused by testicular torsion. The diagnosis is either confirmed or excluded by urgent operation ('Look and see' rather than 'Wait and see').

General/Specific Objectives

- Through efficient, focused data gathering:

  - Distinguish testicular torsion from acute epididymitis by:

    * Operative findings (operation mandatory if any doubt exists).

    * Rapidity of onset (minutes versus hours).

    * Age group (children or young adults versus older patients).

    * Absence of urinary symptoms.

    * Ultrasound, nuclear scan (occasionally helpful with equivocal presentations, must not delay urgent surgery).

  - Elicit history of dysuria, sexual contacts; examine genitalia, prostate and abdomen.

  - Distinguish true scrotal masses from inguinoscrotal masses.

- Interpret critical clinical and laboratory findings which were key in the processes of exclusion, differentiation, and diagnosis:

  - Define indications and contraindications for nuclear medicine blood flow or Doppler ultrasound studies.

- Develop an algorithm outlining a plan of management for a patient with scrotal pain:

  - Outline natural history of testicular torsion and predisposing factors, and time limits of ischaemia tolerated before infarction.

  - Outline management of epididymitis.

Overview

Seizures are an important differential diagnosis of syncope. A seizure is a transient neurological dysfunction, with symptoms and signs resulting from excessive, abnormal electrical discharge of cortical neurons. Clinical manifestations include disturbances of consciousness, emotion, sensations, motor functions and behaviour. Epilepsy is a chronic condition characterised by recurrent seizures, comprising a heterogeneous group of disorders with multiple causes and manifestations. Most patients with epilepsy have more than one type of seizure. A precise diagnosis of epilepsy requires the integration of all clinical data including seizure type; electroencephalographic and imaging findings; age of onset; aetiology; family history; precipitating factors and pathophysiology.

The International League Against Epilepsy Classification

1) Partial (focal, local) seizures

a) **Simple partial seizures (consciousness not impaired)**
- ❏ With motor symptoms
- ❏ With somatosensory or special sensory symptoms
- ❏ With autonomic symptoms
- ❏ With psychic symptoms

b) **Complex, partial seizures (with impaired consciousness)**
- ❏ Beginning as simple partial, with or without automatisms, and progressing to impairment of consciousness
- ❏ With no other features
- ❏ With features as in simple partial seizures
- ❏ With automatisms

c) **With impairment of consciousness at onset**
- ❏ With no other features
- ❏ With features as in simple partial seizures
- ❏ With automatisms

d) **Partial seizures evolving to secondarily generalised seizures**
- ❏ Simple partial seizures evolving to generalised seizures
- ❏ Complex partial seizures evolving to generalised seizures
- ❏ Simple complex seizures evolving to complex partial seizures to generalised seizures

2) Generalised seizures (convulsive or nonconvulsive)

a) **Absence seizures; either typical or atypical**

b) **Myoclonic seizures**

c) **Clonic seizures**

d) **Tonic seizures**

e) Tonic-clonic seizures

f) Atonic seizures

3) Unclassified epileptic seizures including neonatal seizures, rhythmic eye movements, chewing and swimming movements

Causes of Seizures

1) Partial seizures (focal seizures)

2) Partial seizures complex (temporal lobe or psychomotor)

3) Generalised tonic-clonic (grand mal) seizure

a) Idiopathic (20%)

b) Trauma

c) Infectious

d) Vascular / Hypertension (malignant, eclampsia)

e) Neoplasia

f) Degenerative

g) Metabolic

❏ Electrolyte abnormalities

❏ Alcohol or drug withdrawal

❏ Renal or liver failure

4) Absence (petit mal) seizure

5) Pseudoseizures

6) Status epilepticus

Key Objective
• Differentiate syncope from disturbances of cerebral function caused by a seizure.

General/Specific Objectives

- Through efficient, focused, data gathering:

  - Differentiate between a true seizure and pseudoseizure.

  - Differentiate between partial seizures and generalised seizures.

  - Determine which seizures may be secondary to co-existing medical problems.

- Interpret critical clinical and laboratory findings which were key in the processes of exclusion, differentiation, and diagnosis:

  - Contrast findings in patients with focal seizures, complex partial seizures, generalised seizures, and petit mal seizures.

  - Compare findings in syncope with cerebral seizures.

- Conduct an effective plan of management for a patient with seizures:

  - Formulate a plan of management for a patient with status epilepticus.

  - Contrast the plan of management of petit mal seizures with grand mal and partial seizures.

  - Select patients in need of specialised care and/or referral to other healthcare professionals.

  - Outline educational and/or supportive counselling for patients with seizure disorders including concerns for psychosocial impact, considerations for employment, and driving.

096A   Sexual Maturation, Normal

Overview
The normal process of sexual maturation, with some acceptable variations, requires the integration of normal central nervous system (CNS) (hypothalamus, pituitary), gonadal, and adrenal function along with a critical body mass and nutrition level. Clinicians familiar with the normal process are in a better position to discern abnormal sexual maturation.

Causes
Processes required for normal growth and maturation in males and females:

Normal sexual maturation results primarily from the integration between the various components of the endocrine system and the gonads.

Key Objective
- Differentiate acceptable variations which occur in male and female progress to puberty and sexual maturation, from abnormal sexual maturation.

General/Specific Objectives
- Through efficient, focused data gathering:
  - Elicit pertinent data regarding birth, infantile growth, and development and its impact upon puberty.
  - Assess the normal sequencing of pubertal development through Tanner stages 1 to 5 for both males and females.
- Interpret critical clinical and laboratory findings which were key in the processes of exclusion, differentiation and diagnosis:
  - Outline the use of growth charts and Tanner staging in the assessment of children.
  - Outline initial evaluation of variations from the expected patterns of sexual maturation.
- Conduct an effective plan of management for a patient with normal or accepted variations of sexual maturation:
  - Counsel adolescents and their parents about the normal progression to sexual maturation.

096B Sexual Maturation, Abnormal

(See also #063A Amenorrhoea (also Oligomenorrhoea))

Overview
Sexual development is important to adolescent perception of self-image and well-being. Many factors may disrupt the normal progression to sexual maturation.

Causes

> **1) Delayed puberty (failure of Stage II: male by 14 years, female by 13 years; or menarche within five years of breast budding)**

a) Growth failure / Delayed puberty overlap
- ❏ Multiple endocrine disorders
- ❏ Variants of normal/constitutional
- ❏ Systemic diseases

b) Central causes
- ❏ Congenital (hypothalamic/pituitary – low gonadotropins or low gonadotropin-releasing hormone (GnRH))
  - • Syndromes (Prader-Willi, Laurence-Moon-Biedl)
  - • Malformations (midline development defects)
  - • Isolated deficiency of gonadotropins / panhypopituitarism
- ❏ Acquired
  - • Infection / Trauma / Tumours (craniopharyngioma, pituitary adenoma)
  - • Malnutrition / Chronic systemic disease

c) Primary gonadal disorders
- ❏ Congenital
  - • Chromosomal (Turner syndrome, Klinefelter syndrome)
  - • Gonadal differentiation / Biosynthetic defects
- ❏ Acquired
  - • Infection (oophoritis, orchitis)
  - • Trauma, torsion

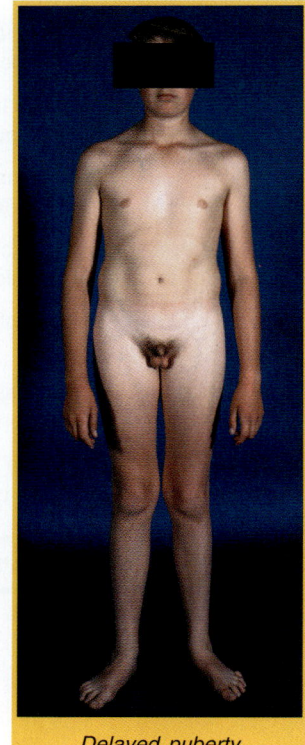

Delayed puberty

- Neoplasms / Neoplasia therapy (irradiation, cytotoxic drugs) / Surgery

d) Interruption / Lack of completion
❏ Testicular feminisation
❏ Müllerian duct abnormalities (absent/hypoplastic uterus/vagina)

2) Precocious puberty (female before 8 years; male before 10 years)

a) Central
❏ Constitutional (gonadotropin dependent / gonadotropin independent)
❏ Central nervous system (CNS) (neoplasms, post-inflammatory, neurofibromatosis, hydrocephalus)
❏ Hypothyroidism, McCune-Albright syndrome

3) Pseudoprecocious puberty (incomplete)

4) Other

Key Objective
- Counsel patients and their families about the need for immediate or delayed screening, referral or careful followup.

General/Specific Objectives
- Through efficient, focused, data gathering:

  - Differentiate between the principal causes of abnormal sexual development.

  - Identify features of delayed and precocious puberty; differentiate delayed puberty versus growth failure.

- Interpret critical clinical and laboratory findings which were key in the processes of exclusion, differentiation, and diagnosis:

  - Evaluate patients with suspected abnormal sexual development with a minimum of investigations.

- Conduct an effective plan of management for a patient with abnormal sexual maturation:

  - Outline initial management and counsel both caregivers and patients with abnormal sexual development.

Overview

The social appropriateness of sexuality is culturally determined. The clinician's own sexual attitude needs to be recognised and taken into account in order for the clinician to deal with the patient's concern in a relevant manner. The patient must be set at ease in order to make possible discussion of private and sensitive sexual issues.

Causes

1)	**Sexual dysfunction in the male or female**

a) **Premature ejaculation / Ejaculatory failure**

b) **Erectile dysfunction (impotence)**

c) **Anorgasmia**

d) **Dyspareunia**

e) **Inhibition of sexual desire**

f) **Vaginismus**

2)	**Sexual paraphilias (exhibitionism, fetishism, voyeurism, transvestism, sadomasochism, paedophilia)**

3)	**Lesbian and gay patients**

4)	**Disabled patients and sexuality**

5)	**Children/Adolescents; sexuality and gender identity**

6)	**Ageing patients and sexuality**

7)	**Gender identity in adults**

Key Objectives

- Elicit factors precipitating and maintaining the sexual concern, effort to escape the concern, and relevant medical history to rule out reversible organic conditions.

- Determine the patient's social and physical sexual development and behaviour as well as the patient's sexual orientation and comfort with it.

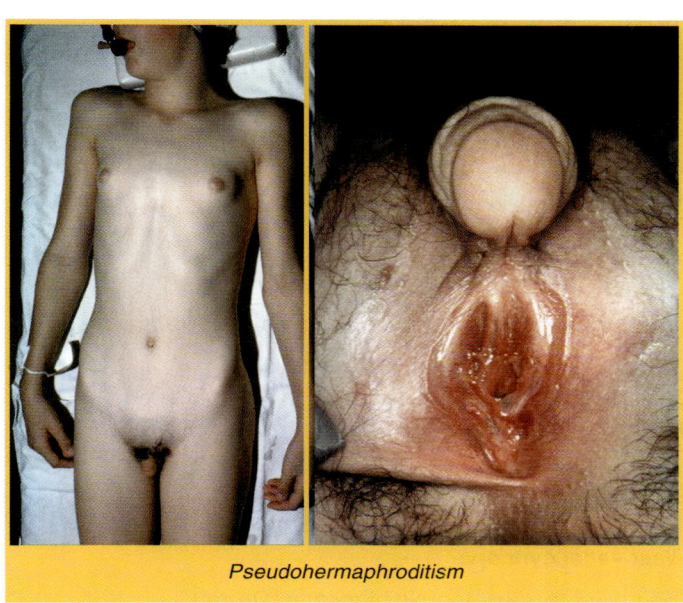

Pseudohermaphroditism

Overview

Shock is an acute and potentially life-threatening clinical emergency with multiple causes leading to broadly similar clinical syndromes associated with failure of vital organ and tissue perfusion. All clinicians must be familiar with principles of recognition, diagnosis and treatment of shock as a life-threatening emergency with plans appropriate to rapid clinical identification and treatment of the most common causes; and selective use of clinical and laboratory investigations to identify those cases refractory to initial management. Hypotension, although common to many types of shock, is one aspect only of the clinical syndrome.

Causes

1) Cardiogenic

a) Myocardial infarction (MI)

b) Cardiomyopathy

2) Hypovolaemic

a) Haemorrhage – overt or concealed blood loss

b) Plasma loss – burns, peritonitis

c) Water and electrolyte loss

❑ Gastrointestinal losses

❑ Interstitial (third space) losses

❑ Skin losses (burns, hyperthermia)

3) Obstructive

a) Pulmonary embolism

b) Tension pneumothorax

c) Pericardial tamponade, constrictive pericarditis

d) Aortic dissection, venacaval obstruction

4) Distributive

a) Septic

b) Anaphylaxis

c) Vasovagal syncope

d) Spinal injury / Autonomic blockade / Drugs

e) Endocrine – pituitary, adrenal, thyroid deficiencies

Key Objectives

- Recognition of key features of shock (pallor, hypotension, thready pulse, oliguria) as a life-threatening acute clinical emergency.

- Ability to formulate rapidly diagnostic and management plans and strategies appropriate to the various causative agencies in a practical and logical sequence.

General/Specific Objectives

- Through rapid, efficient, focused data gathering:

  - Recognise and diagnose shock states.

  - Formulate integrated diagnostic and management plans to differentiate and deal with the various causes.

- Identify critical clinical and investigational findings which are key in the process of diagnosis, exclusion, differentiation, and monitoring of response to treatment.

- Use the above to formulate a flow chart covering the effective diagnosis, management and monitoring of a patient with shock.

- Outline the principles and specifics of the management plans of a patient with:

  - Hypovolaemic shock.

  - Cardiogenic shock.

  - Septic shock.

  - 'Refractory' shock.

- Identify patients with shock requiring use of central venous pressure or pulmonary wedged capillary pressure monitoring.

098A Anaphylaxis

Overview

Anaphylaxis causes a significant number of fatalities per year, and occurs in 1 in 5,000 hospital admissions. Children most commonly are allergic to foods.

Causes

1)	**Drugs**

   a) *Beta*-lactam antibiotics

   b) Nonsteroidal anti-inflammatory drugs (NSAIDs)

   c) Anti-neoplastic medications

   d) Angiotensin-converting enzyme (ACE) inhibitors

2)	**Hymenoptera (bees, wasps) envenomation**

3)	**Radiographic contrast media**

4)	**Blood products**

5)	**Foods (seafood, milk, nuts)**

6)	**Latex**

Key Objectives

• Differentiate anaphylaxis from conditions which are similar such as shock from other causes, other flush syndromes, 'restaurant syndrome', increased endogenous histamine production, acute respiratory failure syndromes, or non-organic syndromes such as panic attacks or Münchausen stridor.

• Initiate therapy by ensuring airway, intubation if necessary, establishing intravenous lines with large bore needles, stop antigen administration, and select pharmacologic agents.

General/Specific Objectives

- Through efficient, focused, data gathering:

  - Perform examination for skin involvement (90% have pruritus, urticaria, angio-oedema, flushing), upper and lower respiratory tract involvement (50%), shock or conduction disturbances (30%), gastrointestinal or nervous system involvement.

- Interpret critical clinical and laboratory findings which were key in the processes of exclusion, differentiation, and diagnosis.

- Conduct an effective plan of management for a patient with anaphylaxis:

  - Outline initial management for anaphylaxis.

  - Outline rationale for use of epinephrine, glucagon, antihistamines, steroids, and *beta*-agonists in aerosols for respiratory symptoms.

  - Discuss biphasic anaphylaxis and protracted anaphylaxis.

  - Select patients in need of specialised care.

Overview

Sudden infant death syndrome (SIDS) and/or acute life-threatening event (ALTE) are devastating events for caregivers and healthcare workers alike. It is imperative that the precursors, probable cause and parental concerns are extensively evaluated to prevent recurrence.

Causes

1) **Idiopathic**

2) **Prolonged apnoea**

3) **Response to hypoxia/hypercarbia**

4) **Upper airway obstruction**

5) **Abnormal sleep patterns**

6) **Cardiac arrhythmias**

7) **Face-down position**

Key Objectives

- Evaluate fully the possible causes of an infant history of ALTE or SIDS.

- Counsel the parents and families of such children.

- Provide management of children who are at risk for ALTE or SIDS.

General/Specific Objectives

- Through efficient, focused, data gathering:

  - Determine whether there is evidence of possible risk factors or causes known to be associated with ALTE or SIDS.

  - Diagnose the infant presenting with ALTE or SIDS.

- Interpret critical clinical and laboratory findings which were key in the processes of exclusion, differentiation, and diagnosis:

  - Evaluate fully, but with compassion and empathy, the possible causes of the infant presenting with ALTE or SIDS.

- Conduct an effective plan of management for a patient with ALTE or SIDS:

  - Perform immediate resuscitative measures.

  - Conduct short/long term bereavement management for parents/family.

  - Select patients in need of referral and/or consultation for infants and families at risk, i.e. bereavement issues, genetic counselling.

  - Select patients who are in need of child protection (if appropriate).

100A Focal Skin Lesions – Benign Lesions

Overview

The majority of focal skin lesions are manifestly benign longstanding lesions of congenital or acquired origin requiring no treatment. An important group of benign lesions are dysplastic and premalignant.

Focal skin lesions can usually be rapidly assessed on clinical grounds into:

- Clearly benign skin lesions.
- 'Suspicious' lesions.

Causes of Clearly Benign Focal Skin Lesions

In Children (macules, nodules or papules):

1) Pigmented lesions

a) Vascular malformation
- ❏ 'Port wine stain' (capillary haemangioma)
- ❏ 'Strawberry naevus' (cavernous haemangioma)

b) Benign melanocytic naevi ('common moles')
- ❏ Junctional
- ❏ Intradermal
- ❏ Compound

c) Common freckle (ephelis)

d) Uncommon lesions
- ❏ 'Blue naevus' (Mongolian spot)
- ❏ Juvenile melanoma

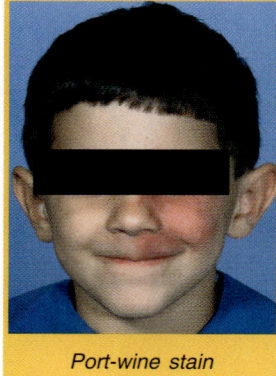

Port-wine stain

2) Other Lesions

a) Viral infective wart – verruca vulgaris

b) Pyogenic granuloma

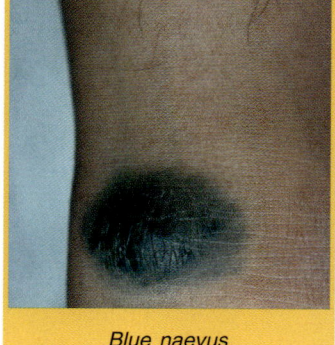

Blue naevus

In Adults (macules, nodules or papules):

1) Pigmented lesions

   a) **Benign melanocytic naevus**

      ❏ Junctional

      ❏ Intradermal

      ❏ Compound

   b) **Seborrhoeic keratosis (seborrhoeic wart)**

   c) **Campbell de Morgan spot (senile haemangioma, cherry angioma)**

   d) **Dermatofibroma (sclerosing haemangioma, histiocytoma)**

   e) **Spider naevus**

   f) **Senile freckle (lentigo) – macular**

   g) **Senile purpura – macular**

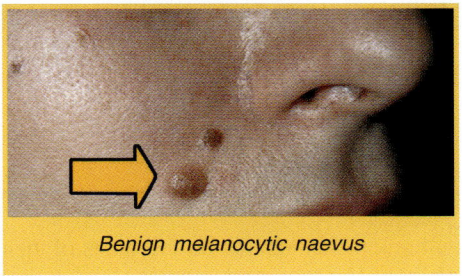

Benign melanocytic naevus

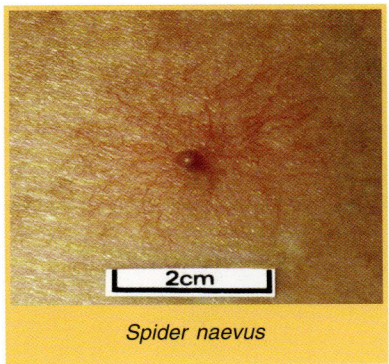

Spider naevus

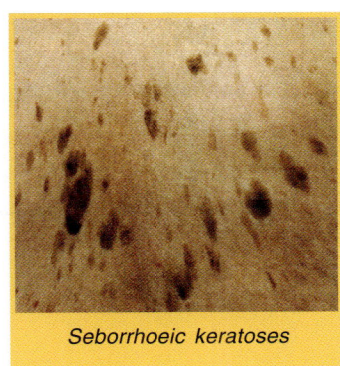

Seborrhoeic keratoses

a) **Skin tag (soft fibroma, benign squamous papilloma)**

b) **Solar keratosis (hyperkeratosis, senile keratosis – premalignant)**

c) **Callosity (callus)**

d) **Xanthoma**

e) **Viral infective wart – verruca vulgaris**

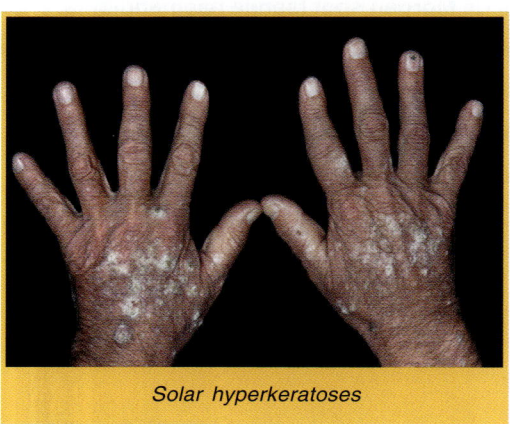

Solar hyperkeratoses

Key Objective

- Identify clearly benign skin lesions on the basis of their clinical features and distinguish between the various types.

General/Specific Objectives

- Through efficient, focused data gathering:

  - Identify clearly benign lesions not requiring treatment and provide appropriate reassurance.

  - Identify premalignant lesions.

  - Discuss risk factors, prevention and treatment of premalignant lesions.

  - Identify lesions requiring treatment and outline management plans.

100B Focal Skin Lesions – 'Suspicious' Lesions

Overview

Malignant and premalignant skin lesions are common in Australia with a susceptible population and excessive solar exposure. Malignant melanoma is virtually unknown in children but occurs throughout adult life; its frequency in Australia and in most other countries is increasing. Basal and squamous cell cancers occur in older patients and multiple lesions are common. Preventive measures against excessive solar exposure (e.g. 'Slip, Slop, Slap' UV-protection campaign) comprise important public health measures.

Causes of 'Suspicious' Focal Skin Lesions

1) Basal cell carcinoma (BCC)

Various morphologic types

a) Nodular

b) Ulcerative

c) Cystic

d) Psoriatic

e) Comedoform

f) Sclerosing/Cicatrising

g) Pigmented

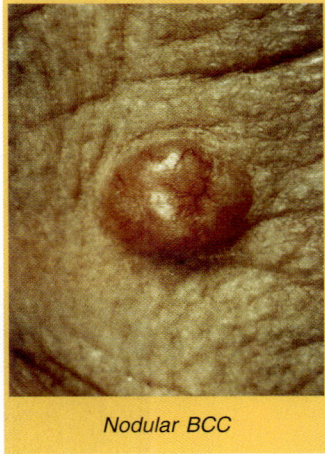

Nodular BCC

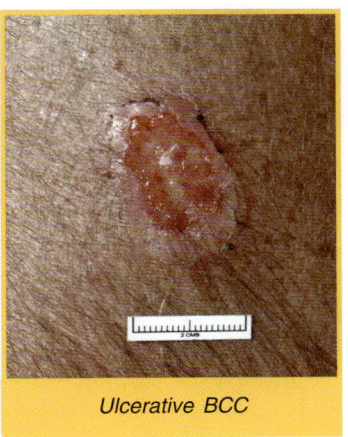

Ulcerative BCC

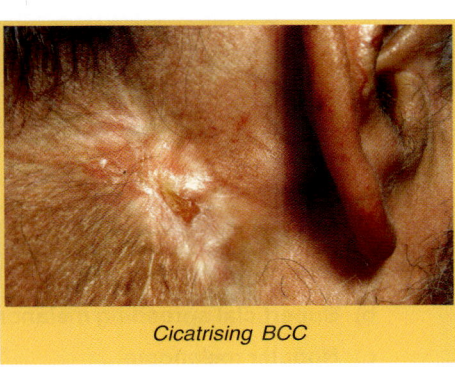

Cicatrising BCC

2) Squamous cell carcinoma (SCC)

a) SCC-*in-situ* (Bowen disease)

b) Invasive SCC

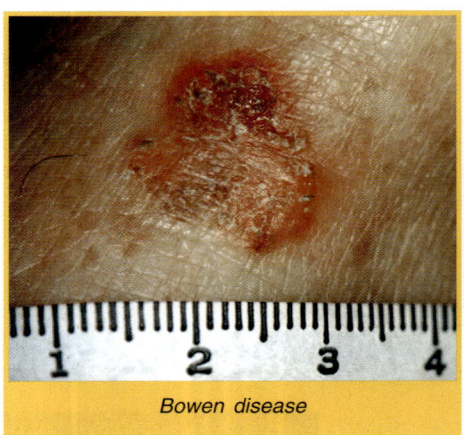

Bowen disease

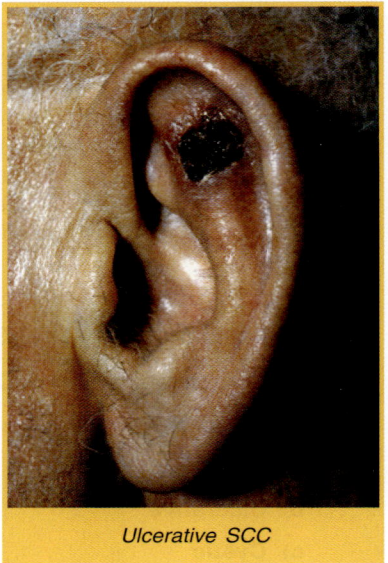

Ulcerative SCC

3) Keratoacanthoma (molluscum sebaceum)

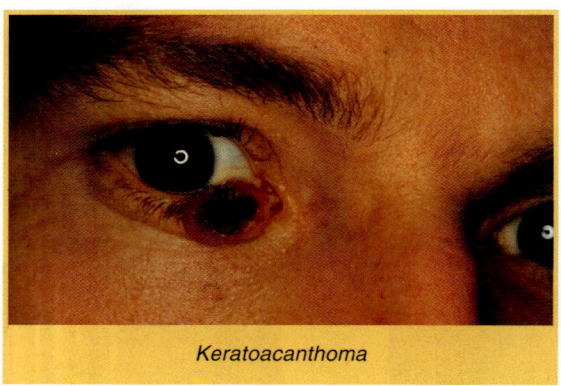

Keratoacanthoma

4) Malignant melanoma

a) Hutchinson melanotic freckle (lentigo maligna)

b) Superficial spreading melanoma

c) Nodular melanoma

d) Amelanotic melanoma

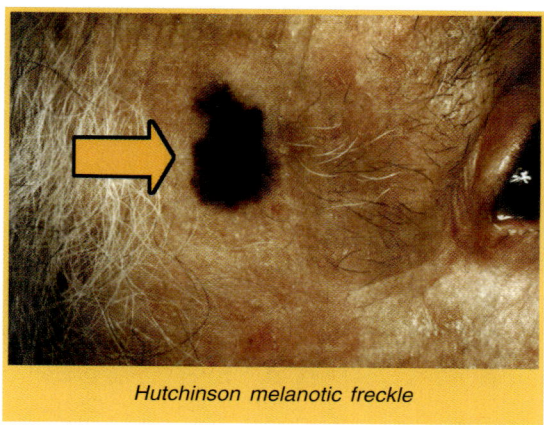

Hutchinson melanotic freckle

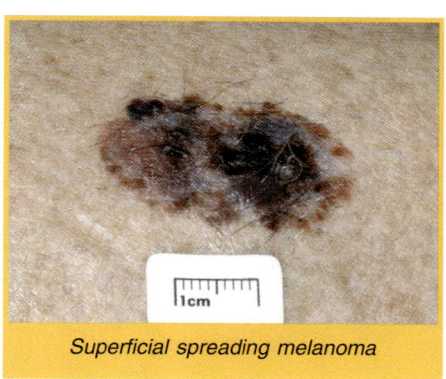

Superficial spreading melanoma

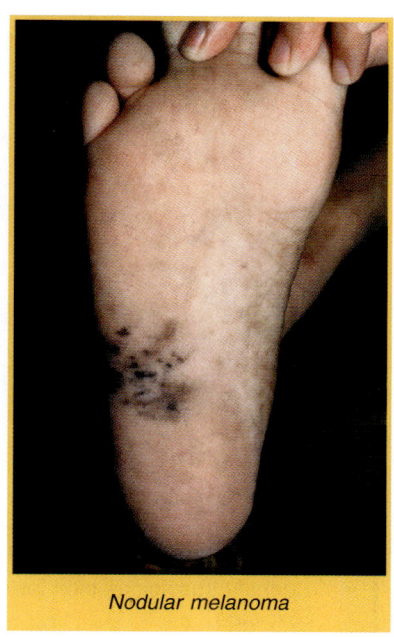

Nodular melanoma

5) Other suspicious lesions

  a) Infected/Traumatised benign lesions

  b) Pyogenic granuloma

  c) Kaposi sarcoma (haemangiosarcoma)

  d) Lymphoma of skin (mycosis fungoides)

  e) Dermatofibrosarcoma protuberans

  f) Cancer – metastatic skin deposits, acanthosis nigricans
     (paraneoplastic skin reaction)

  g) Merkel cell tumour (rare malignancy from sensory dermal cells)

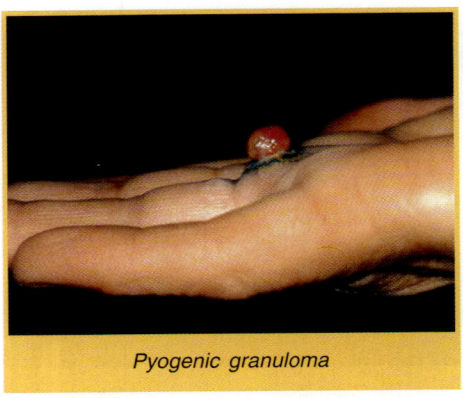
Pyogenic granuloma

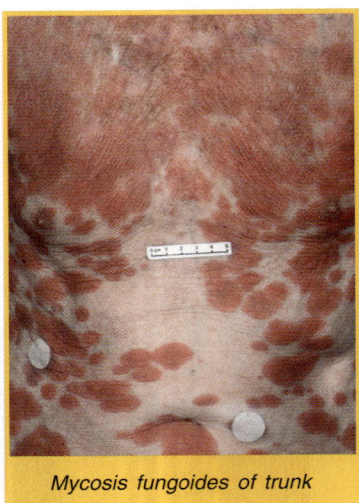
Mycosis fungoides of trunk

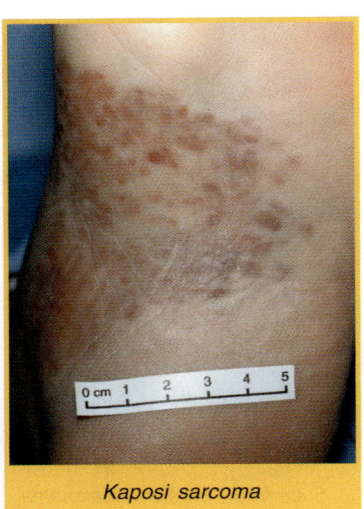
Kaposi sarcoma

Key Objectives
- Identify suspicious skin lesions and refer appropriately for diagnostic excision.
- Differentiate between different types on basis of history and examination.

General/Specific Objectives
- Discuss natural history and spread of common skin malignancies.
- Discuss management plans by surgery and adjuvant means.
- Discuss indications for and technique of biopsy of suspicious skin lesions.
- Discuss indications for surgical excision of skin lesions (cosmetic, irritative, prophylactic, suspicion of malignancy).
- Discuss pathology of malignant melanoma.
- Discuss types of benign and malignant pigmented lesions and indications for excision.

100C Focal Subcutaneous Lumps

Overview

A subcutaneous lump is a very common clinical problem. Most are of longstanding; the vast majority are benign lesions. Distinction on clinical grounds alone can almost always be made between the four most common lesions: **lipomas**, **cysts**, **ganglia** and **bursae**.

Causes

1) Lipomas

Very common. Present as benign slow-growing, soft, painless lobulated subcutaneous swellings occurring anywhere there is fat.

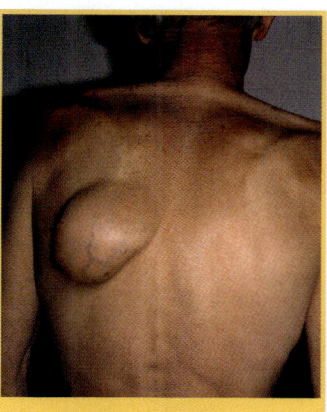

Subcutaneous lipoma

Variants

a) **Unusual sites – sub-fascial, intramuscular (IM), breast, bowel (submucosal)**

b) **Multiple painless subcutaneous lipomas of limbs or trunk (sometimes familial)**

c) **Retroperitoneal liposarcoma – locally invasive and malignant**

2) Cysts

a) **Keratinous ('sebaceous' or 'epidermoid') cysts**

Very common. Derived from pilosebaceous follicle – found anywhere there is hair: particularly scalp, scrotum. Rounded, smooth contour and skin attachments (not always with a punctum) distinguish cysts from lipomas.

Variants and complications:

❏ Infection – Cock peculiar tumour

❏ Accretion – 'seborrhoeic' horn

❏ Desiccation and plaque formation – pilomatrixoma (Malherbe calcifying epithelioma)

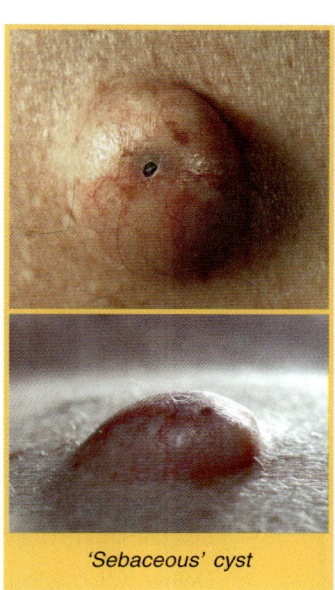

'Sebaceous' cyst

b) **Implantation 'dermoid' cyst – traumatic**

❏ Overlying puncture wound or scar

c) **Inclusion 'dermoid' cyst – developmental**

❏ In ventral midline head and neck, and at lateral angles of eyes

3) Ganglia

Common deeper subcutaneous swellings around joints or tendon sheaths of the wrists, fingers and ankles.

Variants:

a) Synovial (mucous) cyst of fingers on dorsum of terminal phalanx

b) Compound palmar and dorsal ganglia of wrist tendon sheaths

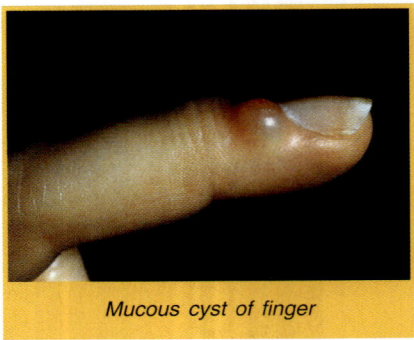
Mucous cyst of finger

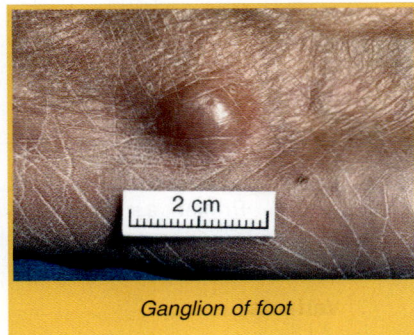
Ganglion of foot

4) Bursae

Sited around tendon insertions or over bony prominences (olecranon, prepatellar, pretibial, ischial, anserine) and may communicate with joints (suprapatellar, subacromial). May develop as adventitious **de novo** swellings at any site of abnormal friction (bunion).

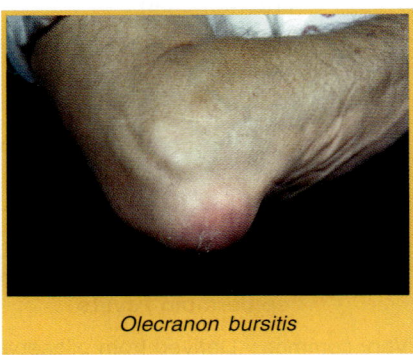
Olecranon bursitis

Key Objective
- Differentiate between most common lesions (lipomas, cysts, ganglia and bursae) from history, physical findings and anatomical localisation.

General/Specific Objectives
- Through efficient, focused data gathering:

    - Compare and contrast physical characteristics of lipomas and keratinous cysts.

    - List common bursae presenting with clinical problems.

    - Define which subcutaneous lumps will require diagnostic investigation to clarify diagnosis.

    - Define which subcutaneous lumps will require surgical excision.

100D   Red, Hot, Tender, Swollen Skin and Subcutaneous Layers

Overview

Red, hot, tender, swollen skin and subcutaneous tissues suggesting cellulitis and other spreading infections of skin and subcutaneous layers comprise important and common clinical presentations in primary care and in hospital emergency departments and wards. Causative organisms are commonly staphylococcal or streptococcal via a skin breach. Oedematous limbs are at increased risk.

Injured and ischaemic tissues predispose to serious necrotising anaerobic infections of skin and deeper tissues, from a wider range of infecting organisms. These infections are more common after devitalising injuries, in diabetic patients and immune-compromised hosts, and as postoperative complications after abdominal and vascular operations. Severe life-threatening infections such as necrotising fasciitis and clostridial myositis ('gas gangrene') require early radical excisional debridement and drainage as well as antibiotics.

Causes

1)   Cellulitis and erysipelas

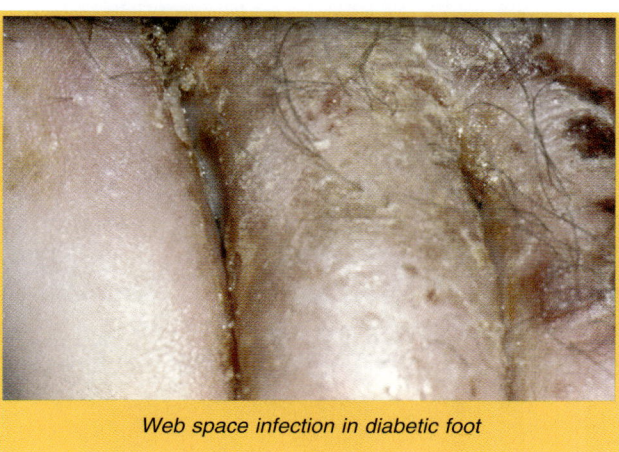

Web space infection in diabetic foot

2) Necrotising infections of skin and subcutaneous tissues

a) Fournier gangrene (spreading necrotising panniculitis)

b) Necrotising fasciitis

c) Clostridial myonecrosis ('gas gangrene')

d) Other (Meleney ulcer / synergistio gangrene, pyoderma gangrenosum, anthrax)

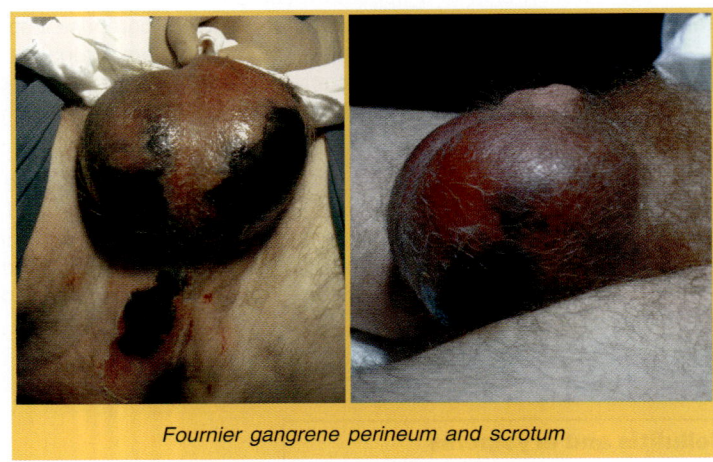

Fournier gangrene perineum and scrotum

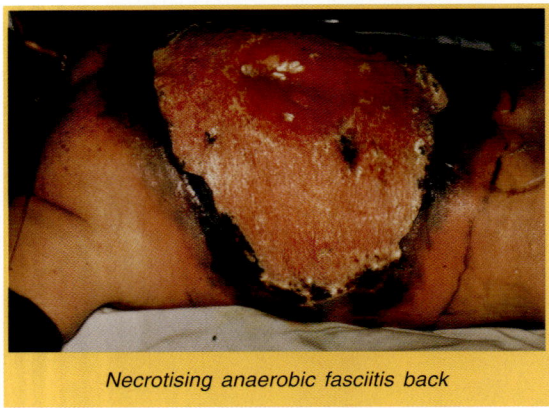

Necrotising anaerobic fasciitis back

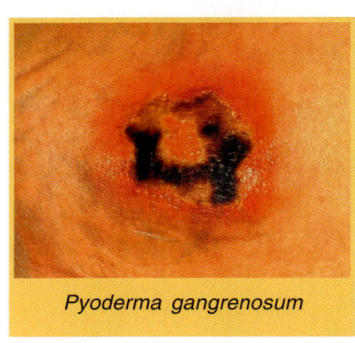

Pyoderma gangrenosum

Key Objectives

- Early recognition of cellulitis/erysipelas and differentiation from other erythematous skin conditions.

- Early recognition of serious necrotising infections.

General/Specific Objectives

- Through efficient, focused data gathering:

  - Identify signs of cellulitis/erysipelas and check for predisposing factors (skin wound/abrasion, chronic venous or lymphatic oedema, arterial insufficiency, underlying osteomyelitis), signs of local spread (ascending lymphangitis, lymphadenopathy) and general effects (fever, tachycardia) (see also #034B Unilateral Limb Oedema (Swollen Limb)).

  - Recognise signs of severe necrotising anaerobic infection (impending skin necrosis, subcutaneous crepitus, generalised toxicity).

- Interpret critical clinical and laboratory findings which were key in the processes of exclusion, differentiation, and diagnosis:

  - Discuss methods of identifying causative organisms.

  - Discuss role of imaging in diagnosis.

- Outline management plans for the effective treatment of infections of skin and subcutaneous tissues.

  - Recognise the vital role of excisional surgery and drainage in management of necrotising infection.

  - Discuss choice of antibiotic and routes of administration.

  - Discuss role of adjuvant hyperbaric oxygen treatment

Overview

Comedones are a feature of the very common skin disorder of acne vulgaris. Acne affects many teenagers and is associated with chronic inflammation of blocked pilosebaceous follicles and seborrhoea. Boils (furuncles) are acute staphylococcal abscesses developing in hair follicles. Carbuncles form more extensive sub-cutaneous abscesses, often with inadequate drainage. Both boils and carbuncles are commoner in diabetic patients. Blistering or vesiculobullous disorders include a wide range of conditions and can be considered according to their incidence. The less common causes may require histology and immunofluorescence studies.

Causes

1) Comedones, papules and pustules

    a) **Acne vulgaris – very common**

    b) **Furuncle/Carbuncle**

    c) **Impetigo**

    d) **Scabies, insect bites, etc.**

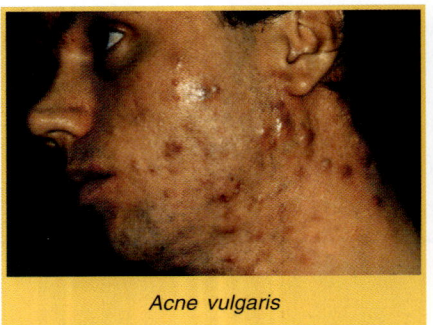

Acne vulgaris

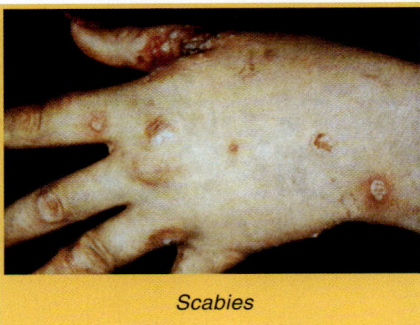

Scabies

2) Vesicles / Vesiculobullous disorders – common

    a) **Herpes simplex**

    b) **Varicella**

    c) **Herpes zoster**

    d) **Contact dermatitis**

        ❏ Plants

        ❏ Industrial agents

        ❏ Other chemicals

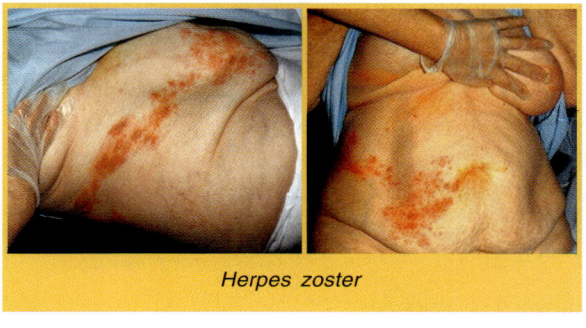

Herpes zoster

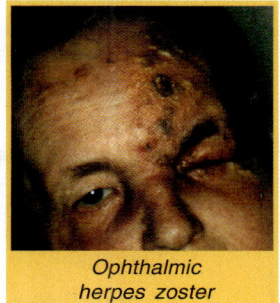

Ophthalmic
herpes zoster

e) **Insect bites**

f) **Dyshidrotic eczema (pompholyx)**

g) **Burns**

3) **Vesicles / Vesiculobullous disorders – uncommon**

a) **Drug eruptions**

b) **Bullous pemphigoid**

c) **Bullous erythema multiforme**

d) **Dermatitis cutanea tarda**

4) **Vesicles / Vesiculobullous disorders – rare**

a) **Epidermolysis bullosa**

b) **Pemphigus**

c) **Linear immunoglobulin A (IgA) disease**

d) **Cicatricial pemphigoid**

e) **Toxic epidermal necrolysis**

f) **Bullae of diabetes, renal failure**

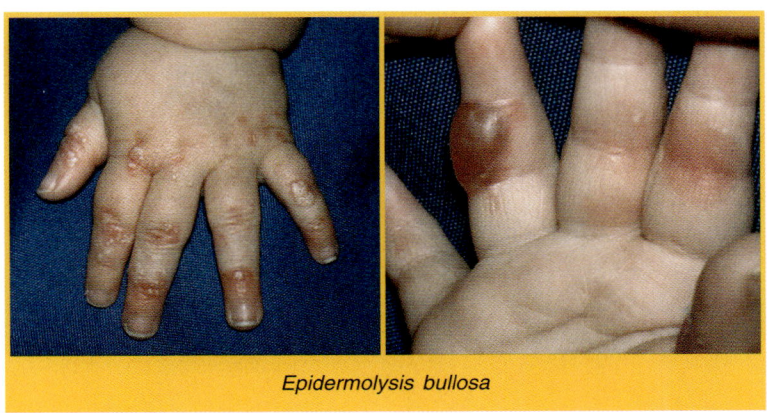

Epidermolysis bullosa

Key Objective

- Recognise and differentiate common and important skin disorders presenting as comedones, papules, pustules, blisters and vesicles.

General/Specific Objectives

- Through efficient, focused data gathering:

  - Determine areas of involvement, type of patient, and associated findings.

  - Differentiate between types of lesion.

- Interpret critical clinical and laboratory findings which were key in the processes of exclusion, differentiation, and diagnosis:

  - Select patients in need of further investigation.

- Conduct an effective plan of management for a patient with skin blisters:

  - Outline management for common and important skin conditions.

  - Select patients in need of specialised care.

- Conduct an effective plan of management for a patient with a furuncle or carbuncle.

- Conduct an effective plan of management for a patient with acne vulgaris.

101A Chronic Leg Ulcer

Overview

Chronic leg ulcers can be due to many causes; but the three most common causes are: chronic deep venous insufficiency ('venous ulcer'), arterial ischaemia ('arterial ulcer') and diabetes mellitus ('diabetic ulcer'). The site and appearance of the ulcer will often establish the diagnosis. A host of less common causes exists. Aims in treatment are initially to heal the ulcer and subsequently to prevent recurrence.

Causes

> **1) 'Venous ulcer' – chronic deep venous insufficiency (post-thrombotic syndrome)**

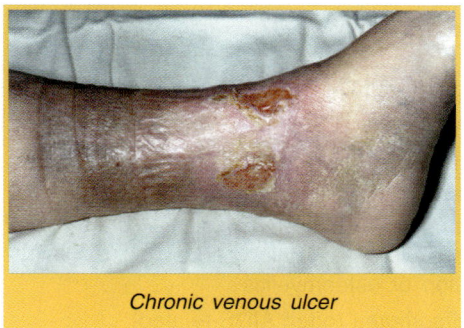

Chronic venous ulcer

> **2) 'Arterial ulcer' – arterial ischaemia (macrovascular/microvascular)**

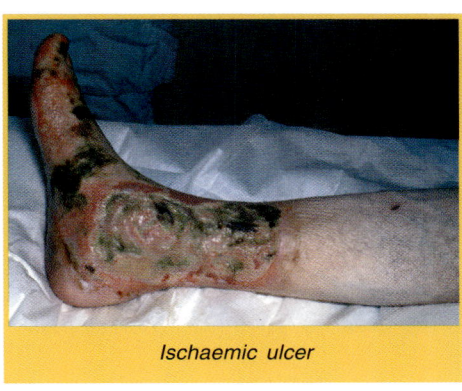

Ischaemic ulcer

3) 'Diabetic ulcer' – usually of primarily neuropathic origin; ischaemia and infection will often also contribute

4) Less common causes

a) **Infective ulcer**
  - ❏ 'Tropical ulcer'
  - ❏ Mycobacterium ulcerans ('Bairnsdale ulcer')
  - ❏ Pyogenic and synergistic infections

b) **Vasculitis complicating systemic and immunodeficiency states**
  - ❏ Rheumatoid arthritis (RA), polyarteritis neurosa
  - ❏ Inflammatory bowel disease (IBD)
  - ❏ Haemoglobinopathies
  - ❏ Severe hypertension ('Martorell ulcer')
  - ❏ Microembolisation from proximal arterial/valvular lesions

c) **Malignant ulcer – squamous cell carcinoma (SCC)**
  - ❏ Complicating chronic burn scar ('Marjolin ulcer'), chronic venous ulceration or osteomyelitis
  - ❏ Kaposi sarcoma (often AIDS-related)
  - ❏ Melanoma

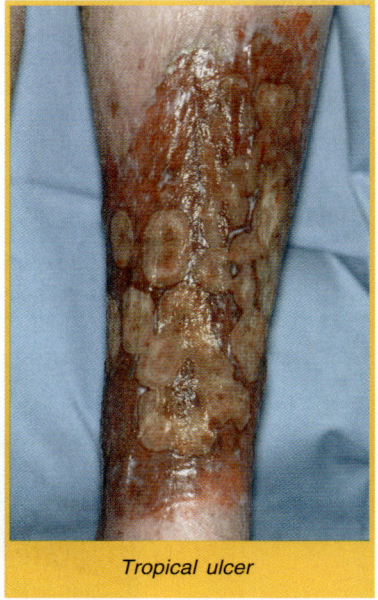
Tropical ulcer

d) **Other neuropathic ulcers**
  - ❏ Alcoholism, peripheral neuropathy, leprosy, syringomyelia, spina bifida

e) **Insect bites (e.g. wolf spider)**

f) **Healing failure of traumatic ulcers**
  - ❏ Skin flap avulsions in elderly
  - ❏ Sites of intravenous drug use

g) **Self-inflicted (factitious) ulceration**

Key Objectives

- Appreciate and recognise the characteristic features from each of the most common causes; venous disease, arterial disease and diabetes.

- Formulate diagnostic and management plans related to individual causes.

General/Specific Objectives

- Through efficient, focused data gathering:

  - Recognise symptoms and signs of chronic venous insufficiency associated with chronic venous ulceration with ambulatory superficial venous hypertension: fibrotic induration, oedema, pigmentation and venous eczema, and ankle flares.

  - Recognise local features of ischaemic arterial ulcers.

  - Perform appropriate assessment of arterial supply of limb by examination of circulation and capillary refilling, aided by clinical tests (Buerger, ankle/arm systolic index).

  - Assess for relative contributions of neuropathy, infection, macrovascular and microvascular disease in patients with diabetes.

  - Be alert to other potential causes of chronic leg ulceration and formulate diagnostic, investigational and management plans for patients with leg ulcers due to various causes.

  - Consider self-inflicted (factitious) ulceration in ulcers with atypical appearance, site or response to treatment.

102A Skin Rash / Dermatitis and/or Fever, Urticaria / Angio-Oedema

Overview

Skin rashes are often identified by their location and distribution as well as their morphology.

Causes

1) Dry/Scaly rash

   a) **Atopic dermatitis**

   b) **Nummular dermatitis**

   c) **Pityriasis rosea**

   d) **Psoriasis**

   e) **Seborrhoeic dermatitis**

   f) *Microsporum canis* infection ('ringworm')

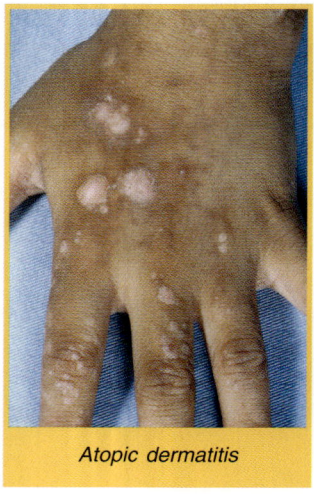

Atopic dermatitis

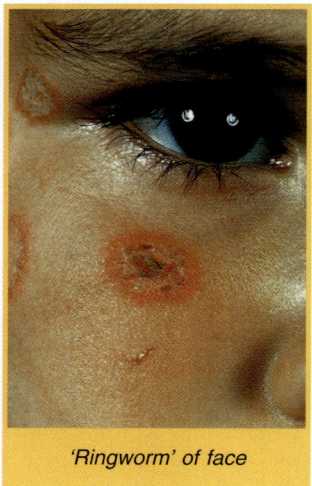

'Ringworm' of face

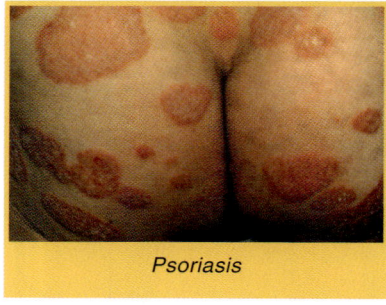

Psoriasis

2) Moist/Macerated rash

a) Candidiasis

b) Tinea cruris

c) Tinea pedis

d) Tinea capitis

e) Contact dermatitis

3) Urticaria / Angio-oedema

a) **Acute urticaria (greater than two-third of cases, self-limited, recurrence lasts less than six weeks)**

b) **Chronic urticaria (one-third of cases, recurrence lasts greater than six weeks)**

❏ Associated with triggers (aetiology not identified in up to 90% of patients)

- Drugs (antibiotics, hormones, nonsteroidal anti-inflammatory drugs (NSAIDs), aspirin, local anaesthetics, opiates, angiotensin-converting enzyme (ACE) inhibitors)

- Physical contact (animal saliva, plant resins, latex, metals, lotions, soap)

- Insect stings – risk of anaphylaxis (bees, wasps, hornets)

- Latex – risk of anaphylaxis if sensitised (gloves, condoms, balloons)

- Aeroallergens (oral allergy syndrome)

- Foods and additives (only 10% if placebo controlled)

- Infections (greater than 80% of urticaria in paediatric patients)

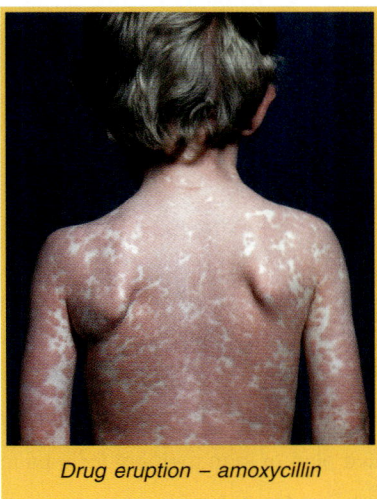

Drug eruption – amoxycillin

- ❏ Associated with angio-oedema (50% of urticaria, both acute and chronic)
- ❏ Associated with systemic disease
  - • Systemic lupus erythematosus (SLE)
  - • Henoch-Schönlein purpura
  - • Cryoglobulinaemia
  - • Autoimmune thyroid disease
  - • Mastocytosis
  - • Urticarial vasculitis

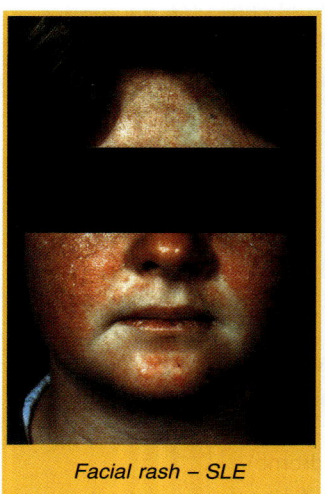

Facial rash – SLE

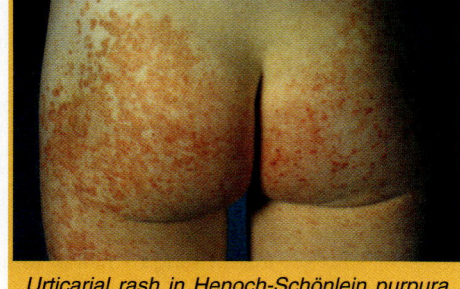

Urticarial rash in Henoch-Schönlein purpura

Key Objectives
- • Categorise skin problems by rash type, configuration and the distribution of the lesion.
- • Determine whether the condition is acute, chronic or a manifestation of a systemic illness based on lesion resolution, length of occurrence, and clinical picture.

General/Specific Objectives
- • Through efficient, focused data gathering:
  - - Elicit a detailed history and physical examination including timing of symptom onset, duration of lesions, identification of precipitants.
- • Interpret critical clinical and laboratory findings which were key in the processes of exclusion, differentiation, and diagnosis:
  - - Select patients in need of further investigation and specialised care.
- • Conduct an effective plan of management for a patient with a skin rash:
  - - Outline management for common skin conditions.
- • Select patients in need of specialised care.

102B Childhood Communicable Diseases with or without Skin Rash

Overview

Communicable diseases are common in childhood and vary from mild inconveniences to life-threatening disorders. Clinicians need to differentiate between these common conditions and initiate management specific to the cause.

Causes

1) Presenting with a rash

    a) Viral (measles, rubella, roseola, varicella, herpes zoster, herpes simplex, molluscum contagiosum ('water warts'))

    b) Bacterial (meningococcal septicaemia, scarlet fever, 'scalded skin' syndrome, impetigo, staphylococcal or streptococcal toxic shock syndrome)

    c) Other (mycoplasma infection)

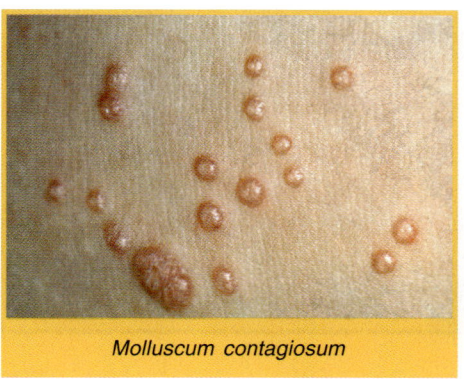

Molluscum contagiosum

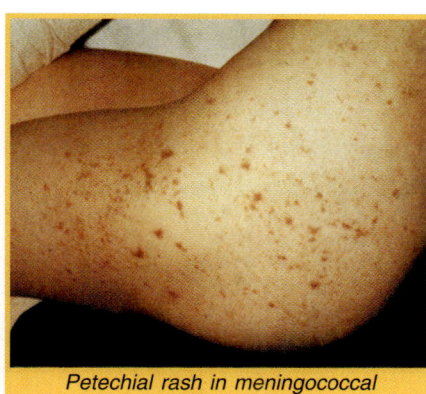

Petechial rash in meningococcal septicaemia

2) Presenting with sore throat

    a) Viral (infectious mononucleosis)

    b) Bacterial (diphtheria, streptococcal)

3) Presenting with diarrhoea

Key Objectives

- Recognise early those life-threatening presentations involving a skin rash.

- Describe the principles of immunisation procedures.

- Determine the incubation period and possible route of communication of the underlying disease.

- Outline measures of prevention to contain the spread of communicable disease.

General/Specific Objectives

- Through efficient, focused, data gathering:

    - Identify the presenting features of the rash, sore throat or diarrhoea; and identify and treat possible cases of meningococcal septicaemia and other life-threatening conditions.

    - Determine the immunisation status of the infants/children.

    - Determine history of contacts, travel, farm visits, ingestion of unpasteurised milk or uncooked meat, source of water supply.

    - When dealing with an infant, consider prenatal issues, especially maternal history of infection.

- Interpret critical clinical and laboratory findings which were key in the processes of exclusion, differentiation, and diagnosis:

    - Evaluate fully the individual and contacts of individuals with sexually transmitted diseases (STDs).

    - Describe rapid viral testing, stool tests, and viral serology.

- Conduct an effective initial plan of management for a patient with a childhood communicable disease:

    - Outline the procedure for immunisation and for immunising an incompletely immunised child.

    - Outline management of specific communicable diseases.

Overview
Speech disorders present in all age groups, central causes being more common in the elderly while non-neurological articulation disorders present more frequently in younger patients.

Causes

1) Receptive disorders (hearing/deafness)

2) Central disorders

   a) **Aphasia – speech apparatus intact**
     (see #050 Hemiplegia / Hemisensory Loss / Stroke with or without Aphasia / Prevention of Stroke)

   b) **Mental retardation**

3) Articulation disorder

   a) **Nasal / Badly articulated / Slurred speech**
- Soft palate with or without other muscles paralysis (myasthenia, multiple sclerosis)
- Bulbar/Pseudobulbar palsy (amyotrophic lateral sclerosis)
- Tongue paralysis / Macroglossia (cranial polyradiculitis, allergic oedema)

   b) **Disorders of speech rhythm/timing/audibility (Parkinson disease, multiple sclerosis, cerebellar lesions, dementia, etc.)**

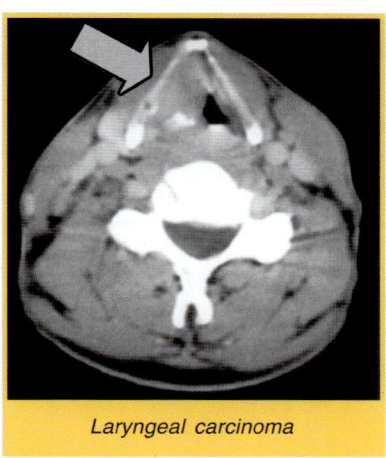

Laryngeal carcinoma

c) Speech apparatus lesions

❏ Hoarseness
   - Inflammation (infection, allergy, abuse/misuse, smoking, alcohol)
   - Neoplasms (laryngeal benign/malignant)
   - Recurrent nerve (thyroidectomy/parathyroidectomy, tumour)

❏ Stammer/Stutter

❏ Open nasal speech (soft palate paralysis, cleft palate)

❏ Dysphasic (in deafness)

d) Silent/Non-speaking (catatonia, depression, brainstem encephalitis, functional)

Key Objectives
- Determine whether the speech apparatus is intact and the speech disorder is centrally determined.
- Determine whether neurological deficits are present.

General/Specific Objectives
- Through efficient, focused data gathering:

   - Elicit information indicative of inflammation/infection, voice abuse or misuse, smoking or alcohol.
   - Determine whether there is dysphagia, cough, haemoptysis, or dyspnoea.
   - Conduct physical examination of head and neck.

- Interpret critical clinical and laboratory findings which were key in the processes of exclusion, differentiation, and diagnosis:

   - Select patients to receive routine investigations or in need for laryngoscopy referral.

- Conduct an effective plan of management for a patient with speech and language abnormalities:

   - Outline management plan for common causes of speech disorders (e.g. voice rest, fluids and humidity, anti-reflux therapy, no smoking).
   - Select patients in need of specialised care.

Overview

The most common spinal fractures are wedge crush fractures of vertebral bodies (osteoporosis, malignancies). Spinal cord injuries from trauma result from motor vehicle accidents (MVA), falls, sports-related trauma, or assault with weapons. The average age at the time of spinal injury is approximately 35 years, and men are four times more likely to be injured than are women. The sequelae of such events have a major impact on society in terms of the cost of rehabilitation and long term care, litigation and liability. Initial immobilisation and maintenance of ventilation are of critical importance.

Causes

1)	**Traumatic or pathological fractures/dislocations of the vertebral column**

2)	**Penetrating injury**

3)	**Acute disc rupture**

4)	**Ruptured arteriovenous malformation**

5)	**Spontaneous epidural haematoma**

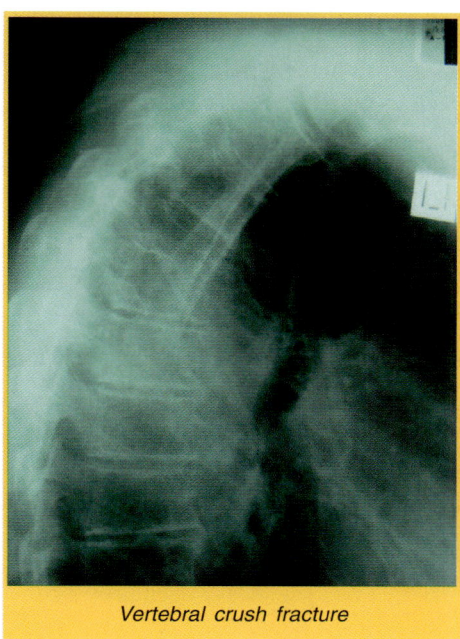

Vertebral crush fracture

Key Objectives

- Understand how to triage and manage patients with potential or actual acute spinal injury and make an appropriate examination of such patients.

- Provide an appropriate plan of management for the patient with acute spinal cord compression or transection.

- Contrast the impairment of ventilatory muscle strength in the case of complete or incomplete cervical spinal cord injury, and explain the effect of denervation of abdominal musculature.

- State that respiratory impairment and susceptibility to respiratory complications are greater with more cephalad injuries of the spinal cord.

General/Specific Objectives

- Through efficient, focused, data gathering:

  - Determine whether there is any impediment of respiratory function.

  - Elicit history about mechanism of injury and examine structures in the spine which have been damaged.

  - Perform examination of spine, motor power in arms and legs, sensation, superficial and deep tendon reflexes.

- Interpret critical clinical and laboratory findings which were key in the processes of exclusion, differentiation, and diagnosis:

  - Select diagnostic imaging for assessment of spinal stability.

  - Outline diagnostic imaging of the lungs in patients with spinal cord injury (e.g. upright films are often contraindicated).

- Conduct an effective plan of management for a patient with spinal injuries:

  - Conduct education of people at risk for prevention of spinal injuries (diving into shallow water, skiing out of control, injuries associated with rugby and Australian League football, cross-checking from behind in hockey, drinking and driving, etc.).

  - List indications for immobilisation; for bladder catheterisation.

  - Initiate and maintain 'spinal precautions' and 'log rolling' of patients; outline methods available for stabilising the spine.

  - List indications for steroid treatment; list analgesic drugs to use.

  - Counsel and support patient and family including access to rehabilitation programmes.

  - Select patients in need of specialised care.

Overview

A normal spleen is not palpable, so that a palpable spleen is virtually always indicative of an underlying problem unless it is confused with the left lobe of the liver or an enlarged left kidney.

Causes

1) Congestive – (liver cirrhosis, portal thrombosis)

2) Infective

    a) Viral – hepatitis, glandular fever (Epstein-Barr virus (EBV)), cytomegalovirus (CMV)

    b) Bacterial – bacterial endocarditis, brucellosis, septicaemia

    c) Protozoal – malaria, leishmaniasis

    d) Fungal – histoplasmosis

3) Neoplastic (chronic leukaemia, lymphoma, myeloproliferative disorders, myelofibrosis)

4) Associated with haemolysis (acquired and congenital haemolytic anaemia)

5) Inflammatory (Still disease, Felty syndrome)

6) Infiltrations – sarcoid, amyloid, lipid storage disorders

Key Objectives

- Perform an abdominal examination for splenomegaly and differentiate an enlarged spleen from the left kidney or left lobe of the liver.

- In a patient with splenomegaly, determine whether it is associated with hepatomegaly.

General/Specific Objectives

- Through efficient, focused, data gathering:

    - Determine whether stigmata of chronic liver disease, an infective process (e.g. fever, chills, lymphadenopathy, Osler nodes, etc.), weight loss, anaemia or jaundice are present in order to differentiate between causes of splenomegaly.

- Interpret critical clinical and laboratory findings which were key in the processes of exclusion, differentiation, and diagnosis; and important in formulating a differential diagnosis:

  - Select and interpret laboratory investigations for various causes of splenomegaly.

- Conduct an effective plan of management for a patient with splenomegaly:

  - Recognise that management depends on the underlying cause.

  - Select patients in need of specialised care.

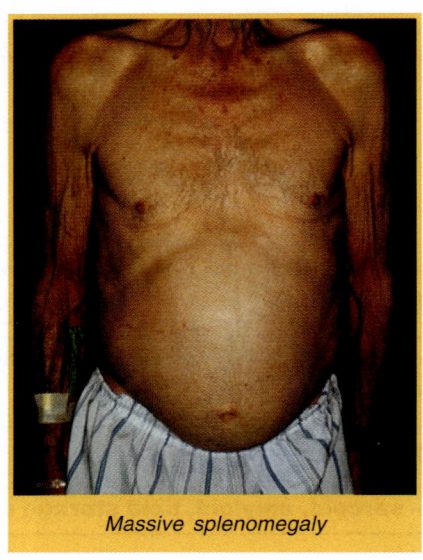

Massive splenomegaly

Overview

'Cross-eye', 'squint' or 'wandering eye' conditions are usually obvious and will often lead to early medical advice being sought. However, poor vision in one eye is often not noted until a much later stage when the possibility of significant visual impairment is high. Both types of presentations require specialist advice.

Causes

1) **Esotropia (convergent, internal, cross-eye) – congenital and acquired**

2) **Exotropia (divergent, external, wall-eye) – congenital and acquired**

3) **Vertical strabismus**

4) **Mechanical restriction**

5) **Convergence insufficiency**

6) **Amblyopia without strabismus**

Key Objectives
- Determine the type of strabismus and the necessary timing of intervention.
- Screening of infants for poor vision as early as possible when suspected.

General/Specific Objectives
- Through efficient, focused data gathering:
    - Identify relevant family history.
    - Differentiate pseudostrabismus (lid configuration or negative angle kappa or markedly positive angle kappa) from true strabismus.
    - Conduct an examination of visual acuity, ocular movement, and failure of alignment by the cover/uncover test.
    - Manage and reassure where appropriate.
- Select patients with true strabismus and/or amblyopia for specialised care.

107A Substance Abuse / Drug Addiction/Withdrawal

Overview
Alcohol and nicotine abuse are such common conditions that virtually every clinician is confronted with their complications.

Causes

1)	**Alcohol**
2)	**Nicotine**
3)	**Benzodiazepines, sedative-hypnotic, anxiolytic**
4)	**Opioids**
5)	**Cannabis**
6)	**Cocaine**
7)	**Hallucinogens**
8)	**Inhalants**
9)	**Amphetamines**
10)	**Performance drugs**

Key Objective
- Determine whether the patient is in need of emergency care because of withdrawal symptoms or other complications.

General/Specific Objectives
- Through efficient, focused data gathering:

    - Determine past and recent quantity and frequency of abuse, severity of abuse and dependence, readiness to change or denial, complications of use, family history, past treatment history, support network, and withdrawal symptoms; identify social problems such as assault and impaired driving.

    - Define limits of non-hazardous alcohol; differentiate social from problem drinking/dependence.

    - Examine for mental function, weight loss, route of administration, neurologic examination, signs of use.

- Interpret critical clinical and laboratory findings which were key in the processes of exclusion, differentiation, and diagnosis:
  - Select patients for toxicology screening, liver function if suspected of alcohol abuse and contrast sensitivity and specificity with 'CAGE' questions:
    * Have you felt the need to _**C**ut_ down on your drinking?
    * Have you felt _**A**nnoyed_ by criticism of drinking?
    * Have you felt _**G**uilty_ about your drinking?
    * Do you feel the need for an _**E**ye_ opener in the morning?
- Conduct an effective plan of management for a patient with substance abuse:
  - Outline spectrum of treatment options including mutual/self-help, low-intensity outpatient treatment, non-medical detoxification and residential treatment, medically supervised detoxification and intensive inpatient treatment.
  - Outline office counselling for mild to moderate alcohol dependence (reviewing assessment findings, set drinking goals, conduct of periodic followup).
  - Outline alcohol withdrawal management, indications and contraindications for disulfiram, and naltrexone, methadone; outline management of withdrawal from opioids and benzodiazepines.
  - Outline management for stopping nicotine including advice to quit, nicotine replacement therapy, setting quitting dates, behavioural counselling, information about community resources.
  - Discuss guidelines for safe prescription writing for benzodiazepines and opioids.
  - Outline management of cardiovascular complications of cocaine and alcohol.
  - Outline prevention, detection and management of infectious complications of intravenous (IV) drug use including hepatitis B, C, and HIV.
  - Select patients in need of specialised care.

107B   Pathological/Problem Gambling

Overview

Gambling is the act of staking money or some other item of value on the outcome of an event determined by chance. It is an accepted leisure pursuit enjoyed by the majority of adult Australians. Problem gambling may affect one to three percent of the adult population. Two-thirds of problem gamblers are men, who typically present in their thirties (women present later) and have problems with continuous forms of gambling such as poker machines (slots), off-course agency betting, casino or internet gaming or the stock market.

Problem gamblers are preoccupied with gambling and have needed to use increasing amounts of money or goods to continue. They have had repeated unsuccessful attempts to cut back, control or stop their gambling. They tend to gamble more when they are losing to chase their losses and then rely on others to provide the money to relieve the desperate financial situations created by their gambling. They gamble to escape personal or work problems or to relieve dysphoria, anxiety or depression. They frequently lie to conceal the extent of their gambling involvement, and many will have jeopardised or lost a significant relationship or career opportunity as a result. Many will have committed illegal acts such as forgery, fraud, theft or embezzlement to finance their gambling, and 20% will make a serious attempt at suicide. Bipolar patients may gamble excessively when in a manic phase. Problem gambling has a strong association with alcohol abuse and antisocial personality.

Key Objective

- Determine whether the pattern of gambling behaviour has disrupted the individual's personal, family or vocational pursuits and impaired social and occupational functioning.

General/Specific Objectives

Through efficient and focused data gathering:

- Elicit history and pattern of gambling behaviour from onset to the present.

- Clarify reasons for current presentation.

- Establish impact of gambling on spouse, family, work and social relationships.

- Identify individual triggers for problem gambling behaviour.

- Elicit associated illegal behaviours to maintain gambling behaviour.

- Recognise and treat comorbid psychiatric disorders, especially mood disorders, substance abuse, attention deficit hyperactivity disorder and personality disorders.

- Refer for appropriate financial and psychological counselling.

- Provide ongoing psychological support to the family.

Overview

Suicidality is a spectrum ranging from suicidal ideation to self-harm to completed suicide. Suicide is a conscious fatal self-destructive act, which although grievous, is relatively rare. Suicidal ideation and intent may fluctuate unpredictably over brief periods of time. Suicidal behaviour has no single cause but a conjunction of many biopsychosocial and cognitive factors. Hypofunction of brain serotonin systems may explain some suicidal behaviour.

About 2,000 Australians commit suicide each year and at least 20,000 deliberately harm themselves annually. Most people who commit suicide have visited a doctor (either clinician or psychiatrist) in the weeks prior to the act. Knowledge of the major risk and protective factors for self-harm, as well as the predisposing and precipitating events, is essential for appropriate early identification and management in primary care. Survivors, including health professionals, are left traumatised and with a confused spectrum of emotions.

Major Causal Risk Factors

1) Previous deliberate self-harm

   a) Organised plan

   b) Access to means

2) Psychiatric disorder

   a) Major depression

   b) Bipolar disorder

   c) Other disorders including dysthymia

   d) Substance abuse

   e) Schizophrenia / Schizoaffective disorder especially command hallucinations

   f) Personality disorder

   g) Panic/Anxiety disorder

   h) Organic mental disorders (delirium, anorexia nervosa)

3) Socio-cultural factors

These include:
Living alone; older age; male; unmarried/separated marital status; family history of suicide; physical illness – terminal disease, chronic pain, HIV-AIDS, chronic neurological disorders; rural versus urban – access to support networks; unemployed/unskilled; indigenous aboriginal Australians; recent or anniversary loss life event; environmental influences.

| 4) | Cognitions of hopelessness and helplessness |

| 5) | Previous history of violence and/or impulsivity |

| 6) | Recent disposal of assets and preparation of a legal will |

Key Objective

- Determine whether suicide or a self-harm attempt is likely by assessing risk factors for suicide and patient's mental state. Suicide prediction has a low degree of sensitivity and specificity.

General/Specific Objectives

- Through sensitive and comprehensive data gathering, which may include interviewing other informants:

    - Elicit history of risk factors, suicidal ideation and intent, content, duration, frequency, plan and rehearsal.

    - Determine current stress factors and recent life events.

    - Determine whether a support network is available and accessible.

    - Recognise that risk of self-harm is increased if the patient is depressed, psychotic or intoxicated and has established a plan with the means available.

- Interpret critical clinical and laboratory findings which were key in the processes of exclusion, differentiation, and diagnosis.

- Conduct an effective plan of management for a patient with suicidal ideation:

    - Outline immediate management of a patient at imminent risk for self-harm (e.g. local crisis psychiatric services, urgent or involuntary hospitalisation, specialist assessment). Patient safety is paramount and continuous observation is essential whilst arrangements are put in place.

    - Outline a contingency plan if a patient refuses to cooperate or demands to leave.

    - Outline management of a patient whose risk for suicide is chronic but not imminent.

    - Discuss appropriate medications for patients at risk of suicide who have a treatable psychiatric disorder.

    - Arrange for drug and alcohol counselling when appropriate.

    - Select patients in need of specialist assessment and treatment.

    - Inform and counsel family and friends.

Overview

Syncope is a transient, self-limiting loss of consciousness, usually leading to falling. Syncopal episodes are common, accounting for 3–5% of attendances at emergency departments and affecting 15–25% of the population over a 10-year period. The prevalence increases with age and syncope causes significant morbidity in the elderly. Clinicians are required to distinguish syncope from seizures; and to distinguish syncope caused by benign causes from syncope caused by serious underlying illness.

Causes

1) Neurally-medicated reflex syncopal syndromes

a) **Vasovagal/Vasodepressor syncope**

b) **Carotid sinus syncope**
   - ❏ Carotid sinus syndrome (elderly subjects with vascular disease)
   - ❏ Situational faint (serious consequences may follow when confined surroundings prevent falling)
   - ❏ Acute haemorrhage
   - ❏ Cough/Sneeze syncope
   - ❏ Gastrointestinal stimulation (defaecation, visceral pain)
   - ❏ Micturition
   - ❏ Post-exercise
   - ❏ Other (weightlifting, brass instrument playing, post-prandial)

c) **Glossopharyngeal and trigeminal neuralgia**

2) Orthostatic

a) **Volume depletion**
   - ❏ Haemorrhage
   - ❏ Diarrhoea
   - ❏ Addison disease

b) **Vasodilator drugs (nitrates, antihypertensives, diuretics, antidepressants)**

c) **Mechanical reduction of venous return**

d) **Autonomic failure**
   - ❏ Primary autonomic failure syndromes (pure autonomic failure, multiple system atrophy, Parkinson disease with autonomic failure)
   - ❏ Secondary autonomic failure syndromes (diabetic autonomic neuropathy, amyloid neuropathy)

3

Cardiac arrhythmia

    a) Sinus node dysfunction (including tachycardia/bradycardia syndrome)

    b) Atrioventricular conduction system disease

    c) Paroxysmal supraventricular tachycardia

    d) Paroxysmal ventricular tachycardia

    e) Inherited syndromes (long QT, Brugada syndromes)

    f) Implanted device malfunction (pacemaker, implantable cardiac defibrillator (ICD))

    g) Drug-induced (pro-arrhythmic drugs)

4) **Structural cardiac or cardiopulmonary disease**

    a) Cardiac valvular disease (aortic stenosis, mitral stenosis, pulmonary stenosis)

    b) Acute myocardial infarction (MI) / ischaemia

    c) Obstructive cardiomyopathy (hypertrophic cardiomyopathy)

    d) Atrial myxoma

    e) Acute aortic dissection

    f) Pericardial disease/tamponade

    g) Pulmonary embolism

    h) Pulmonary hypertension

    i) Inflow obstruction (to systemic circulation)

5) **Cerebrovascular causes**

    a) Vascular steal syndromes

Key Objectives
- Differentiate syncope from disturbances of cerebral function caused by a seizure.

- Determine the severity of the complaint and categorise syncope according to severity of underlying cause.

General/Specific Objectives
- Through efficient, focused data gathering:

    - Differentiate between cardiac and non-cardiac causes.

    - Determine volume status.

- Interpret critical clinical and laboratory findings which were key in the processes of exclusion, differentiation, and diagnosis:
    - Identify patients who require tilt table testing.
    - Diagnose disturbances of cardiac rhythm with the assistance of electrocardiography (ECG) and Holter monitoring.
    - Select laboratory investigations most useful in assessment of volume status and interpret the results.
- Conduct an effective plan of management for a patient with syncope / pre-syncope / loss of consciousness:
    - Outline the plan of initial management.
    - Select patients in need of specialised care and/or consultation.
    - List patients who may require cardiac pacing.
    - Evaluate patients for fitness to drive or work; be aware of Australian guidelines.
    - Conduct counselling for patients with syncope.

Overview

To define any growth point, children should be measured accurately and each point (height, weight, and head circumference) plotted. One of the more common causes of abnormal growth is mismeasurement or aberrant plotting.

Causes

1) Tall stature (children develop pituitary gigantism; adults are not taller, but have acromegaly)

a) **Excess growth hormone (GH)**
   - ❑ Pituitary adenoma (98%)
   - ❑ Extrapituitary tumour (very rare)

b) **Excess GH releasing hormone secretion / growth factor activity**

c) **Other (Klinefelter syndrome, precocious puberty)** – it should be remembered that children with precocious puberty are tall at an early age, but often finish up short due to premature bony fusion.

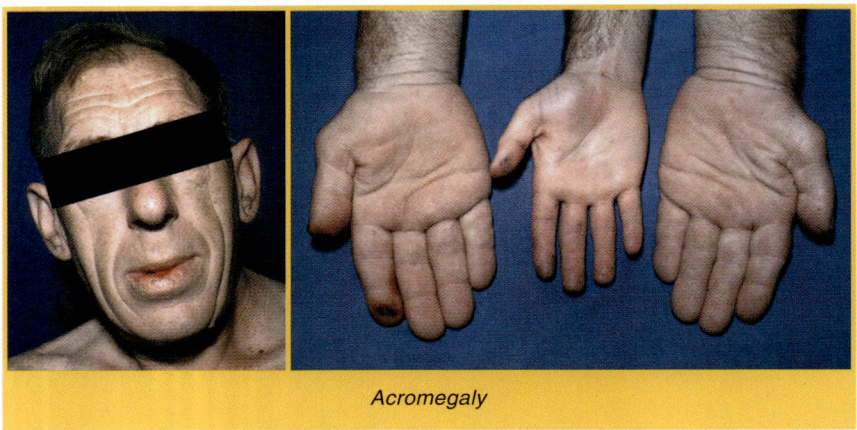

Acromegaly

2) Short stature

a) **Intrinsic shortness (familial, Turner syndrome)**

b) **Delayed growth (constitutional, under-nutrition, underlying disease)**

c) **Attenuated growth**
   - ❑ Chronic renal failure / Metabolic acidosis
   - ❑ Cancer / Chemotherapy / Glucocorticoid excess
   - ❑ Pulmonary/Cardiac/Gastrointestinal disease
   - ❑ Metabolic / Endocrine
     - • Vitamin D deficiency/resistance
     - • GH deficiency

- Hypothyroidism
- Cushing syndrome

❑ Intra-uterine growth retardation (IUGR) (see #123 Weight (Low) at Birth / Intra-uterine Growth Aberration)

d) Accelerated early growth, more accelerated epiphyseal closure (precocious puberty)

Key Objectives
- Determine whether growth progressively deviates from previously defined percentiles.
- Determine whether the child has dysmorphic features.

General/Specific Objectives
- Through efficient, focused data gathering:

  - Elicit history of uterine growth rate, intra-uterine infections, maternal exposure to toxins, smoking, alcohol, or systemic illness.

  - Determine the presence of underlying medical problems (e.g. rickets, hypothyroidism).

  - Calculate growth velocity, and relationship between chronological age, height age, and bone age.

  - In a patient with tall stature, determine the presence of soft tissue overgrowth (macrognathia, swollen hands and feet, nose, frontal ridges).

  - Elicit information about joint symptoms (hypertrophic arthropathy), headaches, visual problems.

  - Determine whether there is hypertension, left ventricular hypertrophy (LVH), cardiomyopathy, cancer (gastrointestinal).

- Interpret critical clinical and laboratory findings which were key in the processes of exclusion, differentiation, and diagnosis:

  - Select diagnostic imaging for bone age and for diagnosis of causes of altered growth.

  - Screen for hormone disorders (particularly GH, thyroxine, corticosteroid) and chromosomal abnormalities.

- Conduct an effective plan of management for a patient with abnormal growth:

  - Counsel families and children with abnormal stature.

  - Select patients in need of specialised care.

Overview

Although tinnitus is mostly harmless it is annoying and difficult to treat. The cause of tinnitus in the vast majority of patients is idiopathic; in some it may be indicative of a serious organic cause which may be reversible. A pulse-related auditory perception suggests a vascular cause.

Causes

1) Auditory

a) **Associated with sensorineural hearing loss**
- ❏ Presbycusis
- ❏ Noise-associated
- ❏ Ménière disease
- ❏ Neoplasms (acoustic neuroma, cerebellopontine tumour)

b) **Drug-related**
- ❏ Aspirin
- ❏ Aminoglycosides
- ❏ Other (chemotherapy, digitalis, quinidine)

c) **Idiopathic**

2) Para-auditory

a) **Pulse-synchronous**
- ❏ Vascular (carotid bruits, hyperdynamic states, aneurysm, venous hum)
- ❏ Glomus tumour

b) **Non-pulse synchronous (temporomandibular joint (TMJ) dysfunction, palatal myoclonus)**

3) Psychogenic (anxiety, depression)

Key Objective
- Recognise that any condition of the ear associated with the ear canal (wax, otitis media), cochlear hearing loss, or central nervous system (CNS) hearing loss can cause tinnitus and the underlying cause must be identified.

General/Specific Objectives

- Through efficient, focused data gathering:

  - Determine whether or not the tinnitus is related to an ear condition or hearing loss.

  - Determine whether the tinnitus is pulsatile or non-pulsatile (vascular causes tend to be pulsatile).

  - Determine whether tinnitus is unilateral or bilateral.

  - Differentiate between drug-related causes, disease-related causes, and tinnitus caused by noise.

- Interpret critical clinical and laboratory findings which were key in the processes of exclusion, differentiation, and diagnosis:

  - Select patients for further investigation based on clinical findings.

- Conduct an effective plan of management for a patient with tinnitus:

  - Select patients in need of specialised care.

  - Identify and counsel patients with causes of tinnitus which are benign.

112 Torticollis

(See #057 Involuntary Movement Disorders / Tic Disorders)

Overview

Trauma is the third most common cause of death worldwide – after cardiovascular disease and cancer. Trauma is the leading cause of death in the age group under 45 years. Deaths from road accidents account for half of all trauma deaths in Australia. Factors involved in motor vehicle deaths include speeding and alcohol; young males contribute most significantly to this mortality. Additional costly morbidity results from non-fatal road crash trauma.

Intense public awareness campaigns aim to decrease the hazards caused from alcohol and other drugs, speeding, fatigue and lack of restraints.

Management principles in traumatised patients are to:

- Check and rapidly restore vital functions (primary survey).
- Diagnose and manage the type and severity of specific injuries (secondary survey).
- Complete rehabilitation after injury.

The level of care is matched to the patient's needs by effective triage.

Causes

Wounds and injuries range from trivial to catastrophic and wounding may be accidental or intentional.

Major categories are:

1) Blunt trauma

a) **Vehicle crash injuries**

b) **Closed bony and soft-tissue trauma from domestic, occupational, sporting and other injuries**

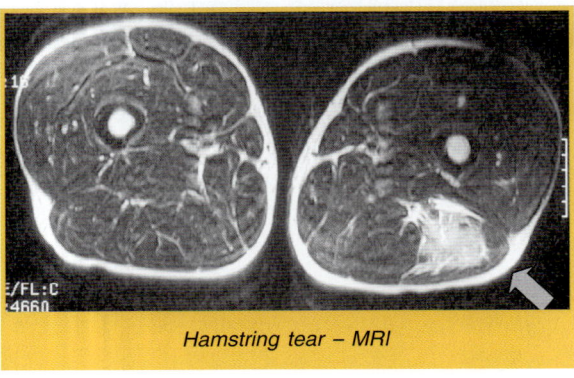

Hamstring tear – MRI

a) Knives

b) Bullets

c) Lacerations and wounds from other causes

Key Objectives

- Match management to type and degree of trauma injury by efficient triage.

- Conduct an efficient primary and secondary survey of all traumatised patients in accord with emergency management of severe trauma (EMST) guidelines.

General/Specific Objectives

- Recognise and conduct an effective initial management plan for the acutely traumatised patient.

- Conduct an effective and rapid primary survey ('ABCDE'):

  - *Airway* – establish patency and adequacy.

  - *Breathing* – check and evaluate breathing (look, feel, listen).

  - *Circulation* – assess for shock, control external bleeding, establish intravenous access.

  - *Disability* – assess neurologic status, record Glasgow Coma Scale.

  - *Exposure* with temperature control – complete exposure and examination which leads into secondary survey.

- Conduct an effective and rapid secondary survey through appropriately focused data collection, while maintaining observations and imaging relevant to primary survey:

  - Head and scalp.

  - Neck.

  - Thorax.

  - Abdomen and perineum.

  - Spine and extremities.

- Use appropriate diagnostic and management aids and adjuncts to primary and secondary surveys appropriate to the type and degree of injury, including:

  - Cardiopulmonary resuscitation (CPR), oxygenation, chin-lift and jaw thrust, endotracheal intubation, cricothyroidotomy, needle and tube thoracentesis, pericardiocentesis, tetanus prophylaxis, blood and urine testing including blood cross match, intravenous access, urinary catheterisation, pulse oximetry, plain X-ray, computed tomography (CT) scan, contrast radiology.

113A   Abdominal Injuries

Overview

Most abdominal injuries in Australia are blunt injuries associated with road crash trauma. Penetrating injuries (e.g. knives, handguns) will usually require surgical intervention. High velocity gunshot wounds are relatively uncommon but carry a higher mortality and morbidity.

Causes

(see #113 Trauma/Accidents/Prevention)

| 1) | **Blunt trauma** |
| 2) | **Penetrating trauma** |

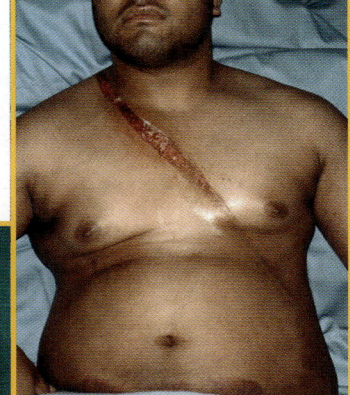

Traumatic laceration of spleen

Key Objective

- Determine which injuries require surgical intervention and active resuscitation.

General/Specific Objectives

- Through efficient, focused data gathering:

  - See #113 Trauma/Accidents/Prevention for initial assessment and resuscitative measures.

  - Determine whether significant blunt or penetrating abdominal injury exists.

- Be aware of further investigations which may be required in management (e.g. computed tomography (CT) scan).

- Interpret critical clinical and laboratory findings which were key in the processes of exclusion, differentiation, and diagnosis.

- Conduct an effective initial plan of management for a patient with abdominal trauma:

  - Outline the principles of management of abdominal trauma.

  - List indications for surgical consultation.

113B   Bone and Joint Injuries

(See also #041 Fractures / Dislocations)

Overview

Major fractures are often associated with other injuries, and priorities must be set for each patient. Control of internal haemorrhage from a ruptured spleen takes precedence over fracture management, but severely injured patients with open fractures should have their fractures dealt with as soon as possible after admission to hospital, if necessary by a combined specialty team. Management of many soft-tissue injuries is facilitated by initial stabilisation of the bone or joint injuries.

Healing of fractures can be expected if the fragments have an adequate blood supply, if the bone surfaces are apposed without soft tissue interposition and if immobilisation of the fracture is adequate. Defective local conditions are far more potent sources of delayed union than are systemic or host factors.

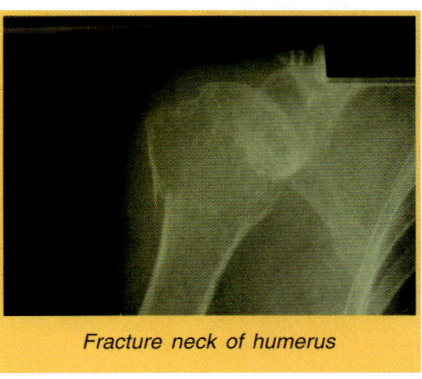

Fracture neck of humerus

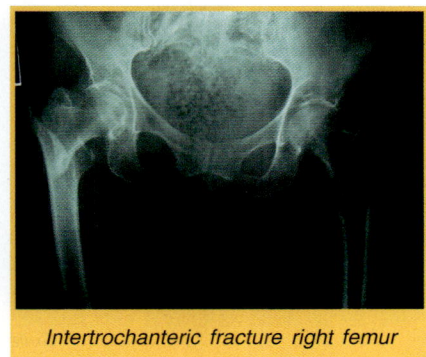

Intertrochanteric fracture right femur

Causes

1)   Varieties of bony injuries

   a) **Complete/Incomplete ('greenstick') fractures**

   b) **Open/Closed injuries**

   c) **Displaced/Undisplaced/Stable/Unstable fractures**

2) Mechanisms of injury

   a) Direct violence (transverse, oblique, 'butterfly', comminuted fractures)

   b) Indirect violence (spiral, compression, avulsion fractures)

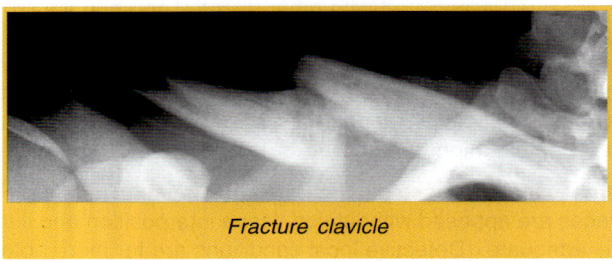

Fracture clavicle

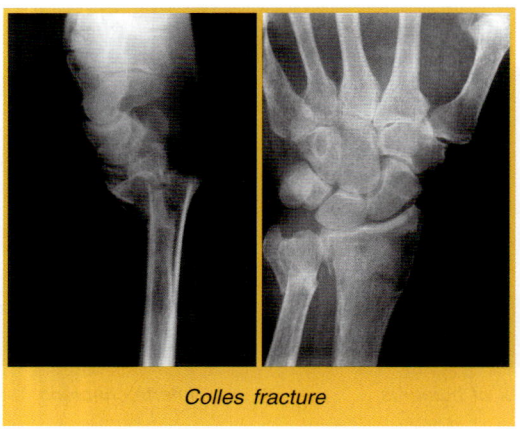

Colles fracture

Key Objectives

- Recognise principles of management as fracture/dislocation **reduction** with restoration of normal alignment and length, **retention** until healing occurs, rapid **restoration** of function, and effective **rehabilitation**.

- Recognition that methods of management used vary according to circumstances between: no immobilisation except a supportive sling, closed reduction and plaster cast immobilisation; closed reduction and continuous traction; external skeletal fixation devices; operative reduction and internal fixation.

113C   Burn Injuries

(See #018 Burns)

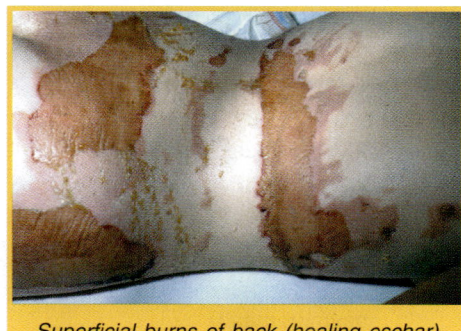

Superficial burns of back (healing eschar)

113D Chest Injuries

Overview

Injury to the chest may be blunt (e.g. motor vehicle trauma, falls, blast and crush injuries) or sharp (knife or bullet). Management of open sucking wounds and of pneumothorax will often need urgent intervention to maintain breathing and adequate oxygenation. Imaging and other diagnostic investigations may need to be delayed until the patient has been resuscitated and stabilised.

Causes

1)   Chest wall / Lung

(see #032B Dyspnoea and/or Cough / Prevention of Cancers and Chronic Respiratory Disese: With Pleural Chest X-Ray Abnormality)

a) **Flail chest**

b) **Haemothorax**

c) **Pneumothorax (open, closed)**

d) **Rib fracture**

2)   Heart injury

a) **Pericardial trauma (pericarditis, acute/delayed tamponade, constrictive pericarditis)**

b) **Myocardial trauma (contusion, coronary vessel injury, traumatic valve injury)**

c) **Aortic rupture**

Key Objective
- Appreciate that patients with chest injuries frequently present with shock or with respiratory compromise. Diagnosis and appropriate emergency treatment depends on suspicion and diagnostic acumen.

General/Specific Objectives
- Through efficient, focused data gathering:

  - Differentiate between hypotension / shock from bleeding and from tamponade.

  - Appreciate that aortic rupture may be present (chest or mid-scapular pain, dyspnoea, hoarseness, dysphagia) although it may be asymptomatic.

  - In patients with lung contusion after blunt injury to the chest, or massive traumatic tissue injury, examine lungs for oedema from acute respiratory distress syndrome.

- Interpret critical clinical and laboratory findings which were key in the processes of exclusion, differentiation, and diagnosis:

  - Select diagnostic imaging of the chest as indispensable for accurate diagnosis.

- Conduct an effective initial plan of management for a patient with chest trauma:

  - Select patients in need of specialised care in an intensive care unit (ICU).

113E Cold Injuries

(See #040D Hypothermia)

113F Eye Injuries

(See also #120 Visual Disturbance/Loss)

Overview
Eye injuries are common. Fortunately the blink reflex and Bell reflex (turning the eyes upward when the lids close) usually protect the globe from blunt trauma. Emergency assessment should check systematically vision, orbital surrounds, lids and eyebrows, and ocular movements. The globe is assessed for lacerating/abrading injury and foreign bodies inspecting sclera/conjunctiva, cornea, pupil size, shape and reaction, iris, and anterior and posterior chambers by direct ophthalmoscopy. Chemical eye burns will require immediate and copious aqueous irrigation. Most uncomplicated 'black eye' injuries will resolve spontaneously with cold compresses. Restricted eye mobility may indicate entrapment of extraocular muscles in a blowout fracture requiring surgery. Penetrating eye injuries require immediate specialist referral.

Causes

1)	**Blunt trauma**

2)	**Burn injuries**

3)	**Penetrating trauma**

Key Objectives
- Ability to assess from history and examination the result of injury, checking systematically vision, orbital surrounds, lids and eyebrows, and ocular movements.
- Ability to recognise serious injuries threatening sight.

113G   Facial Injuries

Overview

Facial injuries are potentially life-threatening because of possible damage to the airway and central nervous system (CNS).

Causes

1)	**Blunt injuries**

2)	**Penetrating (open) injuries**

Key Objective

- Assess and control vital functions and give management priority to life-threatening injuries. Definitive treatment of the facial injury is relatively less urgent, but of major cosmetic importance.

General/Specific Objectives

- Through efficient, focused data gathering:

  - Elicit a history about the nature of the injury.

  - Evaluate airway, cardiopulmonary and neurologic status.

- Interpret critical clinical and laboratory findings which were key in the processes of exclusion, differentiation, and diagnosis:

  - List the most appropriate investigations used to determine the nature and severity of facial injuries.

- Conduct an effective initial plan of management for a patient with facial injury:

  - Outline the priorities in the management of a patient with a facial injury.

  - Outline and provide the initial management of patients with facial injuries.

  - List indications for specialised care.

113H   Hand/Wrist Injuries

Overview
Hand and wrist injuries are common problems presenting to emergency departments. The ultimate function of the hand depends upon the quality of the initial care and the severity of the original injury.

Causes
Hand injuries commonly follow injuries associated with occupational, domestic, sporting and other recreational activities.

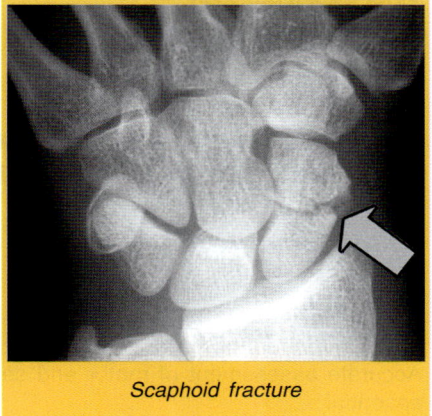

Scaphoid fracture

Key Objective
- Demonstrate the assessment of the nature and extent of hand injuries.

General/Specific Objectives
- Through efficient, focused data gathering:
    - Appreciate the differing mechanisms of injury.
    - Appreciate the distinction between 'tidy' and 'untidy' hand injuries.
    - Elicit history of antecedent trauma and type, and assess the nature and extent of injury. Diagnose damage to tendons, nerves, bones and joints, skin and soft tissues.
    - Determine active and passive range of motion, inspect and palpate joints for deformity, and differentiate between radial, ulnar, and median nerve sensory and motor deficit.
- Interpret critical clinical and laboratory findings which were key in the processes of exclusion, differentiation, and diagnosis:
    - Select patients whose trauma suggests risk of fractures for radiographs of the affected bones and joints.
- Conduct an effective initial plan of management for a patient with a hand injury:
    - Outline initial management for injuries of the hand/wrist.
    - Select patients in need of splints, conservative management, referral for occupational or physiotherapy, or surgery.

113I   Head Injuries

(See #045 Head Injuries / Brain Death / Transplant Donation and #104 Spinal Injuries)

113J Nerve Injuries

Overview

As a component of major injury, damage to peripheral nerves may go unrecognised. Accurate assessment of motor and sensory function of a limb involved in injury is essential.

Causes

1)	Compression/Stretch

2)	Contusion

3)	Laceration/Division

Key Objective

- Identify the peripheral nerve involved, the level and type of involvement.

General/Specific Objectives

- Through efficient, focused data gathering:

    - Elicit and interpret information from the history and physical examination to distinguish a peripheral nerve injury from other non-traumatic neuropathies or central lesions.

- Interpret critical clinical and laboratory findings which were key in the processes of exclusion, differentiation, and diagnosis:

    - Differentiate between injuries causing neurapraxia, axonotmesis, and neurotmesis.

    - Outline the methods used to diagnose the presence of a traumatic peripheral neuropathy.

- Conduct an effective initial plan of management for a patient with nerve injury:

    - List indications for specialised care.

113K   Skin Injuries

Overview

Wounds are open injuries of tissue. The morbidity associated with skin wounds is determined by the severity and site of the injury and the overall state of health of the patient. Severity of skin wounds depends on the extent of penetrating and disrupting skin and soft tissue injury, and of the degree and duration of bacterial contamination prior to treatment. Many skin and subcutaneous wounds are superficial and can be repaired under local anaesthesia. Differentiation between 'tidy' and 'untidy' wounds is crucial to management.

Causes

1)   **'Tidy' wounds (e.g. sharply-incised and penetrating wounds, damage restricted to wound path, contamination minimal and brief)**

2)   **'Untidy' wounds (e.g. lacerations, high-velocity missile wounds, widespread tissue damage, contamination severe and prolonged). Examples include avulsions, bites and crush injuries as well as gunshot and missile wounds**

Key Objectives
- Prior to wound closure, examine all patients thoroughly for evidence for injuries involving important underlying structures (tendon, nerve, vessel).

- Appreciate principles of adequate wound debridement for traumatic wounds.

- Appreciate principles of infection prophylaxis, including recognition and treatment of tetanus-prone wounds.

General/Specific Objectives
- Through efficient, focused data gathering:

  - Elicit and interpret information from history and physical examination to determine the nature and severity of the skin wound, time since injury (more than 24 hours or less than 24 hours), presence of infection.

  - In all cases of human bites, elicit information about HIV status, hepatitis status.

- Interpret critical clinical and laboratory findings which were key in the processes of exclusion, differentiation, and diagnosis:

  - Select patients whose HIV and hepatitis status requires investigation.

- Conduct an effective initial plan of management for a patient with skin injury:

  - Provide definitive care of superficial wounds involving the skin and subcutaneous tissues.

  - Identify wounds that require specialised care; list indications for specialised care.

  - Discuss prophylaxis to prevent infection.

  - Outline principles of wound management.

  - List indications and contraindications of primary versus delayed closure.

  - Select the appropriate suture material and closure technique.

  - Outline management of a human bite if the assailant is HIV/hepatitis positive; if the puncture is caused by a syringe needle or contaminated knife.

113L Spinal Injuries

(See #104 Spinal Injuries)

113M Urinary Tract Injuries

Overview
Closed injuries of the urinary tract are more common than penetrating injuries. Injuries are classified into kidney injuries, ureteric injuries, and bladder and urethral injuries.

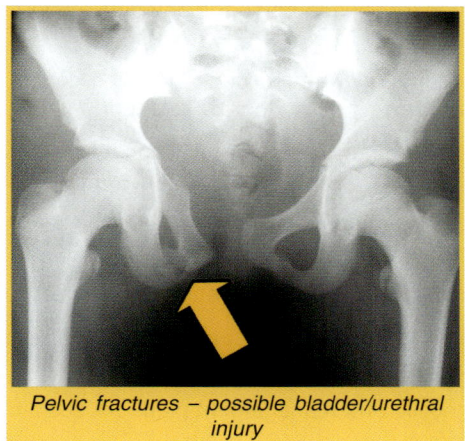

Pelvic fractures – possible bladder/urethral injury

Causes

1) Kidney injuries – associated rib fractures are common from motor vehicle injuries, falls, sporting injuries and blows

2) Ureteric injuries (surgical division or injury)

3) Bladder and urethra

   a) **Bladder and posterior (prostatomembranous) urethra – associated with pelvic fracture or abdominal injury. Full bladder at time of injury increases risk of intraperitoneal or extraperitoneal bladder rupture**

   b) **Anterior urethra – associated with falls astride, kicks to perineum and instrumental damage**

Key Objectives
- Early recognition and treatment of kidney injuries aided by urine examination and imaging.

- Rupture of bladder or posterior urethra must always be suspected in patients with pelvic fractures.

- Recognition that bleeding occurring at the external urethral meatus after injury is the cardinal sign of urethral injury and requires urgent ascending urethrography.

  - Select computed tomography (CT) scanning with intravenous contrast as appropriate investigation for renal injury.

  - Identify patients with renal injury requiring early angiography imaging.

  - Select ascending urethrogram as appropriate initial investigation for urethral injury.

  - Outline diagnostic and management plans for suspected urinary injury.

General/Specific Objectives

- Through efficient, focused data gathering:

  - Recognise urinary injuries early and categorise into renal, ureteric or urethral injuries.

  - Recognise haematuria (macroscopic or microscopic), bleeding from urethral meatus and inability to void as important diagnostic features.

- Interpret critical clinical and laboratory findings which were key in the processes of exclusion, differentiation, and diagnosis:

- Select computed tomography (CT) scanning with intravenous contrast as appropriate investigation for renal injury.

  - Identify patients with renal injury requiring early angiography imaging.

  - Select ascending urethrogram as appropriate initial investigation for urethral injury.

  - Outline diagnostic and management plans for suspected urinary injury.

113N   Vascular Injuries

Overview

Vascular injuries of blunt trauma often involve vessels near joints (e.g. knee, elbow) where vessels are relatively fixed and vulnerable to the shearing forces of fractures and dislocations. Complete or partial transection of the vessel can result in significant local haematoma; alternatively, thrombosis may be due to intimal rupture and elastic recoil without significant blood loss. Penetrating vascular injuries result usually from stab, gunshot or other missile wounds and are more likely to involve segmental loss of artery and vein, especially with high-velocity missile injuries. Although haemorrhage, haematoma, a pulse deficit and distal ischaemia are cardinal signs of vascular injury, a high index of suspicion is required as, in nearly one-third of patients with penetrating arterial injuries of limbs, signs of distal ischaemia are absent and distal pulses are palpable.

Common Causes of Vascular Injury

1)   Closed injury (e.g. motor vehicle accidents (MVA))

a) Head and neck injuries (epidural haemorrhage, carotid occlusion)

b) Supracondylar humeral fracture, fracture/dislocation of the elbow (brachial artery occlusion)

c) Fractured pelvis (major iliac venous and arterial bleeding)

d) Closed chest injuries (aortic tear)

e) Supracondylar femoral fracture, dislocated knee (popliteal artery occlusion)

f) Hyperextension lumbar spine injuries (renal arteries)

2)   Open injury (penetrating knife or gunshot wounds of neck, abdomen, groin, iatrogenic injury)

Key Objectives
- Diagnose major vascular injuries early by appropriate assessment and high index of suspicion.
- Provide initial management and obtain consultation when indicated.
- Classify whether injury is occlusive or haemorrhagic with open vessel.

- Through efficient, focused data gathering:

  - Elicit and interpret information from the history and physical examination to diagnose an arterial injury.

  - Elicit and interpret information from the history and physical examination to diagnose compartment syndromes.

- Interpret critical clinical and laboratory findings (ultrasound, imaging with and without contrast, haematology and biochemistry) which were key in the processes of exclusion, differentiation, and diagnosis:

  - List the most appropriate investigations used in the diagnosis of vascular injury.

- Conduct an effective and rapid initial plan of management for a patient with vascular injury:

  - List risks in the use of tourniquets and clamps.

  - Outline the initial management of arterial injuries.

  - List indications for specialised care.

114A Urinary Frequency: Associated with 'Dysuria and/ or Pyuria / Urethral Discharge'

Overview

Patients with urinary tract infections (UTIs), especially the very young and the very old, may present in an atypical manner. Appropriate diagnosis and management may prevent significant morbidity. Dysuria can mean either pain on micturition or difficulty with micturition. Pain usually implies infection and difficulty is usually related to mechanical obstruction at some point distal to the bladder neck, most commonly from prostatic enlargement.

Causes

1)	Urinary frequency (volume greater than 2 ml/minute)

2)	Urinary frequency (normal or decreased volume) associated with dysuria and/or pyuria

a) **External to urinary tract (infectious vulvovaginitis, colovesical fistula)**

b) **Irritable bladder (psychogenic)**

c) **Urinary tract involved**

- ❏ Urethritis (e.g. gonococci, acute urethra syndrome, *Trichomonas*)
- ❏ Prostatitis
- ❏ UTIs
  - Cystitis
  - Pyelonephritis

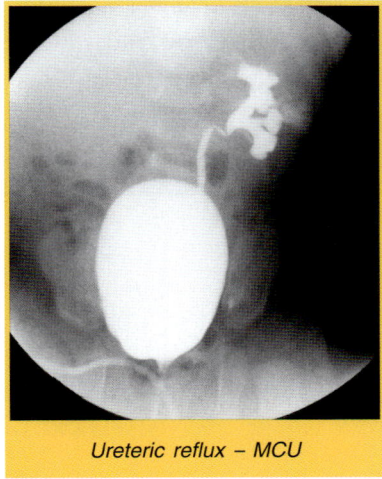

Ureteric reflux – MCU

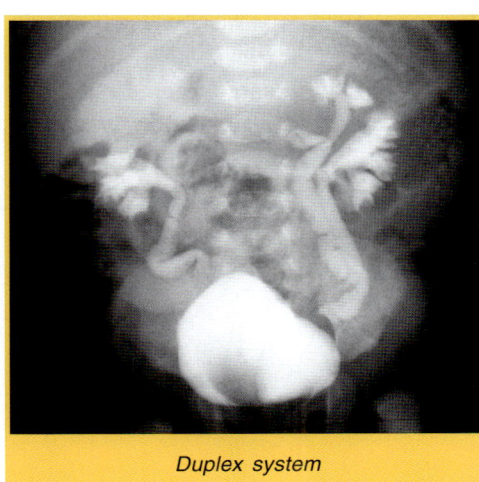

Duplex system

Key Objectives

- Differentiate between UTIs and conditions outside the urinary tract with similar presentation; determine which infections require treatment, and select the appropriate treatment.

- Consider factors predisposing to infection in patient with recurring UTIs (obstruction and stasis, calculi, reflux).

General/Specific Objectives

- Through efficient, focused data gathering:

    - Interpret urinalysis and clinical findings in order to diagnose problems external to urinary tract.

    - Evaluate examination findings so that problems involving the urethra or prostate are identified.

    - Determine whether cystitis or pyelonephritis is the more likely diagnosis.

- Interpret critical clinical and laboratory findings which were key in the processes of exclusion, differentiation, and diagnosis:

    - Outline significance of patient's age, gender, and lifestyle on diagnostic possibilities.

    - State or select findings which are best for differentiating cystitis from pyelonephritis.

    - Describe the collection of samples to be sent for culture and sensitivity; state their interpretation.

- Conduct an effective plan of management for a patient with urinary frequency associated with dysuria and/or pyuria:

    - Determine which patients require additional investigation and/or referral.

    - Determine which patients require hospitalisation.

    - Determine which patients should be on prophylactic treatment and the type of treatment.

    - Select the most appropriate treatment for the underlying condition.

    - List conditions which predispose to UTIs.

    - Outline strategies for prevention of recurrent UTIs.

114B   Urinary Frequency: Associated with 'Polyuria/ Polydipsia'

Overview
Urinary frequency, a common complaint, can be confused with polyuria, a less common, but important complaint. Diabetes mellitus is a common disorder with morbidity and mortality that can be reduced by preventive measures. Intensive glycaemic control during pregnancy will reduce neonatal complications.

Causes

1)   Urinary frequency (volume greater than 2 ml/minute)

a) **Water diuresis**
- ❑ Polydipsia
- ❑ Diabetes insipidus (central or nephrogenic)

b) **Osmotic diuresis**
- ❑ Diabetes mellitus
- ❑ Chronic renal disease

2)   Urinary frequency (normal or decreased volume) associated with dysuria and/or pyuria

Note: Decreased bladder capacity may produce no symptoms apart from urinary frequency.

Key Objective
- Evaluate diabetic patients and determine whether diabetic ketoacidosis or hypoglycaemia is present; formulate a management plan for diabetic emergencies.

General/Specific Objectives
(see #053 Hyperglycaemia / Diabetes Mellitus)

- Through efficient, focused data gathering:
  - Differentiate urinary frequency from polyuria.
  - Contrast water diuresis and osmotic diuresis.

- Interpret critical clinical and laboratory findings which were key in the processes of exclusion, differentiation, and diagnosis:
  - Select and interpret laboratory tests which distinguish between water and osmotic diuresis.

- Conduct an effective plan of management for a patient with polyuria/ polydipsia:
  - Select patients in need of specialised care.

115A Urinary Incontinence, Paediatric Enuresis

Overview

Enuresis is the involuntary passage of urine into bedclothes or undergarments. At least 90% of presenting children will have primary nocturnal enuresis. Diurnal and secondary enuresis is much less common, but requires differentiating between underlying organic diseases and stress-related conditions.

Causes

1) Primary enuresis

    a) Idiopathic/Familial

    b) Anatomic abnormality

2) Secondary enuresis

    a) Urinary tract infection (UTI)

    b) Diabetes mellitus/insipidus / Primary polydipsia

    c) Neurologic disorder

    d) Psychogenic / Stress

Key Objective

- In a child five years of age or older, determine whether a physical abnormality is causing the involuntary passage of urine.

General/Specific Objectives

- Through efficient, focused, data gathering:
  - Determine whether medical reasons underlie the enuresis.
  - Determine whether a stressful event preceded the occurrence of enuresis.
- Interpret critical clinical and laboratory findings which were key in the processes of exclusion, differentiation, and diagnosis:
  - Select patients who require investigation.
- Conduct an effective plan of management for a patient with acute enuresis:
  - Counsel, educate and reassure the parents of a child with primary nocturnal enuresis.
  - In a child with primary enuresis, discuss treatment options including family education and observation of the problem, reward systems, behavioural strategies, conditioning alarm system, medication (1-desamino-8D-arginine vasopressin (DDAVP), imipramine).
  - In a child with secondary enuresis, outline a management plan to treat the underlying cause.

115B Urinary Incontinence, Elderly

Overview
Because there is increasing incidence of involuntary micturition with age, incontinence will increase in frequency as our population continues to age.

Causes

1) Stress incontinence

- a) Women after the menopause when oestrogen deficient (especially multiparae)
- b) Post hysterectomy / Prostatectomy
- c) Bladder tumour

2) Urgency incontinence

- a) Cystitis, urethritis
- b) Vesical polyps, carcinoma, stones
- c) Psychogenic
- d) Dementia

3) Reflex incontinence

- a) Spinal transverse paralysis above T12
- b) Spinal tumour
- c) Syringomyelia

4) Overflow incontinence

- a) Prostatic obstruction
- b) Urethral stricture
- c) Diabetes mellitus
- d) Multiple sclerosis

5) True incontinence – urinary fistulas (including postoperative)

Key Objective
- Contrast between the two most common causes of incontinence, **stress incontinence** and **urgency incontinence** (insufficient sphincter closure in stress incontinence versus excessive detrusor contraction with urgency).

General/Specific Objectives

- Through efficient, focused data gathering:

    - Differentiate between stress, urgency, reflex, and overflow and true incontinence, especially in the female.

    - Perform a pelvic examination and rectal examination for prostate size in the male.

- Interpret critical clinical and laboratory findings which were key in the processes of exclusion, differentiation, and diagnosis:

    - Perform urinalysis.

    - Select patients in need of cystoscopy and other specialised tests such as urodynamic studies.

- Conduct an effective plan of management for an elderly patient with urinary incontinence:

    - Outline a plan of management for cystitis and urethritis.

    - Counsel patients with stress incontinence / urge incontinence.

    - Select patients in need of referral for urodynamic studies, physiotherapy or surgical treatment.

Overview

Urinary tract obstruction, either upper or lower tract, is a relatively common problem. The obstruction may be complete or incomplete. The most common cause in an elderly male is prostatomegalic. Obstruction may be unilateral in the upper tract and asymptomatic. The consequences of the obstruction depend on its onset, nature and overall renal function.

Prostate cancer is usually found in older men (median age at diagnosis is 71 years). One in ten Australian males may develop prostatic cancer at some stage of life; as the growth pattern is usually slow, perhaps one in 50 males will die from, rather than with, prostatic cancer.

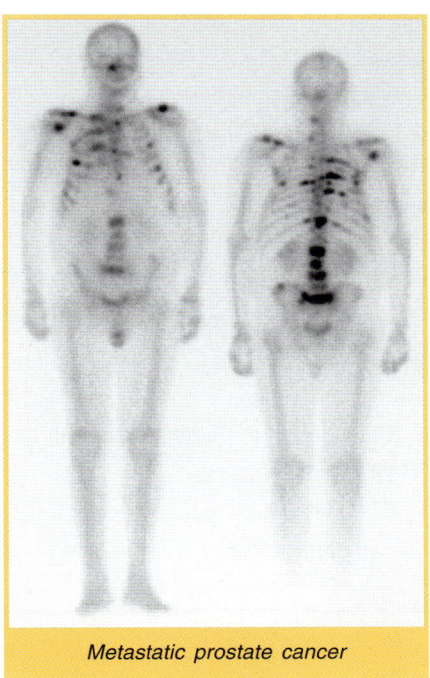

Metastatic prostate cancer

Causes

1) Child (anatomic abnormalities)

a) Urethra (stricture, valve)

b) Junctions (ureterovesical, ureteropelvic)

2) Adult (calculi)

   a) **Prostatomegaly**
      (benign hyperplasia, cancer)

   b) **Calculi**

   c) **Retroperitoneal neoplasm**

   d) **Pelvic neoplasm**

Key Objectives

- Determine the site and duration of the obstruction.

- Determine when acute obstruction requires urgent management.

General/Specific Objectives

- Through efficient, focused data gathering:

  - Determine whether the obstruction is acute or chronic, complete or partial, and unilateral or bilateral.

- Interpret critical clinical and laboratory findings which were key in the processes of exclusion, differentiation, and diagnosis:

  - Select ultrasonography as the diagnostic imaging tool to diagnose obstruction.

  - List indications for other types of diagnostic imaging.

  - Select and interpret tests of renal function.

- Conduct an effective plan of management for a patient with urinary tract obstruction:

  - Perform catheterisation of the bladder for both therapeutic and diagnostic reasons.

  - Select patients for referral to specialised care.

- Discuss methods, advantages and disadvantages of screening for prostatic cancer.

Overview

Vaginal bleeding is considered abnormal when it occurs at an unexpected time (before menarche or after menopause) or when it varies from the norm in amount or pattern.

Causes

1) Not related to pregnancy – gynaecologic

a) Hypothalamic-pituitary-ovarian dysfunction
- ❏ Anovulatory/Ovulatory
- ❏ Functioning ovarian cysts/tumours
- ❏ Emotional stress, drugs, hormones, oral contraceptives

b) Outflow tract conditions
- ❏ Uterus (infection, trauma, cancer/benign masses)
- ❏ Cervix (cervicitis, trauma, carcinoma)
- ❏ Vagina/Vulva (infection, trauma, cancer)

2) Related to pregnancy – non-gynaecologic

a) Less than 20 weeks
- ❏ Miscarriage-threatened, inevitable, incomplete, complete, missed, septic
- ❏ Ectopic pregnancy
- ❏ Gestational trophoblastic disease

b) Twenty weeks
- ❏ Placental abruption
- ❏ Placenta praevia
- ❏ Incidental bleeding – i.e. non-pregnancy causes which occur in pregnancy
- ❏ Bleeding from a vasa praevia – fetal bleeding

Key Objectives
- Determine whether the patient is haemodynamically stable prior to any other task.
- State that history is important, but diagnosis depends on hormonal/cytologic studies.
- Determine the difference between pregnancy related and non-pregnancy related causes.

General/Specific Objectives

- Through efficient, focused data gathering:

  - First differentiate between bleeding related to or unrelated to pregnancy.

  - If age or clinical information makes pregnancy unlikely, differentiate between causes of gynaecologic bleeding.

  - State that pelvic examination is not indicated in a woman more than 20 weeks pregnant with bleeding until ultrasound has been performed and excluded placenta praevia.

  - Perform pelvic and rectal examination.

- Interpret critical clinical and laboratory findings which were key in the processes of exclusion, differentiation, and diagnosis:

  - List indications for hormonal studies, and select tests.

  - List indications for ultrasonography.

  - List indications for cytologic/biopsy studies and select patients to be referred for investigation.

- Conduct an effective plan of management for a patient with vaginal bleeding:

  - Select patients in need of specialised care.

  - Outline management of patient with threatened and other forms of miscarriage.

  - Outline followup of patient after treatment of ectopic pregnancy; gestational trophoblastic disease.

  - Where sexual abuse is suspected, outline legal implications and requirement for support.

  - Discuss the use of oral contraceptives for regulating hypothalamic-pituitary-ovarian dysfunction.

Overview

Vaginal discharge, with or without pruritus, is one of the most common problems seen in the clinician's office.

Causes

1)   Physiologic discharge, and cervical mucus production

2)   Genital tract infections – vulvovaginitis – infectious

    a) **Polymicrobial superficial infection**

    b) **Moniliasis (candidiasis)**

    c) **Trichomoniasis**

    d) **Bacterial vaginosis**

    e) **Human papilloma virus (HPV)**

    f) **Herpes genitalis**

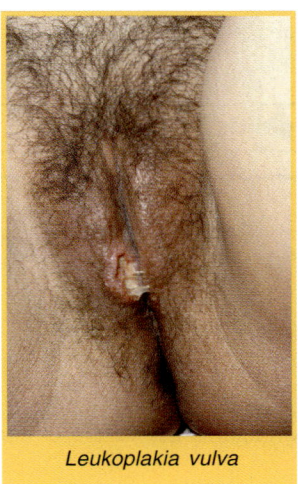

Leukoplakia vulva

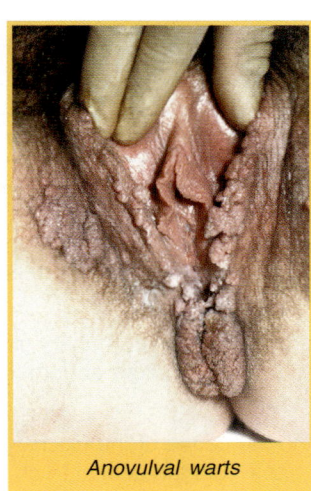

Anovulval warts

a) **Bubble baths, chemical irritants, douches, sprays**

b) **Foreign body**

c) **Atrophic vaginitis / Atrophic or hypertrophic vulvar dystrophy**

d) **Vulvar intraepithelial neoplasia / Vaginal, genital neoplasia**

e) **Systemic process (toxic shock syndrome)**

4) Other genital tract causes – uterine and tubal

a) **Infections**
- ❏ Gonorrhoea and *Chlamydia*
- ❏ Intra-uterine device
- ❏ Pyosalpinx
- ❏ Salpingitis

b) **Vulval, cervical, endometrial and tubal neoplasia**

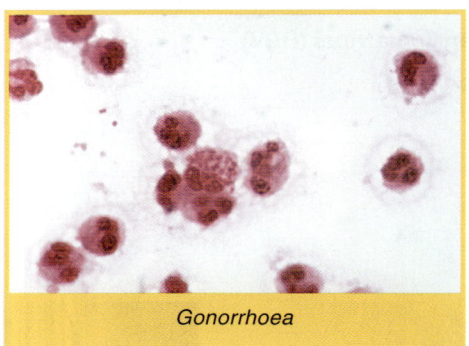

Gonorrhoea

5) Desquamative inflammatory vaginitis / Focal vulvitis

Key Objectives

- Determine the appearance of the discharge, but state that appearance may be misleading, and up to 20% of patients may have two coexistent infections.

- Differentiate between urinary tract infections (UTIs) and vaginal infections (dysuria is a symptom of both, so determine whether vaginal discharge is present).

- Define the cause of the discharge – whether inflammatory or neoplastic, and site within the genital tract.

General/Specific Objectives

- Through efficient, focused data gathering:

  - Differentiate between 'external' and 'internal' dysuria.

  - Elicit information about precipitating or aggravating factors (oral contraceptives, antibiotics, pregnancy, sexual activity, diabetes, genital hygiene, chemical irritants, etc.).

  - Perform genital and pelvic examination; determine whether pelvic inflammatory disease is present.

- Interpret critical clinical and laboratory findings which were key in the processes of exclusion, differentiation, and diagnosis:

  - Contrast pH and wet or potassium hydroxide smear findings in vaginitis of yeast, bacterial, *Trichomonas*, or atrophic type.

  - Select patients with purulent discharge for a Gram stain and cervical culture.

  - Perform Papanicolaou (Pap) smear to evaluate cervix (may also pick up carcinoma of the endometrium or tube).

- Conduct an effective plan of management for a patient with vaginal discharge:

  - List screening of populations at high risk for sexually transmitted diseases (STDs).

  - List types of vulvovaginitis associated with sexual activity and discuss risk reduction.

  - Outline preventive measures for STDs (e.g. limiting number of sexual partners, barrier contraceptives, especially condoms); for prevention of noninfectious vaginitis.

  - Outline a management plan for moniliasis, trichomoniasis, and for vaginitis due to gonorrhoea and/or *Chlamydia* including role of local hygiene in prevention.

Overview
Aggression is any form of behaviour intended to harm or injure other people against their wishes. Violence is a deliberate attempt to inflict physical harm. Dangerousness refers to the likelihood of whether individuals present a risk of harming themselves or others. Clinicians are confronted with the direct and indirect consequences of violent behaviour and will be increasingly expected to make risk assessments of future dangerousness. Although comorbidity of some mental illnesses increases the risk of violence, most episodes of violence are not committed by mentally ill people. The best predictor of future violence is past violence, but violent behaviour is usually the result of the interaction of many factors.

Predisposing Causal Factors

1) Pre-existing vulnerabilities (gender, age, personality, impulsivity, intellectual functioning, neurobiology, individual sensitivity, conduct disorder, family and cultural influences)

2) Psychiatric disorders

   a) Schizophrenia (with active paranoid, or grandiose ideation or command hallucinations, treatment resistance and impaired insight)

   b) Delusional disorder (particularly morbid jealousy)

   c) Substance abuse (intoxication, withdrawal)

   d) Major depression with delusions

   e) Personality disorder (antisocial, borderline, conduct disorder)

   f) Intermittent explosive disorder

   g) Bipolar affective disorder (manic phase)

   h) Cognitive disorders (delirium, dementia)

3) Situational triggers (loss, actual or threatened; confrontation; availability of weapons and presence of a potential victim)

Key Objectives
- List risk factors for dangerousness.
- Recognise signs of imminent violence: threats, paranoid ideas, shouting and pacing, agitated behaviour.

- Through efficient, focused and tactful data gathering:

  - Elicit a history of violence in the distant and recent past, violence against animals and property, forensic history, current thoughts or threats of violence against named victims; degree of insight and ability to maintain control.

  - Assess and document mental state for cognitive, intellectual and psychotic features and degree of intoxication.

  - Determine presence of support systems and recent stressors.

  - Determine the ability and willingness to cooperate with management.

- Conduct an effective plan of management for a patient who may be violent:

  - Outline how to conduct the initial interview with an agitated and potentially violent patient.

  - Outline a safe psychopharmacological management strategy for treating a violent patient.

  - Understand clinician's responsibility to warn police or potential victims in contrast to strict doctor-patient confidentiality.

  - Select patients in need of specialist referral and treatment.

  - Provide counselling and debriefing to victims and onlookers in the aftermath of an episode of violence.

119A   Child Abuse

Overview

Child abuse is part of the spectrum of family dysfunction and leads to significant morbidity and mortality (recently, sexual attacks on children by groups of other children have increased). Abuse causes physical and emotional trauma, and may present as **neglect**. The possibility of abuse must be in the mind of all those involved in the care of children who have suffered traumatic injury or have psychological or social disturbances (e.g. aggressive behaviour, stress disorder, depressive disorder, substance abuse).

Causes

(see #119 Violence/Aggression and Mental Illness)

Types of Abuse:

| 1) | Physical abuse (pushing, hitting, biting, burning, locking out of home, abandoning in an unsafe place) |

| 2) | Sexual abuse (forced unwanted sexual activity: rape, sex with objects, friends, animals, mimic pornography, wear more provocative clothes, etc.) |

| 3) | Emotional or psychological abuse (constant criticism; threats to hurt, kill; extreme jealousy; denying friendships, outside interests or activities; time accounting, etc.) |

| 4) | Economic (not allowing money, deny improvement in earning capacity, accounting of every cent, etc.) |

| 5) | Other |

   a) Münchausen syndrome by proxy

   b) By nurses, medical practitioners, social workers

Key Objective
- Identify the characteristics of families at risk of abusing their children (physical, sexual or emotional abuse) and screen.

General/Specific Objectives

- Through efficient, focused, data gathering:

  - Determine the family dynamics, and parental characteristics.

  - Differentiate abuse by commission from abuse by omission.

  - Determine social correlation.

  - Determine whether the child has signs of physical, sexual, or other abuse (e.g. cutaneous markings, burns), or emotional and behavioural signs of abuse.

- Interpret critical clinical and laboratory findings which were key in the processes of exclusion, differentiation, and diagnosis:

  - List investigation for a child with sexual abuse.

- Conduct an effective initial plan of management for a child who may have been abused:

  - Outline strategies for securing the child's safety.

  - List indications for reporting to appropriate social service department or referral to child welfare.

  - List potential physical and psychological sequelae of physical and sexual abuse.

  - Outline treatment options for victims and perpetrators and outline outcomes of treatment.

  - Outline strategies for prevention of child abuse.

119B Elder Abuse

Overview

The American Medical Association defines elder abuse ('granny battering') as:

> 'an act or omission that results in harm or threatened harm to the health or welfare of an elderly person. Abuse includes intentional infliction of physical or medical injury; sexual abuse; or the withholding of necessary food, clothing and medical care to meet the physical and mental needs of an elderly person by one having the care, custody or responsibility for an elderly person'.

There are no reliable estimates on the incidence or prevalence of elder abuse in Australia, but international experience suggests that about 1 in every 25 elderly may be victims, with only one in five cases reported. The typical victim is an increasingly dependent, cognitively impaired woman, over 75 years, with problem behaviours including shouting and wandering. The typical abuser is a close relative in a long term relationship (spouse or child), who is under increasing stress, socially isolated and abusing alcohol or drugs. There is no provision for mandatory reporting of elder abuse in Australia.

Causes (Frequently in Combination)

1) **Physical dependency**

2) **Caregiver stress**

3) **Pattern of family violence**

4) **Pathological alcohol/drug abuse**

Types of Abuse:

1) **Physical/Sexual**

2) **Emotional/Psychological**

3) **Medical**

4) **Economic exploitation**

5) **Neglect**

Key Objective

- Identify both abused elderly patients and those at risk of abuse; and differentiate abuse from organic brain disorders and dementia.

General/Specific Objectives

- Through efficient, focused data gathering which involves talking to both the alleged victim and the caregiver separately:

  - Determine whether the explanations for illnesses or injuries are consistent or implausible. Denial may be the initial response.

  - Conduct a thorough physical examination of the patient and document bruises, bites, burns, lacerations and other injuries present, especially in areas usually covered by clothing and on the scalp.

  - Determine the period of time between the injury and accessing the medical system, since long delays are usual with elder abuse.

- Interpret critical clinical and laboratory findings which were key in the processes of exclusion, differentiation, and diagnosis.

- Develop an effective initial plan of management for an elderly person who may have been abused, which may involve initial hospitalisation, respite care or long term alternative accommodation if there is concern for the patient's physical health or safety:

  - Understand the legal implications of elder abuse.

  - Counsel and help caregiver by providing information and education and accessing community options.

  - Outline the multidisciplinary approach to intervention and become aware of local resources.

119C   Violence: Domestic/Family

Overview

Domestic and family violence are major public health concerns which affect about three percent of the Australian population annually. They can affect anyone irrespective of economic, social, geographic or racial background, resulting in significant morbidity and mortality. From a health perspective, domestic violence is a chronic syndrome characterised not only by physical violence, but also by emotional and psychological abuse. It is the abuse of power in a relationship involving domination, coercion, intimidation and the victimisation of one person by another, typically a male partner. Women are eight times more likely to be victims than males. The perpetrators are often young, troubled, unemployed men with low self-esteem, who have been abused themselves. Shame and isolation militate against disclosure, but health professionals have responsibility to break the silence. Depression and post–traumatic stress disorder are common sequelae for victims, as are alcohol and drug abuse, self-harm and suicide. Barriers to disclosure often lie with the clinician and not the victim. Programmes for stopping domestic violence can be effective for those who are motivated to change their behaviour.

Classification of Domestic/Family Violence

1)   **Physical: resulting in pain, injury, denial of sleep, warmth or nutrition, denial of medical care, violence to animals and property, disablement and murder: dowry and honour killings**

2)   **Sexual: coerced sex, rape, harassment, incest, pornography**

3)   **Verbal: designed to humiliate, degrade, demean, intimidate, subjugate, including the threat of physical violence**

4)   **Economic: deprivation of basic necessities, seizure of income or assets, unreasonable denial of the means to participate in social life**

5)   **Social: isolation, control of social activity, deprivation of liberty or the deliberate creation of unreasonable dependence**

Key Objectives
- Recognise the typical symptoms and signs, both physical and psychological, which may indicate domestic violence.

- Assess immediate and short term risks to the victim.

- Know the common myths about domestic violence, namely that it is rare, and only involves physical violence; that the perpetrators are mentally ill and cannot control their anger and are always provoked by their victims; that it is a problem only amongst the disadvantaged and minority groups and that it is a private matter between individuals.

General/Specific Objectives
- Through efficient, sensitive and focused data gathering:
    - Include enquiries about possible domestic violence when patients present with obvious physical injuries and bruising in multiple areas or the head and neck; with chronic pain syndromes; insomnia, depression, suicidal ideation; panic/anxiety; eating disorders; drug and alcohol abuse, somatoform disorders; and also during pregnancy and childbirth associated with unwanted pregnancy, miscarriage; antepartum haemorrhage; avoidance of antenatal care or low infant birthweight.

    - Consider the possibility in women with a past history of child abuse or a child who is currently being abused; who have recently undergone separation or divorce; who are socially isolated; who present frequently or with an overly attentive partner; who delay in seeking treatment for injuries or who do not comply with treatment.

    - Be aware that women who have been abused want to be asked about domestic violence and are more likely to disclose if asked. Most women do not openly admit they are victims of abuse unless asked: out of fear, shame, denial, loyalty to their partner and family, or that they will not be believed.

    - Document history, extent and type of abuse and injuries in detail and provide appropriate treatment.

    - Assess the victim's immediate and short term safety and establish if the perpetrator has a gun or other weapon at home.

    - Implement an effective plan of management for a victim of domestic violence which may include supportive and educational counselling and the provision of information about support services and resources and sexual assault centres.

- Assist in devising a safety plan in advance for a worst-case scenario.

- Establish presence and attitudes of other potential support persons towards the victim.

- Refer patients for legal and police advice if necessary.

- Select patients in need of specialist referral for social work, psychological or psychiatric counselling.

- If the victim and perpetrator are both your patients, issues of confidentiality and disclosure arise.

- Respect the patient's autonomy and right to remain in an abusive relationship, even if you do not agree.

- Remember that doctors are obliged to report situations where children are at risk of violence or abuse.

119 Violence/Aggression and Mental Illness

119D Rape / Violence Against Women

(See #119C Violence: Domestic/Family)

120 Visual Disturbance/Loss

Overview

Loss of vision is a frightening symptom that demands immediate attention, particularly if acute. However, patients with neurological lesions may not be aware of visual loss; and patients with a pituitary adenoma rarely present with symptoms of visual loss.

Causes

Acute:

1) **Corneal (oedema)**

2) **Glaucoma (acute angle closure)**

3) **Vitreous haemorrhage (may be traumatic, penetrating, hyphaema)**

4) **Retinal / Macular / Optic disc problems**

    a) Acute macular lesion

    b) Retinal detachment (may be traumatic)

    c) Retinal artery occlusion

    d) Optic neuritis

    e) Amaurosis fugax

    f) Anterior ischaemic optic neuropathy

5) **Nervous system**

    a) Occipital infarction/haemorrhage

    b) Functional visual loss

6) **Migraine**

    (see #046 Headache)

Chronic:

1)   **Corneal disorders (dystrophy, scarring, oedema)**

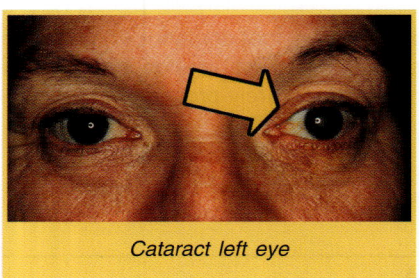

Cataract left eye

2)   **Lens disorders (age related, traumatic, steroid-induced, ultra violet light exposure)**

3)   **Glaucoma (primary, secondary)**

4)   **Retinal dysfunction**

    a) Diabetic (retinal oedema, retinopathy)

    b) Vascular insufficiency

    c) Tumours

    d) Macular degeneration or dystrophy

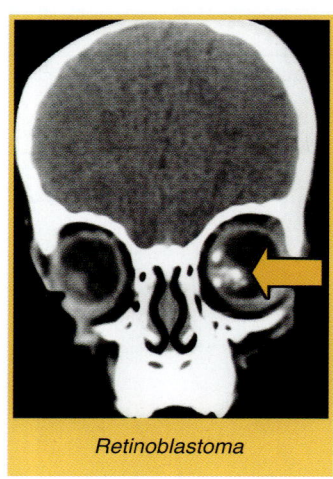

Retinoblastoma

5) Optic nerve lesions

a) **Compressive optic neuropathy**
  - ❏ Intracranial (masses)
  - ❏ Orbital (thyroid disease)

b) **Toxic/Nutritional (nutritional deficiencies, tobacco-alcohol amblyopia, methanol)**

c) **Hereditary optic neuropathies**

6) Pituitary adenoma

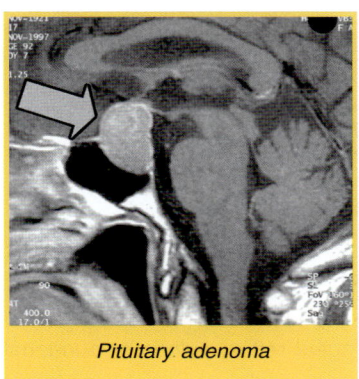

Pituitary adenoma

Key Objectives
- Determine whether the loss of vision is acute or chronic (at times, the loss of monocular vision is noted incidentally when the other eye is covered so that a chronic loss presents acutely).
- Perform direct ophthalmoscope examination of the eye.

General/Specific Objectives
- Through efficient, focused data gathering:

  - Determine whether the visual loss is monocular or binocular.

  - Differentiate causes of visual loss by examination of cornea, lens, retina, and optic disc.

  - Determine the presence of a foreign body, abnormal extraocular musculature or pupillary reflex.

- Interpret critical clinical and laboratory findings which were key in the processes of exclusion, differentiation, and diagnosis:

  - Perform visual acuity and field testing.

  - List indications for fluorescein angiography.

- Conduct an effective plan of management for a patient with chronic loss of vision:

  - Select patients in need of specialised care.

Overview

Nausea may occur alone or along with vomiting (powerful ejection of gastric contents), dyspepsia (see #003C Chronic Recurrent Abdominal Pain), and other gastrointestinal complaints. Vomiting may be a manifestation of a systemic, central or local problem. There is a continuum of severity from a minor inconvenience (and accompaniment to a systemic illness) to a major life-threatening symptom in conditions such as gastric obstruction. When prolonged or severe, vomiting may be associated with disturbances of volume, water and electrolyte metabolism that may require correction prior to other specific treatment.

Causes

1) Gastrointestinal system

a) **Stomach**
   - ❏ Gastroenteritis
   - ❏ Postoperative
   - ❏ Acid peptic disease
   - ❏ Gastroparesis / Obstruction
   - ❏ Gastro-oesophageal reflux, pyloric or duodenal stenosis

b) **Small bowel / Colon**
   - ❏ Obstruction
   - ❏ Acid peptic disease
   - ❏ Appendicitis

c) **Hepato-biliary disease**

d) **Pancreatic disease**

e) **Peritoneal irritation**

2) Central nervous system (CNS)

a) **Infections**

b) **Tumours**

c) **Multiple sclerosis**

d) **Vestibular nerve lesions**

e) **Brain stem lesions**

f) **Migraine**

g) **Psychiatric/Psychologic problems**

h) **Travel sickness**

3) Endocrine-metabolic (diabetes, uraemia, hypercalcaemia, pregnancy)

4) Cancer (paraneoplastic syndromes, ovarian, hypernephroma, gastric)

5) Systemic

    a) Sepsis (pyelonephritis, pneumonia, any infection in childhood)

    b) Drugs (chemotherapy)

    c) Food poisoning

    d) Alcohol intoxication

Key Objectives

- Contrast vomiting and regurgitation, which is return of oesophageal contents into the hypo-pharynx with little effort, such as with gastro-oesophageal reflux.

- Determine severity of volume and electrolyte abnormalities in a patient with vomiting.

General/Specific Objectives

- Through efficient, focused data gathering:

  - Determine whether there is a secondary cause for the vomiting, delayed gastric emptying is present, or the vomiting is in response to other agents.

- Interpret critical clinical and laboratory findings which were key in the processes of exclusion, differentiation, and diagnosis:

  - Select patients requiring investigation since laboratory testing may be unnecessary in many.

  - Select patients in need of endoscopic examination.

- Conduct an effective plan of management for a patient with vomiting and nausea:

  - Outline management plan for patients with vomiting caused by documented diseases, as contrasted to delayed gastric emptying, or other causes (e.g. chemotherapeutic drugs).

  - Calculate volume and electrolyte deficit and outline management (see #005B Metabolic Alkalosis and #008A Hypokalaemia).

Overview

Many patients who complain of weakness are not objectively weak when muscle strength is formally tested. A careful history and physical examination will permit the distinction between functional disease and true muscle weakness.

Causes

(see #038 Fatigue)

1) Myopathies

   a) Genetic (e.g. muscular dystrophy)

   b) Inflammatory (e.g. polymyositis, vasculitis, collagen-vascular)

   c) Infectious (e.g. HIV, influenza, cytomegalovirus (CMV))

   d) Neoplastic (e.g. malignancy-associated myositis)

   e) Toxic/Drug (e.g. steroids, 3-hydroxy-3-methylglutaryl coenzyme A (HMG-CoA) reductase inhibitors, alcohol)

   f) Metabolic/Endocrine (e.g. hypothyroidism, Cushing syndrome, electrolyte disorders)

2) Neuromuscular junction

   a) Genetic (e.g. myasthenia gravis)

   b) Inflammatory (e.g. myasthenia gravis)

   c) Infectious (e.g. botulism)

   d) Neoplastic (e.g. Eaton-Lambert syndrome)

   e) Toxic/Drug (e.g. organophosphate poisoning)

3) Peripheral neuropathies

   a) Genetic (e.g. peroneal muscular atrophy)

   b) Inflammatory (e.g. Guillain-Barré syndrome)

   c) Infectious (e.g. leprosy)

   d) Neoplastic (e.g. myeloma/amyloid)

   e) Toxic/Drug (e.g. lead)

   f) Metabolic/Endocrine (e.g. diabetes mellitus)

   g) Idiopathic (e.g. Bell palsy)

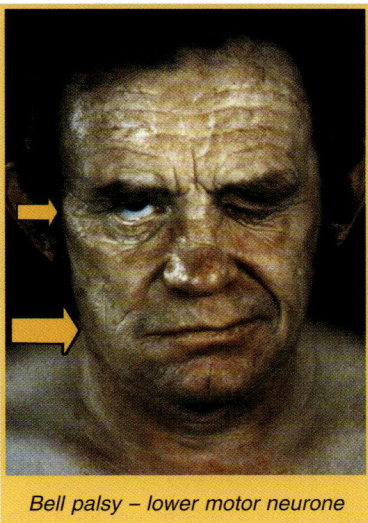

Bell palsy – lower motor neurone

4) Anterior horn cell

    a) Genetic (e.g. spinal muscular atrophy)

    b) Inflammatory (e.g. amyotrophic lateral sclerosis)

    c) Infectious (e.g. poliomyelitis)

    d) Neoplastic (e.g. paraneoplastic syndromes)

    e) Toxic/Drugs (e.g. lead)

5) Upper motor neuron

    a) Genetic (e.g. leucodystrophy)

    b) Inflammatory (e.g. vasculitis)

    c) Infectious (e.g. brain abscess)

    d) Neoplastic (e.g. brain tumour)

    e) Toxic/Drug (e.g. radiation)

    f) Metabolic/Endocrine (e.g. vitamin B_{12} deficiency)

6) Functional

Key Objectives

- Differentiate between patients who complain of generalised weakness (usually functional) compared to patients who complain of inability to perform specific tasks.

- Differentiate between weakness due to an upper motor neuron lesion and weakness due to a disturbance affecting the lower motor neuron or motor unit.

- Determine the cause of the lesion.

General/Specific Objectives

- Through efficient, focused data gathering:

    - Determine whether the weakness is localised or generalised, assess muscle strength, tone, bulk/atrophy, fasciculation, tremor, myoclonus, tendon reflexes, and plantar reflexes.

    - Determine whether the weakness occurred as a result of an abnormality in the cerebral cortex, descending motor pathways, brain stem, spinal cord, anterior horn cells, nerve roots and plexuses, peripheral nerves, neuromuscular junction, or skeletal muscle.

- Interpret critical clinical and laboratory findings which were key in the processes of exclusion, differentiation, and diagnosis:

    - List the physiologic principles and indications for electromyelography (EMG), muscle enzymes.

    - List indications for muscle biopsy.

- Conduct an effective plan of management for a patient with weakness, paresis, or paralysis:

    - Outline an initial plan of management for Guillain-Barré syndrome.

    - Outline an initial plan of management for myasthenia gravis.

    - Outline an initial plan for rehabilitation of patients with hemiplegia and paraplegia.

Overview

Intra-uterine growth restriction (IUGR) is often a manifestation of congenital infections, poor maternal nutrition or maternal illness. In other patients, the infant may be large for the gestational age. There may be long term sequelae for both.

Causes

1) Newborn infant small for gestational age (growth restricted)

a) **Maternal**

- ❏ Social and/or economic status
- ❏ Drugs (cigarettes, alcohol, narcotics, cocaine)
- ❏ Illness (pregnancy-induced hypertension / 'HELLP' (**H**aemolysis, **E**levated **L**iver enzymes, **L**ow **P**latelets) syndrome, diabetes, malnutrition, systemic lupus erythematosus (SLE), lupus anticoagulant)

b) **Fetal**

- ❏ Multiple gestation
- ❏ Intra-uterine infections ('TORCH' – **T**oxoplasmosis, **O**ther, **R**ubella, **C**ytomegalovirus, **H**erpes simplex virus)
- ❏ Chromosomal abnormality

c) **Placental insufficiency – infarction, previous placental abruption**

2) Newborn infant large for gestational age

a) **Maternal (familial, diabetes)**

b) **Fetal (e.g. Beckwith syndrome, transposition of great vessels)**

Key Objective

- Determine the most probable diagnosis by clinical means.

General/Specific Objectives

- Interpret critical clinical and laboratory findings which were key in the processes of exclusion, differentiation, and diagnosis:

  - List indications for investigations such as fetal ultrasound, and blood biochemistry.

- Conduct an effective initial plan of management for an infant with intra-uterine growth aberration:
  - Discuss the complications associated with IUGR and outline the management of such an infant.
  - Outline management and complications that can occur in large-for-gestational-age infants.
  - Outline preventive strategies of large-for-gestational-age infants.
- Outline the management in late pregnancy when IUGR or fetal macrosomia has been diagnosed; including fetal assessment, mode of delivery and potential problems in labour and at delivery.

Overview

Obesity is a chronic condition that is increasing in prevalence. It is contributed to by lifestyle changes including inactivity and dietary changes, and may result in diabetes, hypertension, atherosclerosis and sleep-apnoea.

Causes

1)   Increased energy intake

    a) Dietary (progressive hyperphagic, frequent eating, high-fat diet, overeating)

    b) Social and behavioural (socio-economic, ethnicity, psychological)

    c) Iatrogenic (drugs, hormones, hypothalamic surgery)

2)   Decreased energy expenditure (sedentary lifestyle, smoking cessation)

3)   Neuroendocrine

    a) Hypothyroidism

    b) Cushing syndrome

    c) Hypothalamic syndrome

    d) Polycystic ovary syndrome

    e) Hypogonadism

    f) Growth hormone (GH) deficiency

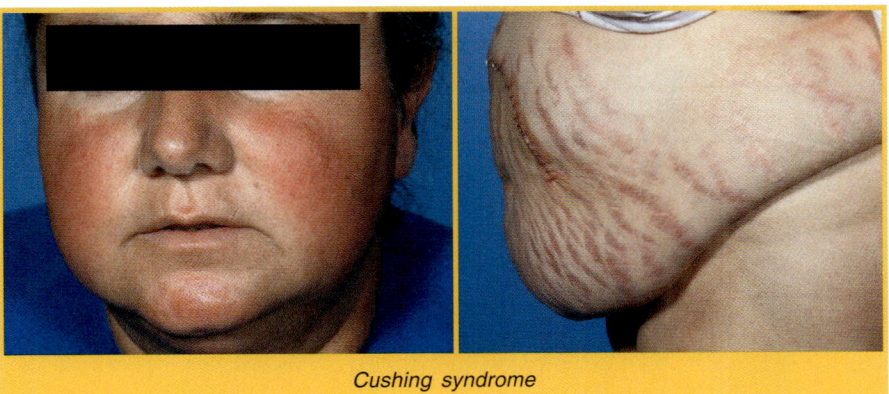

Cushing syndrome

4)   Genetic (dysmorphic)

Key Objectives

- Recognise that the sequelae of obesity may be life-threatening.

- Determine whether obesity is the result of lifestyle changes or neuroendocrine disorder.

General/Specific Objectives

- Through efficient, focused data gathering:

  - Determine the degree and type of obesity.

  - Determine whether a treatable cause of obesity (secondary or neuroendocrine) is present.

  - Describe the risk of morbidity and mortality.

  - Perform a measurement of waist-to-hip ratio and determine body-mass index (BMI).

  - Determine whether comorbid conditions are present (hypertension, diabetes mellitus, dyslipidaemia, sleep-apnoea, etc.).

- Interpret critical clinical and laboratory findings which were key in the processes of exclusion, differentiation, and diagnosis:

  - Select patients who require investigation for a neuroendocrine cause of obesity.

- Conduct an effective plan of management for a patient with weight gain / obesity:

  - Formulate a plan of management consistent with the reality that the great majority of patients require chronic long term treatment since obesity cannot be cured.

  - List the modalities of treatment for obesity including increased energy expenditure through exercise, decreased energy intake through healthy diets, and behaviour modification.

  - Contrast advantages and disadvantages of anorectic drugs and surgery for the treatment of obesity.

125 Weight Loss / Eating Disorders / Anorexia / Nutritional Disorders

125A   Weight Loss / Eating Disorders / Anorexia

Overview
Involuntary weight loss is nearly always a sign of serious medical or psychiatric illness and should be investigated.

Causes

1)   Involuntary weight loss

a) **Decreased energy intake**
   - ❏ Malignancy decreasing appetite
   - ❏ HIV
   - ❏ Endocrinopathies (adrenal insufficiency, hypercalcaemia, diabetes mellitus)
   - ❏ Chronic illness (chronic obstructive pulmonary disease (COPD), congestive cardiac failure (CCF))
   - ❏ Gastrointestinal disease (obstruction and malabsorption)
   - ❏ Intercurrent illness (hepatitis, glandular fever, chronic fatigue syndrome)
   - ❏ Psychiatric disease (bipolar disorder, personality disorder, paranoia/delusion)
   - ❏ Drugs (alcohol, opiates, cocaine, amphetamines, anticancer)

b) **Increased energy expenditure**
   - ❏ Hyperthyroidism
   - ❏ Phaeochromocytoma
   - ❏ Chronic illness (COPD, CCF)
   - ❏ Malignancy (hypercatabolic)
   - ❏ Infection (presence of fever indicative of hypercatabolic state)

c) **Energy loss**
   - ❏ Urine (uncontrolled diabetes mellitus)
   - ❏ Stool (malabsorption)

2)   Voluntary weight loss

a) **Decreased intake**
   - ❏ Diet for treatment of obesity
   - ❏ Anorexic drugs
   - ❏ Anorexia / Bulimia
   - ❏ Psychological

b) **Increased energy expenditure (distance runners, models, ballet dancers, gymnasts)**

Key Objectives
- Determine extent of weight loss in relation to previous weight, whether voluntary or involuntary, whether with increased appetite or decreased appetite, and if fluctuations in weight are usual or unusual.

General/Specific Objectives
- Through efficient, focused data gathering:

  - Differentiate involuntary weight loss from voluntary.

  - Contrast weight loss associated with increased appetite from that with decreased appetite.

- Interpret critical clinical and laboratory findings which were key in the processes of exclusion, differentiation, and diagnosis:

  - Conduct an investigation of involuntary weight loss, whether appetite is decreased or increased.

- Conduct an effective plan of management for a patient with weight loss / eating disorder / anorexia:

  - State that management is dependent on the underlying condition.

  - Counsel patients with voluntary weight loss on healthy diets and lifestyle changes.

  - Select patients in need of specialised care.

125B Nutritional Disorders and Deficiencies

Overview

No clinical assessment is entirely complete without an assessment of the patient's nutritional status. Nutritional disorders present from infancy through to old age. They may involve disorders of energy-yielding macronutrients (carbohydrate/fat/protein) or of essential organic/inorganic micronutrients (vitamins / trace elements).

Serious illness, prolonged hospitalisation and inanition are likely to be associated with varying degrees of protein-energy malnutrition (PEM) from negative energy balance, particularly in the presence of uncontrolled chronic sepsis.

Vitamin and trace element deficiencies cause syndromes relating to their specific metabolic effects. For example zinc, a predominantly intracellular cation, is a component of important enzyme systems involved in active cellular proliferation and repair. Zinc deficiency gives clinical manifestations which include an exanthematous rash, gastrointestinal symptoms, and problems with wound healing.

Causes of Nutritional Deficiencies

1) Energy-yielding macronutrients

    a) **PEM (undernutrition, starvation, marasmus/kwashiorkor)**

2) Inorganic nutrients

    a) **Calcium and phosphorous**
       (see also #004 Abnormal Serum Calcium/Phosphate, #064 Menopause and #077 Periodic Health Examination / Growth and Development)

    b) **Iron**
       (see also #012 Anaemia and Pallor)

    c) **Iodine**
       (see also #068 Neck or Facial Mass / Goitre / Thyroid Disease)

    d) **Zinc and other trace elements (zinc, manganese, beryllium, boron, selenium, cobalt, etc.)**

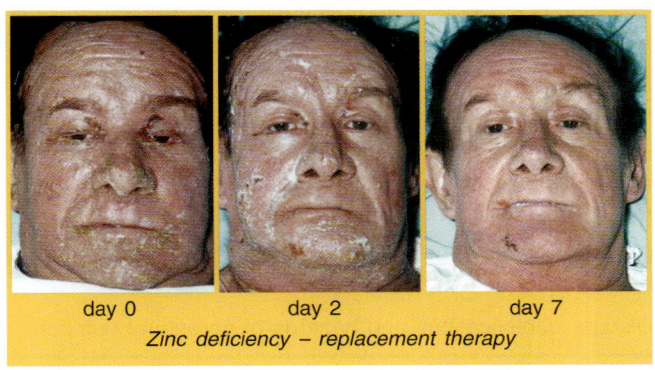

day 0   day 2   day 7
Zinc deficiency – replacement therapy

a) Fat-soluble vitamins (A, D, E, K)

b) Water-soluble vitamins (B complex, C)

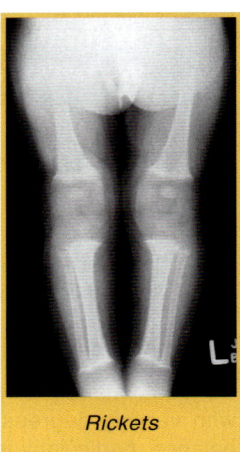

Rickets

Key Objectives
- Identify those patients liable to develop syndromes of nutritional deficiencies.

- Recognise clinical features of major deficiencies.

General/Specific Objectives
- Through efficient, focused data gathering:

  - Conduct a clinical assessment of nutritional status from history, physical examination and appropriate office tests.

  - Diagnose syndromes of PEM; compare and contrast features applicable to children and to adults.

  - Appreciate principles of normal energy balance and of dietary requirements of major energy sources.

  - Appreciate principles of micronutrient requirements.

  - Appreciate risk factors for nutritional depletions and institute preventive measures where appropriate.

  - Diagnose trace element and vitamin deficiencies in patients at risk.

- Select appropriate investigations which were key in the processes of exclusion, differentiation and diagnosis, recognising that serum or urinary measurements of vitamins and trace elements are not routinely done and may not be available or diagnostically helpful at short notice.

- Outline effective plans of management for patients with PEM, vitamin deficiency or trace element deficiencies:

  - Outline basal requirements of energy intake and expenditure (kilojoules/calories) and daily requirements and proportions of macronutrients and essential micronutrients.

  - Outline methods and principles of formulation of enteral and parenteral nutrition regimens.

  - Discuss complications and hazards of parenteral nutrition.

126A *Upper Respiratory Tract Disorders*

Overview

Wheezing, a whistling sound, is produced by vibration of opposing walls of an airway that is narrowed almost to the point of closure. It can originate from airways of any size, from upper airways to intrathoracic small airways. Stridor is an even more strident, urgent, harsh noise indicating extreme difficulty with breathing.

Causes

1) Extrathoracic upper airway obstruction

    a) Sleep-apnoea syndrome / Obesity

    b) Goitre

    c) Postnasal drip

    d) Vocal cord dysfunction (nodule, paresis)

    e) Epiglottitis

    f) Laryngeal oedema/stenosis

    g) Anaphylaxis

    h) Retropharyngeal mass (abscess, neoplasm)

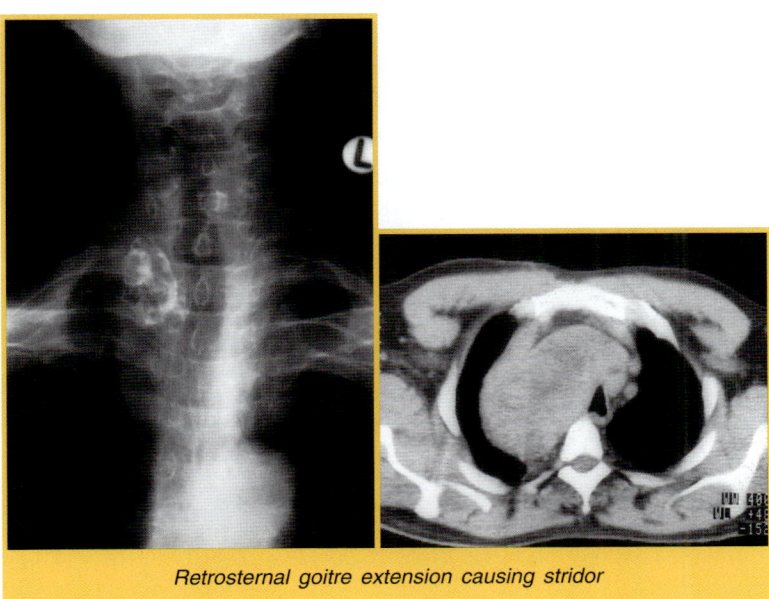

Retrosternal goitre extension causing stridor

2) Intrathoracic upper airway obstruction

a) Tracheobronchitis

b) Tracheal obstruction (stenosis, compression, e.g. retrosternal thyroid mass)

c) Foreign body aspiration

d) Tracheal or bronchial tumours (benign, malignant)

Key Objectives

- Determine whether the wheezing is associated with chronic dyspnoea and cough, because this triad is highly suggestive of asthma.

- Appreciate that asthma is **not** the sole or most common cause of wheezing; identify extrathoracic/intrathoracic upper airway obstruction (e.g. from thyroid).

General/Specific Objectives

- Through efficient, focused, data gathering:

  - Determine whether the wheezing is polyphonic, since if so it is more likely to originate from more central airways.

  - Determine if wheezing is maximum in inspiration or expiration, and whether accompanied by stridor.

  - Determine the most likely site of obstruction, whether large or small intrathoracic airway or extrathoracic airway.

  - From history and clinical examination, determine the most likely cause and the urgency of management.

- Interpret critical clinical and laboratory findings which are key in the processes of exclusion, differentiation, and diagnosis:

  - List indications for diagnostic imaging.

  - Select pulmonary function studies as one means to differentiate between causes once diagnostic possibilities have been narrowed by clinical means.

- Conduct an effective plan of management for a patient with upper respiratory tract disorders:

  - Outline the use of bronchodilator therapy for diagnostic purposes.

  - Select patients in need of specialised care.

126B   Lower Respiratory Tract Disorders

Overview

Individuals with episodes of wheezing, breathlessness, chest tightness, and cough usually have limitation of airflow. The most common cause of airflow limitation is **asthma** which is reversible with treatment. Without treatment it may be lethal.

While the prevalence of asthma is rising (asthma affects an estimated 2,000,000 Australians), the mortality from asthma has fallen dramatically – deaths in Australia yearly have decreased from around 1,200 a decade ago to around 400 currently.

Causes

1)   Obstructive lung disease

   a) Asthma

   b) Chronic obstructive pulmonary disease (COPD)

   c) Bronchiectasis

   d) Cystic fibrosis

2)   Small airway disorder

   a) Aspiration

   b) Bronchiolitis

   c) Cystic fibrosis

3)   Cardiovascular

   a) Pulmonary oedema

   b) Pulmonary embolism

Key Objectives

- Determine the severity of the airway obstruction and use this to guide therapy.

- Distinguish respiratory and cardiac causes of respiratory symptoms.

General/Specific Objectives

- Through efficient, focused, data gathering:

  - Elicit information about intermittency, seasonal waxing and waning, nocturnal episodes, exacerbation on exposure to exercise, cold air, allergens, air pollutants, or upper respiratory tract infections (URTIs) (suggestive of asthma, but also found in COPD and bronchiectasis).

  - Determine whether the wheezing is polyphasic (multiple pitches, start and stop at various points in respiratory cycle).

- Interpret critical clinical and laboratory findings which are key in the processes of exclusion, differentiation, and diagnosis:

  - Examine and discuss evaluation of sputum.

  - Understand that pulmonary function tests are key to diagnosis and management of asthma. Select spirometry and FEV_1 (forced expiratory vital capacity in one second) before and after bronchodilator inhalation, to quantify severity of airway narrowing and to define reversibility.

  - Discuss the use of provocative testing for diagnosis of asthma if lung function is normal.

  - Select diagnostic imaging to detect complications of asthma and to exclude alternative diagnoses.

  - List indications for allergy testing for asthma.

- Conduct an effective plan of management for a patient with lower respiratory tract disorders:

  - Outline an initial plan of management for a patient with asthma.

  - Select patients in need of specialised care.

Overview

Allergic reactions are common in all age groups. They exhibit a variety of clinical responses and are considered individually elsewhere under the appropriate presentation. The rationale for considering them together is that in some patients with one response (e.g. atopic dermatitis), other atopic disorders such as asthma or allergic rhinitis may occur at other times. Moreover, 50% of patients with atopic dermatitis report a family history of respiratory atopy. The child of a mother with atopy is at high risk for atopic diseases.

Clinical Presentations

1) Allergic rhinitis, rhinorrhoea, hay fever

(see #092 Rhinorrhoea / Sore Throat)

2) Eye redness

(see #035 Eye Redness)

3) Anaphylaxis

(see #098A Anaphylaxis)

4) Skin rash / Dermatitis

(see #102A Skin Rash / Dermatitis and/or Fever, Urticaria/Angio-Oedema)

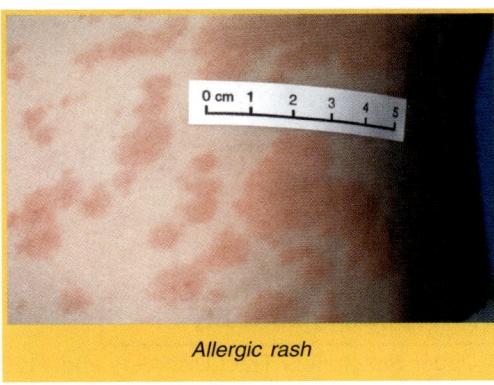

Allergic rash

5) Urticaria/Angio-oedema

(see #102A Skin Rash / Dermatitis and/or Fever, Urticaria/Angio-Oedema)

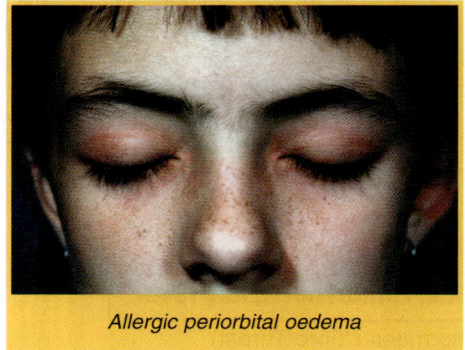

Allergic periorbital oedema

6) Atopic dermatitis

(see #102A Skin Rash / Dermatitis and/or Fever, Urticaria/Angio-Oedema)

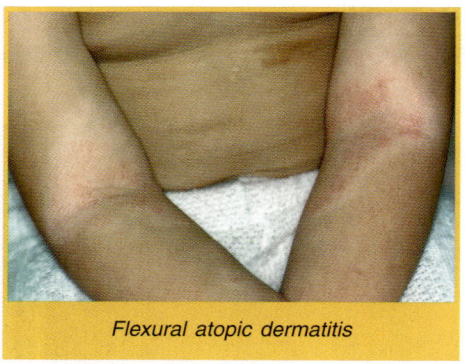

Flexural atopic dermatitis

7) Wheezing / Respiratory difficulty

(see #126A Upper Respiratory Tract Disorders and #126B Lower Respiratory Tract Disorders)

Key Objectives
- Recognise allergy as the probable basis of a variety of clinical presentations.
- Familiarity with common allergens.
- Diagnose potentially lethal anaphylaxis and initiate immediate treatment.

General/Specific Objectives

- Through efficient, focused data gathering:

    - Elicit a history or identify the possible causes of an anaphylactic reaction.

    - Differentiate between food intolerance and food allergy.

    - Identify common allergens and their possible effects on susceptible individuals.

- Interpret critical clinical and laboratory findings which were key in the processes of exclusion, differentiation, and diagnosis:

    - List cost-effective use of tests designed to identify allergens.

    - Interpret results so as to differentiate the allergic from the non-allergic individual.

- Conduct an effective plan of management for a patient with allergies:

    - Outline emergency management of anaphylaxis, with and without shock.

    - Discuss skin testing in allergic patients.

    - Outline the immediate and long term management of the child with allergies including education and counselling for the child, parents, school and the community.

    - Identify the social and psychologic impact of allergic disease on the child and its family.

Overview

Bites and stings in Australia from land, air and marine creatures are commonplace but serious and fatal bites are uncommon. Knowledge of first aid measures and early treatment is required for all clinicians; effective first aid using the pressure-immobilisation technique lowers risks of envenomation and can be life-saving. Polyvalent and specific anti-venoms are available for most snake, spider and marine bites and stings and have significantly reduced mortality and morbidity.

Fatalities from predators such as crocodiles and sharks are horrifying and invoke headlines, but are rare compared to other causes of death. In a 10-year period between 1980 and 1990, in rounded figures there were 5 fatal crocodile and 10 fatal shark attacks in Australia. In the same period, 20 people died from bee stings, 20 people were fatally struck by lightning, 3,000 people drowned and 30,000 people died in accidents involving motor vehicles.

Causes

1)   Snake bites

Venomous Australian snakes include taipan and small-scaled snake, tiger snake, brown and black snakes, copperhead, death adder and others. The comparative lethal effects in mice of small-scaled snake ('fierce snake') venom is 50 times greater than Indian king cobra venom and 1,000 times greater than American rattlesnake venom.

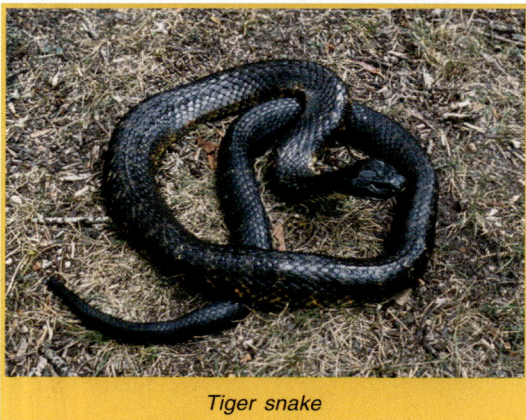

Tiger snake

2)   Spider bites

Toxins of a few species (funnel-web, red-back) can cause severe systemic and local symptoms, and deaths from envenomation can occur. Painful necrotising arachnidism is a feature of some species (white-tailed spider, wolf spider). Most species evoke local pain and inflammation only.

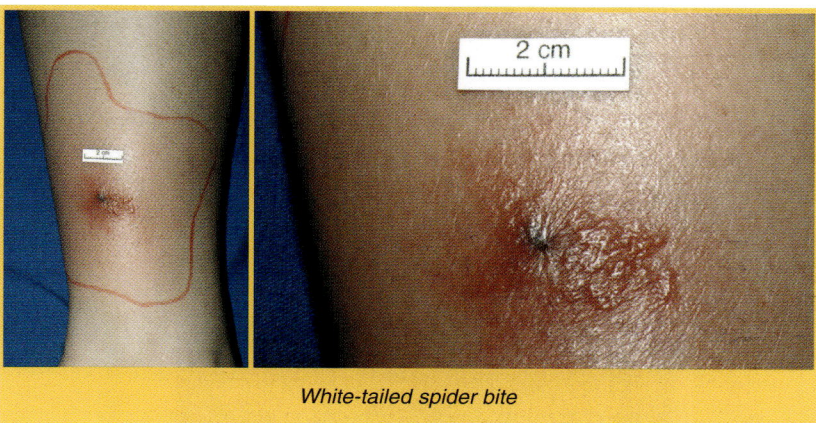

White-tailed spider bite

3) Marine bites, stings and attacks

a) **Sandfly bites:**

These are the most common beach irritant.

b) **Blue-ringed octopus and cone shell venoms:**

These can cause respiratory paralysis.

c) **Stonefish, scorpion fish and stingray:**

These have venomous spines and injuries can cause intense pain.

d) **Box jellyfish (*Chironex fleckeri* – 'seawasp'):**

Stings can occur in northern coast areas in summer and are intensely painful; occasional fatalities have occurred.

e) **Other northern jellyfish carybdeid species ('Irukandji' syndrome: *Carukia barnesi*):**

These can cause severe systemic effects and hypertension.

f) **'Bluebottle', and other jellyfish species**

g) **Attacks by estuarine crocodiles and sharks:**

These can cause gross wounding and death.

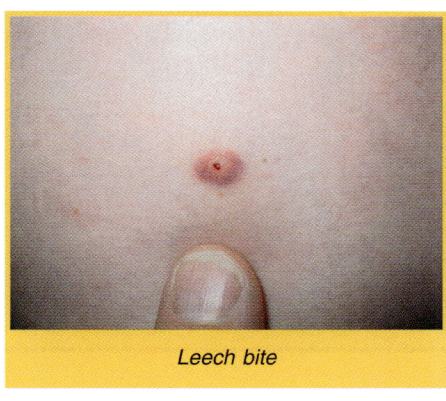

Leech bite

a) Ticks (Australian paralysis tick – 'bush tick': *Ixodes holocyclus*)

b) Ants, bees, wasps, mosquitoes, scorpions, caterpillars, leeches

c) Domestic animals (dog and cat bites, etc.)

d) Human bite injuries

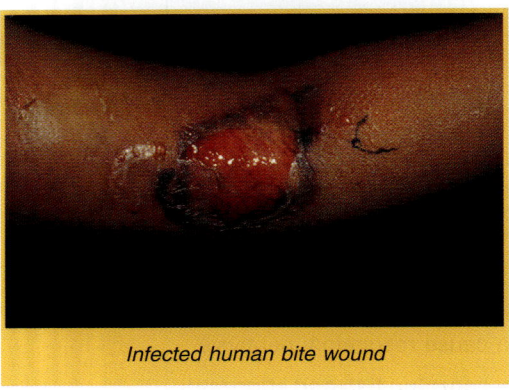

Infected human bite wound

Key Objectives

• Appreciate principles of first aid management for bites and stings by pressure-immobilisation, and of local management of the wound for specific causes.

• Recognise symptoms of envenomation and institute treatment.

General/Specific Objectives

• Construct an algorithm for management of a bite from an unidentified snake.

• Describe principles of local and general treatment of stings from:

- A bee.

- A wasp.

- A box jellyfish.

- A funnel-web spider.

- An unidentified spider bite.

• Demonstrate the technique of effective pressure-immobilisation for a snake bite to a limb.

129A Congenital Malformations

(See also #043 Genetic Concerns, Dysmorphic Features)

Overview

Management of malformations is a very important component of paediatric care. Some of the more common conditions encountered in Australia are summarised here. Many will also have been discussed in relation to specific conditions. No system is exempt from either single or multiple malformation. Causes include exogenous teratogens, chromosomal abnormalities, and an abnormal dominant or recessive gene; but in most instances the cause is unknown. Incidence of inguinal hernia in liveborn children is approximately 1:70; of more serious lesions such as tracheo-oesophageal fistula approximately 1:5,000.

Predisposing Causal Factors

These include parental age, consanguinity, race, maternal diseases, birth rank and sex of child.

Common Malformations:

1)	**Cleft lip and palate**

2)	**Umbilical or inguinal hernia**

3)	**Club foot (talipes)**

4)	**Developmental dysplasia of hip (DDH, CDH)**

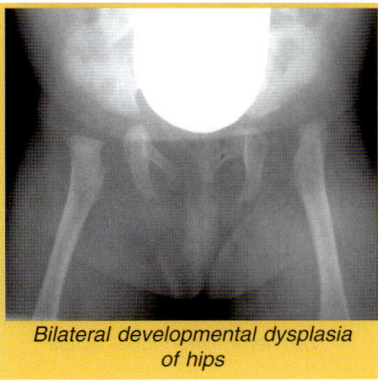

Bilateral developmental dysplasia of hips

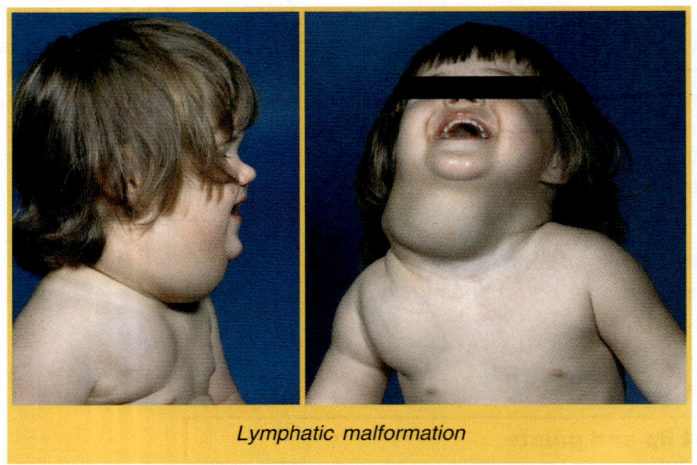

Lymphatic malformation

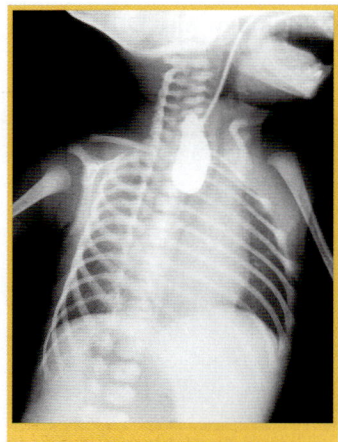

Tracheo-oesophageal fistula

13) **Hydrocephalus**

14) **Urinary tract anomalies**

15) **Anal atresia**

16) **Exomphalos**

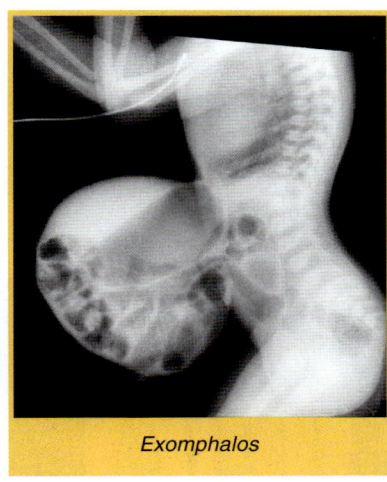

Exomphalos

17) **Hypospadias**

18) **Ambiguous genitalia**

Precipitating Teratogens:

1) **Physical (ionising radiation)**

2) **Chemical/Pharmacological (thalidomide, folic acid antagonists, etc.)**

3) **Infections (rubella, etc.)**

4) **Dietary deficiency (goitre)**

Key Objectives
- Be able to advise about known preventive factors, especially periconceptual folate in prevention of neural tube defects.
- As well as preventive measures:
    - Diagnose malformations as early as possible after birth.
- Provide empathetic counselling and appropriate referral.

129B Hand Deformities

Overview

Structural abnormalities and deformities in adults are common consequences of disease of bones or soft tissues; many are described with the relevant causative condition. The more common hand deformities are grouped as an illustrative example.

Causes

1) Congenital contractures

    a) Congenital contracture of little finger (camptodactyly, clinodactyly – approximately 1:200 incidence)

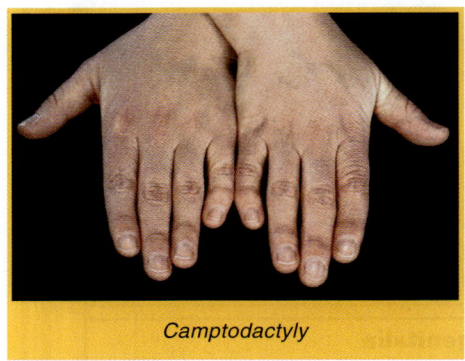

Camptodactyly

2) Dupuytren disease (nodule, contractures – palmar fasciae)

3) Muscle contracture

    a) Long flexor forearm muscles (Volkmann ischaemic contracture)

    b) Short hand muscles ('intrinsic plus' deformity – rheumatoid arthritis (RA), cerebral palsy hypertonicity)

4) Tendon deformities

    a) Trigger finger (stenosing tenosynovitis)

    b) Mallet finger

    c) Boutonnière deformity

    d) Swan neck deformity

    e) Spontaneous tendon rupture (dropped finger, thumb)

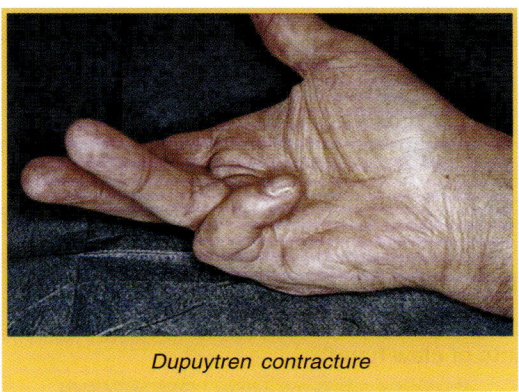

Dupuytren contracture

Bone and joint deformities

a) **Osteoarthritis**
   - ❏ Distal interphalangeal joints (Heberden nodes)
   - ❏ Proximal interphalangeal joints (Bouchard nodes)
   - ❏ Carpo-metacarpal joint of thumb

b) **RA**
   - ❏ Wrist deformity, metacarpo-phalangeal joint subluxations, ulnar deviation fingers, Z-thumb deformity, etc.

c) **Gout – tophaceous arthropathy**

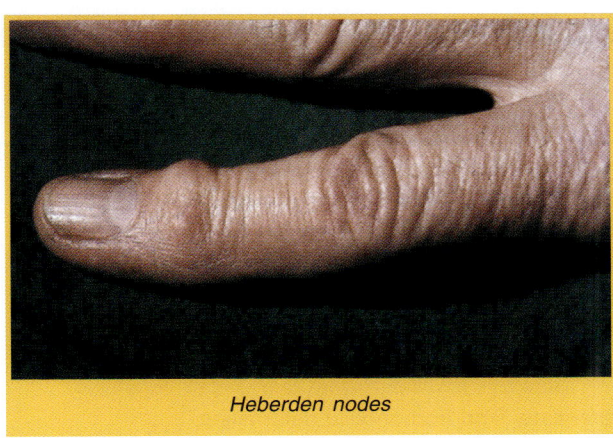

Heberden nodes

a) Radial or posterior interosseous nerve – wrist and finger drop

b) Ulnar nerve palsy – ulnar claw hand

c) Median nerve palsy – 'simian' hand, 'accoucheur' hand, pseudo-opposition

d) Upper brachial plexus lesion (C5, C6 nerve roots – Erb paralysis)

e) Lower brachial plexus lesion (T1 nerve root – Klumpke paralysis (complete claw hand))

f) Others (syringomyelia, leprosy, motor neurone disease, poliomyelitis – variants of claw hand)

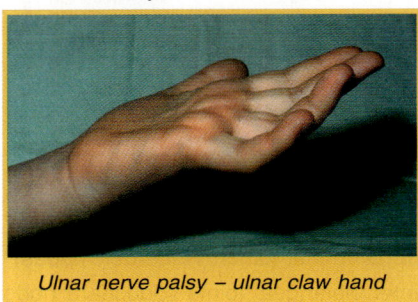

Ulnar nerve palsy – ulnar claw hand

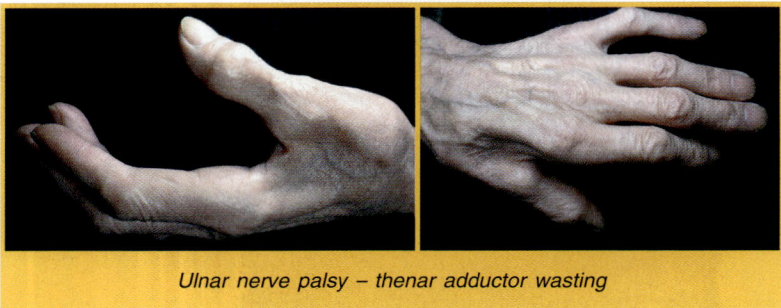

Ulnar nerve palsy – thenar adductor wasting

Key Objective
- Diagnose individual deformities and causative conditions from careful history and physical examination.

General/Specific Objectives
- Through efficient, focused data gathering:

  - Appreciate mechanisms of deformity resulting from individual causes.

  - Differentiate fixed from mobile deformities.

  - Conduct focused examination of hand status, and assess effect of deformities on hand function.

  - Discuss appropriate medical and surgical methods for correcting/coping with individual deformities.

Overview

A number of tropical infections is prevalent in the Australian Far North.

Additionally, international air travel and tourism have facilitated the spread of infectious diseases worldwide; and the potential spectre of bio-terrorism is relevant to all countries. All medical practitioners require basic knowledge of diseases not normally native to their own country, including those likely to cause fatal epidemics.

Travellers are exposed to the ubiquitous risks of traveller's diarrhoea, to diseases prevalent in the visited countries, and to sexually transmitted diseases (STDs) including AIDS.

Causes

1)   Tropical and specific fevers

    a) Brucellosis (*Brucella abortus*)

    b) Q fever (*Coxiella burnetii*)

    c) Malaria (*Plasmodium falciparum*, etc.)

    d) Dengue (arbovirus)

    e) Amoebiasis (*Entamoeba histolytica*)

    f) Melioidosis (*Pseudomonas pseudomallei*)

    g) Leptospirosis (*Leptospira pomona*)

    h) Ross River fever (arbovirus)

    i) Murray Valley encephalitis (arbovirus)

    j) Listeriosis (*Listeria monocytogenes*)

2)   Zoonoses/Ornithoses (infections transmitted between animals or birds and humans)

    a) Bovine tuberculosis (TB), brucellosis, listeriosis, Lyme disease, plague, psittacosis, rabies, typhus, etc.

    b) Schistosomiasis (bilharziasis) / Trypanosomiasis

3)   Biological agents as weapons

    a) Anthrax (*Bacillus anthracis*)

    b) Plague (*Yersinia pestis*)

131A Life-Threatening Emergencies

(See also #019 Cardiac Arrest / Respiratory Arrest)

Overview

Life-threatening medical emergencies require early recognition and prompt treatment to avert death. Treatment and diagnostic plans must proceed simultaneously and rapidly if success is to be achieved. Competence in dealing with primary care of each of the following emergencies is a basic clinical skills requirement for all medical practitioners. Most are also dealt with under headings of the causal conditions. Some of the most seriously life-threatening causes of medical emergencies are grouped below.

Causes

1) Cardiac emergencies

   a) Cardiac arrest

   b) Cardiac dysrhythmias

   c) Acute cardiac failure

   d) Acute pericardial tamponade

2) Ventilatory/Respiratory emergencies

   a) Respiratory arrest

   b) Airway obstruction / Asphyxiation

   c) Tension pneumothorax

   d) Flail chest

3) Circulatory emergencies

   a) Haemorrhage
- Overt/Concealed
- Primary / Reactionary / Secondary
- Arterial/Venous/Capillary

   b) Shock
- Hypovolaemic
- Cardiac
- Obstructive (thromboembolism, air embolism, tamponade)
- Septic
- Anaphylactic

4) Overwhelming sepsis (e.g. meningococcal septicaemia)

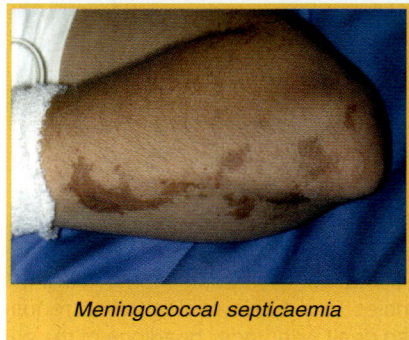

Meningococcal septicaemia

5) Cerebral emergencies

a) Disturbed consciousness
- ❑ Coma/Stupor (meningitis/encephalitis, traumatic cerebral compression)
- ❑ Acute brain syndrome (delirium)

b) Convulsions/Seizures

6) Multisystem/Organ failure

a) Acute renal failure (ARF) (oliguric/nonoliguric) with severe hyperkalaemia

b) Acute haematologic failure (disseminated intravascular coagulation (DIC)) with massive bleeding

c) Acute gastrointestinal failure (stress ulcer syndrome/necrotising enteritis) with massive bleeding or peritonitis

d) Acute metabolic emergencies (acid-base disequilibrium, water-electrolyte disturbance)

7) Drowning/Electrocution

Key Objectives
- Demonstrate competence in primary care of medical emergencies.
- Recognise life-threatening medical emergencies and their causes as early as possible.
- Appreciate principles and practice of combined therapeutic and diagnostic plans for initial management of such emergencies.

General/Specific Objectives
- Appreciate the specific treatment and diagnostic plans for individual emergencies.
- Construct algorithms to deal efficaciously with each emergency, including specific diagnostic tests.

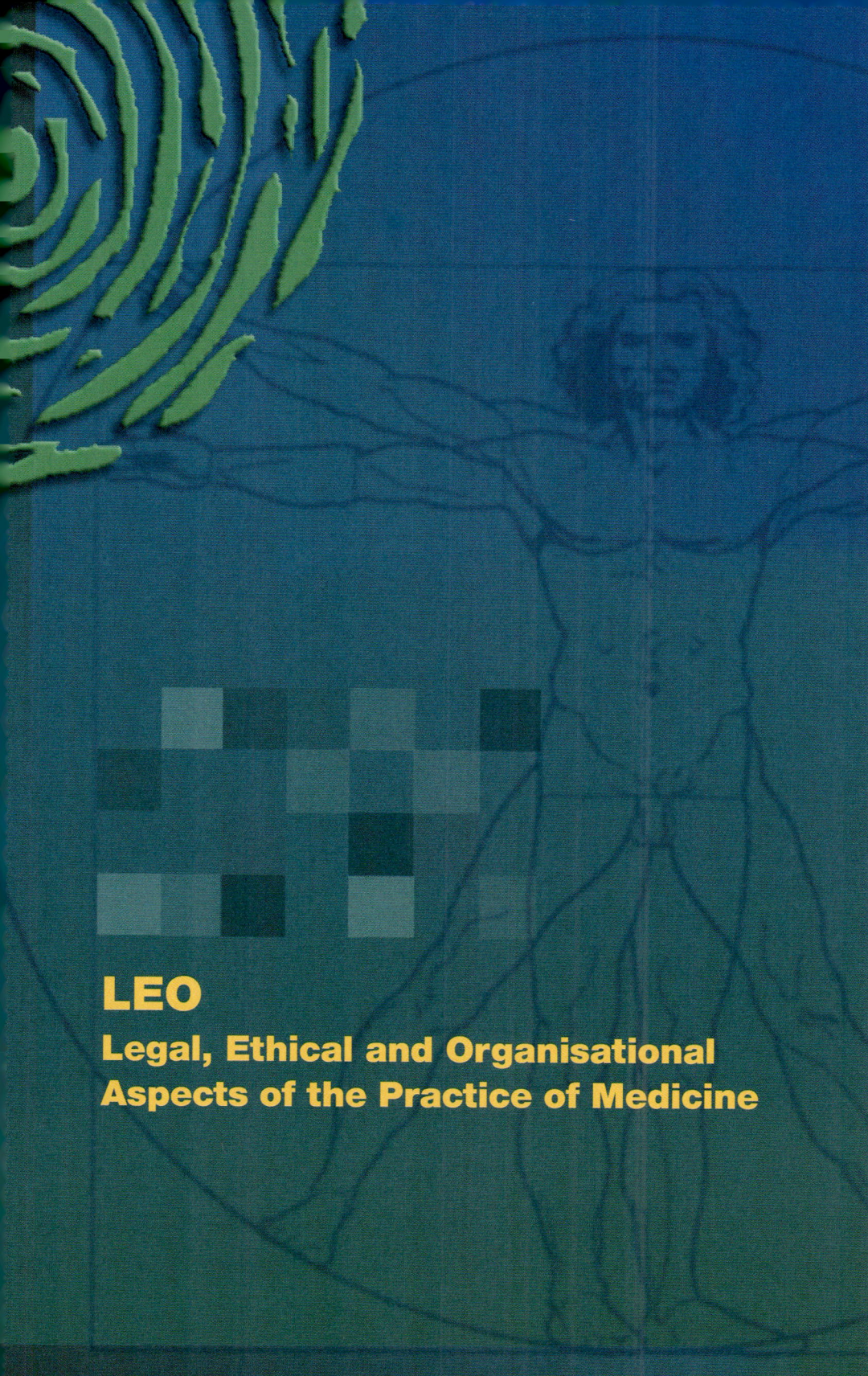

LEO
Legal, Ethical and Organisational
Aspects of the Practice of Medicine

Contents

1 Introduction

The three distinct sections of Legal, Ethical and Organisational Aspects of the Practice of Medicine (LEO) focus in turn on the **legal**, the **ethical** and the **organisational** aspects of the practice of medicine. Although there is considerable overlap between topics covered in the three sections, they are able to be approached separately, and are cross-referenced with each other where appropriate. Each section has its own contribution to make to medical professionalism and to the practice of safe and effective medicine. For each section, there are also important differences in how professional conduct is taught, fostered, monitored and where necessary investigated. Understanding the differences between the legal, the ethical and the organisational segments will help you to get the most out of this document.

Medical **ethics** arise from the traditions of the profession, its philosophy, and our social standards and mores. Ethics are expressed as principles and concepts, which lead to more specific guidelines or codes for particular situations. Ethical problems tend to be resolved through prolonged public debate and discussion. Breaches of the ethical guidelines of medical practice are generally dealt with within the profession, but may also be the concern of healthcare institutions as well.

The **legal** section is based on the statutory and case laws relevant to the practice of medicine. Laws are specific, not conceptual. Legal requirements may be set out by the state and federal parliaments or determined by the courts as they make rulings on particular cases. This document discusses the area of law that is in effect in most areas, although occasional reference is made to notable laws that may only apply in an identified state or territory. Clinicians entering medical practice will want to be sure of the specific legal requirements of the state or territory in which they are registered to practise. A breach of a relevant law would be dealt with legally.

Registration to practise medicine in Australia is conferred by state and territory medical boards of: Australian Capital Territory (ACT); New South Wales (NSW); Northern Territory (NT); Queensland (QLD); South Australia (SA); Tasmania (TAS); Victoria (VIC); and Western Australia (WA).

The third section is on **organisational** aspects of the practice of medicine. Clinicians in Australia practise within a complex healthcare system. They have numerous professional obligations, and interact with many other groups responsible for various aspects of healthcare. This section is written from the point of view of what the clinician entering medical practice will need to know. Breaches of expected standards in these aspects may be the concern of the appropriate colleges, the medical boards, the courts, or the healthcare institutions, or may simply result in inefficiencies and frustrations.

The Australian Medical Council (AMC) hopes that medical practitioners will be familiar with much of LEO, though these areas may not have been formally taught. To assist in understanding the basis of these objectives, references to key print and electronic resources are included either in the preambles or following each set of objectives.

Please take time to become familiar with the layout and the content of LEO and its appendices.

AMA: Australian Medical Association.

AMC: Australian Medical Council.

ARPNSA: Australian Radiation Protection and Nuclear Safety Agency.

Autonomy: The moral right to choose and follow one's own plan of life and action, including the right to refuse treatment.

Beneficence: The moral duty to help persons in need.

Capacity: The patient's ability to understand information relevant to making a decision. Capacity determinations are made by medical practitioners, sometimes using the help of psychiatrists and other members of the healthcare team.

Clinician: A registered medical practitioner engaged in clinical practice.

Clinician-assisted suicide: The act of intentionally killing oneself with the assistance of a clinician who deliberately provides the knowledge, means, or both.

CME: Continuing medical education.

Competence: This term is frequently used interchangeably with capacity. Strictly speaking it is a legal term denoting the right to make a decision. The legal presumption is that all adults are competent, and only a judge can rule a person incompetent.

Conflict of interest: A set of conditions in which professional judgement concerning a primary interest (such as a patient's welfare or the validity of research) tends to be unduly influenced by a secondary interest (such as financial gain). (Thompson DF. Understanding financial conflicts of interest. N Engl J Med 1993;329:573-576.)

Consent: The autonomous authorisation of a medical intervention by individual patients. Consent has three components: disclosure, capacity, and voluntariness.

Disclosure: The provision of relevant and material information regarding a decision by a doctor to a patient (and its comprehension by the patient).

Discrimination: An act, practice or policy that differentiates between, or otherwise treats persons in a different way, on the basis of such status as gender, age, nationality, religion, race, financial means or sexual orientation.

Distributive justice: The obligation of clinicians to make appropriate healthcare available to their patients in a fair and equitable manner.

Doctor: A registered medical practitioner.

Ethics: The discipline dealing with principles and values defining what is good (acceptable/appropriate/reasonable) and bad (unacceptable/inappropriate/ unreasonable), and with duties and obligations for various groups. In medicine, application of ethical principles to complex and controversial issues and to evolving therapies can lead to consensus codes of practice in specific areas.

Euthanasia: A deliberate act undertaken to end the life of another person in order to end suffering; the act is the cause of death.

Fiduciary: Person to whom property or power is entrusted for the benefit of another.

Fiduciary obligation: The obligation to promote the best interests of persons who have entrusted themselves to the fiduciary (e.g. the clinician); an obligation of the highest loyalty, fidelity and trust.

HIC: Health Insurance Commission.

Justice: The fair distribution of benefits and burdens within a community.

Material risks: Those that are common, and those that are serious, even if uncommon.

MJA: Medical Journal of Australia.

Morals: The practice of ethics in everyday life. The nouns ethics and morals can be concisely separated by defining ethics as the science of morals and morals as the practice of ethics. The adjectives ethical/moral, and unethical/immoral in everyday speech have additional nuances. We tend to speak of the ethical rather than the moral bases of society or of medicine and of unethical breaches of these; whereas immoral is commonly associated with sexual morality. These nuances can be influenced by a perception that the words 'right' and 'wrong' and 'good' and 'bad' may seem old-fashioned.

NGO: Non-governmental organisation.

NHMRC: National Health and Medical Research Council.

Non-maleficence: The duty to refrain from doing harm.

OH&S: Occupational health and safety.

PBS: Pharmaceutical Benefits Scheme.

Profession: A self-regulating organisation that controls entry by certifying that medical practitioners have necessary knowledge and skills used to benefit society. (Beauchamp T, Childress J. Principles of biomedical ethics. Oxford: Oxford University Press; 1994. p. 4-7.)

QA: Quality assurance.

Resource allocation (and rationing): The distribution of goods and services to programmes and people; rationing is the systematic distribution of goods to specific individuals in conditions of scarcity.

Security of the person / inviolability: The fundamental right of individuals to expect respect for their bodies and persons and non-violation of their bodies and persons, be it through physical, psychological or other means.

VMO: Visiting medical officer.

Voluntariness: The patient's right to come to a decision freely, without undue pressure including force, coercion, or manipulation.

3.1   Doctor-Patient Relationship

Overview

The doctor-patient relationship is the fundamental basis of the therapeutic relationship. The relationship is based on ethical and legal principles. These describe the quality of the relationship, and the obligations and restrictions inherent to it. Both the medical practitioner and the patient enjoy certain rights, responsibilities, and freedoms which determine the doctor-patient relationship and the need for this relationship to be kept in appropriate balance.

Issues

- Obligations and restrictions
- Conflict of interest, disclosure of personal or moral limitations
- Professional boundaries
- Clinician's and patient's rights
- Care of friends and family

General/Specific Objectives

- To recognise and demonstrate the elements in current codes which define the doctor-patient relationship.
- To recognise that the clinician will place the best interest of the patient as first priority.
- To establish a relationship of trust between the clinician and the patient.
- To maintain confidentiality of information proffered by the patient.
- To follow through on undertakings made to the patient, in good faith.
- To accept or refuse patients requesting care:
  - without consideration of race, gender, age, sexual orientation, financial means, religion or nationality;
  - without arbitrary exclusion of any particular group of patients, such as those known to be difficult, or afflicted with serious disease; and
  - except in emergency situations, in which case care must be rendered.
- Once having accepted a patient into care, the clinician may terminate the relationship, providing:
  - care has been transferred; or
  - adequate notice has been given to allow the patient to make alternative arrangements.
- The clinician will not exploit the doctor-patient relationship for personal advantage: be it financial, academic or otherwise.

- To disclose the limitations to the patient where personal beliefs or inclinations limit the treatment a clinician is able to offer.
- To maintain and respect professional boundaries at all times:
  - including physical, emotional, and sexual boundaries; and
  - regarding treatment of themselves, their families, or friends.

References

- *AMA Code of Ethics*
  Australian Medical Association:
  http://www.ama.com.au

3.2   Personal and Professional Conduct

Issues

- Personal conduct:
  - competence
  - impairment
- Professional conduct

Key Objective

- Clinicians should be aware of the professional conduct expected of them, and should recognise their responsibilities if a colleague demonstrates unprofessional conduct.

General/Specific Objectives

3.2.1 Personal conduct

- To conduct oneself in a professional manner, characterised by honesty, respect, integrity, and dignity:
  - to possess and maintain medical expertise; and
  - to practise competently without impairment by substances, ill health, or other incapacity.

3.2.2 Professional responsibilities

- To recognise responsibility of the profession in self-regulation via:
  - maintenance of appropriate standards of the profession; and
  - participation in peer review.
- To participate in learning with peers and others who may include:
  - students and postgraduate trainees;

- - other healthcare professionals; and
- - community or patient groups.
- To assist peers and others in achieving effective methods of care, in the best interests of patient well-being.
- To recognise the role of the medical boards in assisting and monitoring impaired medical practitioners.

3.2.3 Payment for uninsured services

Definitions

Uninsured services are:

- Those which are not covered under the state schedules of medical benefits as amended from time to time.
- Services to unregistered patients who are ineligible for state health coverage or for coverage under the reciprocal agreement among states.

Principles

- Consider, in determining professional fees, both the nature of the service provided and the ability of the patient to pay, and be prepared to discuss the fee with the patient.
- Avoid any personal profit motive in ordering drugs, appliances or diagnostic procedures from any facility in which the clinician has a financial interest.
- The patient's best medical interest must always be foremost.

3.2.4 Advertising professional services

When advertising professional services avoid:

- misrepresenting fact;
- comparing either directly, indirectly or by innuendo, services or abilities with those of any other clinician or clinic, or promising or offering more effective services or better results than those available elsewhere;
- deprecating another clinician or clinic;
- creating an unjustified expectation as to the results the clinician can achieve;
- taking advantage of the vulnerability of patients; and
- disclosing the identity of patients.

References

- *AMA Code of Ethics*
  Australian Medical Association:
  http://www.ama.com.au
- Medical boards (various states and territories) – see Appendix 1

3.3   Ethics of Medicine

Overview

Medicine is an ethical profession. It is based on ethical principles and bound by codes, both explicit and implicit, regarding the relationships between clinicians and their patients, their profession, and society at large.

Clinicians should be familiar with codes set out by the Australian Medical Association (AMA) and the various states and territories, and understand their ethical foundation.

The key ethical principles, which provide the foundation of these ethical codes and may be invoked in the resolution of ethical dilemmas, include: respect for autonomy, justice, beneficence and non-maleficence, among others. Clinicians should be able to identify the relevant principles at issue in the analysis or resolution of an ethical dilemma.

Ethical dilemmas faced by clinicians are often matters of social interest and controversy. An ethical clinician must be prepared to consult and seek input or guidance into such decisions, including the participation of formal bodies, such as ethics committees, to assist in resolution of situations where the principles are in conflict.

References

* *AMA Code of Ethics*
  Australian Medical Association:
  http://www.ama.com.au

* National Health Medical Research Council (NHMRC):
  http://www.nhmrc.gov.au/issues/index.htm

* *The Duties of a Doctor Registered with the New South Wales Medical Board*
  The New South Wales Medical Board:
  http://www.nswmb.org.au
  > Duties of a doctor registered with the NSWMB

* Various national specialty and subspecialty colleges and associations – see Appendix 2

3.4   Confidentiality and Privacy

Overview

Clinicians receive confidential information from and regarding their patients, and are legally bound not to disclose such confidences. This obligation is the foundation of confidence in the doctor-patient relationship. The clinician is obliged to recognise the legitimate interests and rights of third parties to patient information in appropriate circumstances, and to disclose this information in an ethical fashion. Electronic communication technology increases the risk of disclosure of confidential information. Clinicians will need to be aware of evolving standards and precautions in this regard.

Issues

* Trust in doctor-patient relationship

- Patient's right to confidentiality and privacy

- Legal obligations to disclose to public authorities

- Disclosure to third parties (see also 3.5 Consent to Investigation or Treatment)

- Rights of minors and incapacitated patients

- Right to access information only of patients under care, and with consent of patient

- Duty to warn individuals discovered to be at risk through disclosures made in confidence

General/Specific Objectives

- To explain the basis for the clinician's obligation to maintain confidentiality.

- To explain reasonable precautions to maintain confidentiality (verbal, telephone, fax or e-mail communication; charts, written or computer-stored; and educational or research rounds or presentations).

- To appreciate sensitivities and special circumstances in case of minors and incapacitated patients.

- To recognise situations in which third parties have a legitimate interest and right to information:

  - legal requirements in the interest of public health;

  - legitimate interest of third parties (e.g. insurance companies, police);

  - duty to warn threatened individuals; and

  - care of minors and incapacitated patients.

- To recognise reasonable limits to disclosure, and reveal only the relevant and necessary information, in a situation requiring disclosure to a third party.

- To recognise duty to advise patients of known risks of voluntary disclosure (e.g. risks of disclosure of HIV status).

- To recognise the need to advise patients of obligatory disclosure of information.

- To transmit required information in a timely fashion.

- To recognise and seek guidance where harm from disclosure balances harm of maintaining confidentiality.

- To recognise and apply the relevant federal and state/territory privacy legislation or codes.

References

- Australian Medical Association:
  http://www.ama.com.au
  > Policy and Issues > Privacy Legislation

- *Handbook for the Management of Health Information in Private Medical Practice*
  The Royal Australian College of General Practitioners:
  http://www.racgp.org.au
  > Your practice > Privacy

- The Office of the Federal Privacy Commissioner:
  http://www.privacy.gov.au
  > Health

3.5   Consent to Investigation or Treatment

Overview

Respect for patient autonomy requires the patient's informed choice, consent, and participation. Conversely, the informed patient's right to refuse treatment must be respected, even when it may seem medically unwise. Individuals must be capable of understanding the relevant risks, benefits, and alternatives, and the consequences of declining. The choice should be made free of any coercion. Patients unable to give informed consent are entitled to have their interests protected through an appropriate substitute decision-making procedure.

Issues

- Expressed consent, oral or written:
  - current
  - advanced directives
- Informed choice (disclosure of material risks and alternatives)
- Voluntariness (freedom from coercion)
- Consent for emergency treatment
- Capacity to give consent:
  - impairment
  - consent by minors
  - assessment of capacity
- Implied consent
- Substitute decision makers or proxies
- Refusal or revocation of consent

Key Objective

- Clinicians should communicate with patients or their legitimate delegates, so as to obtain their consent or refusal to a given investigation or treatment.

General/Specific Objectives

- To explain the legal and ethical basis for consent.
- To demonstrate awareness of the process for the assessment of capacity to give consent, and to be able to conduct such an assessment.

- To recognise factors which can alter capacity (e.g. disease, drugs, depression).

- To identify an appropriate substitute decision-maker, or to establish the process to determine an appropriate decision-maker.

- To clearly communicate information relevant to informed consent (what a reasonable person would want to know in a given circumstance).

- To identify reasonable steps to ensure understanding of information: can the patient explain the medical problem, and the proposed treatment or test.

- To determine free choice, and absence of coercion.

- To recognise the patient's right to refuse or revoke consent without prejudice to subsequent treatment.

- To recognise and identify ways of determining the appropriate balance between the emerging autonomy of a minor with the legitimate interests of parents or child welfare authorities.

- To recognise legal requirements in such cases.

- To recognise the legitimacy of the intentions of impaired patients as they may have been expressed (advanced directives).

- To recognise the duty to provide necessary emergency care where consent is unavailable.

- To recognise the need to provide non-consensual treatment in the public interest; e.g. involuntary admission for patients whose conditions possess an unacceptable risk to themselves or others.

- To recognise the role of religious belief in obtaining patient consent and the provision of treatment.

References

- *AMA Code of Ethics*
  Australian Medical Association:
  http://www.ama.com.au

3.6   Disclosure

Overview

Respecting patient autonomy and avoiding paternalism, clinicians should disclose to their patients relevant information regarding their diagnosis, prognosis, or the implications of diagnostic tests. This follows from principles of truthfulness and of maintenance of a relationship of trust.

Issues

- Ethical basis for a patient's right to know

- Consequences of violating a patient's right to know

- Disclosure of relevant information

- Prohibition from transmitting false information
- Incomplete disclosure
- Exceptions (cultural, potential harm)

Key Objectives

- Clinicians should recognise that their duty is to speak truthfully and appreciate that imparting the truth may conflict with their duty to 'do no harm'.
- Make sure when telling the 'truth' to a patient that you know what the 'truth' is; and that the patient wants and needs to hear it.

General/Specific Objectives

- To understand and explain the ethical and legal basis for disclosure:
  - respect for patient's autonomy;
  - situations of inevitable disclosure;
  - provision of support with disclosure of difficult news; and
  - respect patient's need to make realistic life decisions.
- To recognise the reasonable rights of patients to know relevant information:
  - purpose and implications of investigations;
  - diagnosis and prognosis of medical condition;
  - risks and benefits of treatment; and
  - health risks to which they are exposed.
- To respect patients' right to not know, and ascertain patients' wishes:
  - identify and respect valid exceptions to disclosure;
  - seek consent for disclosure;
  - be aware of specific personal and cultural contexts and how these may influence a patient's choice; and
  - respect a patient's choice above that of family members.
- To recognise and seek guidance in situations of conflict between disclosure and other ethical duties, particularly the duty to do no harm.

References

- *AMA Code of Ethics*
  Australian Medical Association:
  http://www.ama.com.au

3.7   Resource Allocation

Overview

Acting in the patient's best interest, the obligation of clinicians is to make appropriate healthcare available to their patients in a fair and equitable manner (distributive justice). An expanding number of treatable patients and an increasing array of expensive technology exist, but healthcare resources are finite. This can lead to an inevitable conflict between the best interest of the patient and the interest of society at large. Ethical principles should guide the orderly resolution of such conflicts.

Issues

- Fair access to healthcare resources
- Obligation to seek the best interests of the patient
- Prudent use of healthcare resources

General/Specific Objectives

- To make healthcare resources available to patients in a manner which is fair and equitable, without bias or discrimination.
- To recognise situations in which allocation of resources is unfair, and to seek resolution.
- To recognise or propose fair means of resolving disputes for resources:
  - recognise the primary obligation is to the patient;
  - rank known patients ahead of unknown or future patients;
  - use morally relevant criteria in allocating resources; and
  - consult hospital ethics committees or other responsible bodies.
- To choose interventions, on the basis of best available evidence, which are:
  - known to be effective; and
  - expected to have anticipated cost benefit.
- To avoid marginally beneficial investigations or treatments.
- To inform patients of impact of cost restraint in a supportive way.
- To be prudent and avoid waste in the utilisation of scarce or costly resources.

References

- *AMA Code of Ethics*
  Australian Medical Association:
  http://www.ama.com.au

3.8   Clinicians and Commerce

Overview

Clinicians will in the course of their practice need to have ethical relationships with industries that may have areas of common interest. Clinicians need to be aware of the potential for a conflict of interest, and of their primary responsibility to the patient.

Issues

*   Conflict of interest
*   To place first the best interests of the patient

Key Objectives

*   Clinicians should be aware of the existence of ethical codes which regulate the relationship between the profession and the pharmaceutical industry, and recognise situations which breach such codes.

*   The primary obligation of clinicians is to their patients. Relationships with industry are appropriate only if they do not impinge upon that responsibility.

*   Any conflicts of interest arising from a relationship with industry must be resolved in favour of the patient.

*   Clinicians in their practice must preserve their professional autonomy. Any potential conflict of interest must be disclosed to the patient.

*   Institutions and organisations in which a clinician works or holds privileges may have additional requirements regarding disclosure of potential conflict of interest.

*   If a conflict of interest cannot be resolved, the clinician may recommend a second opinion or refrain from offering an opinion.

References

*   *AMA Code of Ethics*
    Australian Medical Association:
    http://www.ama.com.au

*   National Health Medical Research Council (NHMRC):
    http://www.nhmrc.gov.au/issues/index.htm

*   *Code of Conduct*
    Medicines Australia:
    http://www.medicinesaustralia.com.au

*   *Ethical Guideline #5 – Guide to Ethical Principles in the Relationship Between Psychiatrists and the Pharmaceutical Industry (Research Activity)*
    The Royal Australian and New Zealand College of Psychiatrists (RANZCP):
    http://www.ranzcp.org/eg/eg5.htm

3.9   Ethical and Professional Issues

Overview

Clinicians will be required to advise their patients on evolving moral and legal issues regarding tests or treatments that may conflict with the clinicians' own values, or with morally prevalent values.

Issues

- Euthanasia
- Clinician-assisted suicide
- Maternal-fetal conflict of rights
- Advanced reproductive technology
- Fetal tissue
- Abortion
- Genetic testing
- Female circumcision (genital mutilation)
- Aspects of transplantation biotechnology (including indications for autograft, isograft, allograft or xenograft tissues and organs)

General/Specific Objectives

- Clinicians should be aware that they may be asked to comment on unresolved or controversial ethical issues, and to name and describe relevant key issues and ethical principles.
- When confronted with such a situation, clinicians should:
  - discuss the matter with patients and others in a nonjudgemental manner;
  - ensure patients have full access to relevant and necessary information;
  - identify if certain options lie outside their own moral boundaries and refer to another clinician if appropriate;
  - be aware that there are legal implications if a procedure such as female circumcision (genital mutilation) is performed in Australia;
  - consult with appropriate hospital and institutional ethics committees or boards where appropriate; and
  - protect freedom of moral choice for students or trainees.

References

- *AMA Code of Ethics*
  Australian Medical Association:
  http://www.ama.com.au

- National Health Medical Research Council (NHMRC):
  http://www.nhmrc.gov.au/issues/index.htm

3.10   Seeking Ethical and Legal Advice

Overview

Clinicians will, from time to time, need to seek advice about specific legal or ethical dilemmas in daily clinical practice.

Issue

- The need to seek advice from colleagues, medical defence associations and professional associations when faced with a legal or ethical problem

Key Objective

- Competent clinicians will recognise the circumstances under which it is appropriate to seek advice and where to seek that advice.

General/Specific Objectives

- To recognise the circumstances under which it is appropriate to seek advice.
- To recognise where to seek advice under specific circumstances.

References

- *AMA Code of Ethics*
  Australian Medical Association:
  http://www.ama.com.au

- National Health Medical Research Council (NHMRC):
  http://www.nhmrc.gov.au/issues/index.htm

- Medical defence organisations – see Appendix 10

3.11   Research Ethics

Overview

Clinicians have a responsibility to contribute to the advancement of medical care, which may involve research participation. They also have an obligation to provide the best available care to their patients, which may be accomplished through participation in research. Clinicians need to be aware of special populations for which the rules may be different, such as children, psychiatric patients, or the cognitively impaired; and for the sensitivities involved with indigenous Australians and people of non-English speaking backgrounds.

The ethics of animal research requires appreciation of possible alternative techniques to the use of animals, as well as appreciation and monitoring of appropriate guidelines for animal care and welfare.

Issues

- Scientific and ethical merits of research
- Conflict of interest
- Full disclosure in obtaining informed consent
- Right of non-participation or withdrawal without prejudice

Key Objectives

- To ensure that any research study in which their patients are involved is scientifically and ethically sound, that their patients have received full disclosure of anticipated risks and benefits, and have made informed choices free from coercion.
- To ensure that animal research conforms to appropriate national standards.

General/Specific Objectives

- To identify reasonable criteria for ethical approval of research involving patients.
- To identify or propose reasonable steps to ensure scientific rigour of research (peer review, expert opinion).
- To refuse to participate or to enrol patients in research which has not been scientifically and ethically evaluated.
- To recognise the need for fully informed and voluntary consent.
- To identify additional information which should be disclosed in the course of research, as opposed to clinical consent.
- To acknowledge and disclose any possible conflict of interest on the part of the investigator.
- To recognise that all human research must have prior approval by an appropriately established human research ethics committee and that all animal research must similarly be reviewed by an animal research ethics committee.

References

- *AMA Code of Ethics*
  Australian Medical Association:
  http://www.ama.com.au
- *Ethical Conduct in Research*
  National Health Medical Research Council (NHMRC):
  http://www.nhmrc.gov.au/issues/researchethics.htm

4.1   Applicable Basic Principles of Law

Overview

The laws of society regulate many aspects of human conduct, including medical practice. The principles and provisions of law applicable to the practice of medicine have a number of sources. There is significant overlap between clinicians' 'generally-recognised' ethical obligations in the Australian context and the requirements of the law with regard to medical practice. (Note: it is recognised that different cultural approaches may lead to differing views regarding applicable ethical mores. The law, however, while always evolving, does not always account for such divergence of ethical views, and seeks to articulate 'universal' standards applicable to a given jurisdiction.)

Issues

*   Relationship between law and ethics

*   Principles and provisions of law also apply to the practice of medicine

General/Specific Objectives

Competent clinicians should be able to identify in a clinical context that:

*   statutes, regulations, by-laws, and the rulings of courts (the 'common law') are applicable in various ways to the practice of medicine and are binding on clinicians;

*   legal principles and provisions often reflect ethical standards, e.g. in the areas of consent, confidentiality, and the duty of care; and

*   Australia is a federal state, in which the federal government has jurisdiction in certain areas (e.g. espionage and certain aspects of criminal law) and the state governments in others (e.g. administration of healthcare and the regulation of professions).

Important note: Australian law applicable to the practice of medicine varies from jurisdiction to jurisdiction and evolves constantly. These objectives are therefore necessarily general and provide an overview only. Clinicians, teachers, and examiners should ensure that information relied upon is up-to-date and appropriate to the applicable jurisdiction.

References

*   Australian Medical Association:
    http://www.ama.com.au
    > Policy and Issues > Legal issues

*   Attorney General's Department:
    http://www.ag.gov.au

4.2 The Patient: A Person with Human and Legal Rights

Overview

The patient is a human being and citizen, and as such, is the beneficiary of many fundamental human and legal rights. The patient's status as the focus and central subject of medical practice, and the requirements of law, dictate that medical practice conforms with current concepts of patients' rights.

Issues

- The patient as a beneficiary of human and legal rights
- The patient as the focus of medical practice
- Clinician practice regulated by patient rights

Key Objective

- Competent clinicians should recognise the patient as a key focus and central subject of medical practice, and understand that the patient is a person with certain fundamental human and legal rights that the clinician is required to respect and uphold.

General/Specific Objectives

- To identify the patient (rather than the clinician or the hospital, for example) as a key focus and central subject of medical practice.
- To identify patients' fundamental human rights relevant to the practice of medicine, such as:
  - the right to security of the person and inviolability; and
  - the right to freedom from discrimination by virtue of age, race, gender, nationality, religion, sexual orientation, financial means, or other status.
- To demonstrate the knowledge that the patient has fundamental legal rights in the medical context, arising under both statutory law and the rulings of the courts, that are binding on the clinician.

References

- Australian Medical Association:
  http://www.ama.com.au
  > Policy and Issues > Legal

4.3 Legal Aspects of Consent

Overview

The right to security of the person / inviolability means that it is legally (and ethically) mandatory that the clinician obtain the consent of his/her patient (or in the case of the incompetent/incapacitated patient, the patient's lawful substitute) for any medical investigation, treatment, or research. This consent must be voluntarily given and fully informed, and may be expressed or implied and given orally or in writing according to the circumstances. Consent may be lawfully withheld and this decision must be respected. The law provides for a limited number of exceptions to the requirement for consent.

Key Objectives

- Voluntary and informed consent as a fundamental legal requirement.

- The elements and practical aspects of consent to investigation, treatment, or research.

- The right to refuse consent.

- Exceptions to the requirement for consent.

(These issues should be considered in conjunction with corresponding objectives concerning the ethical aspects of medical practice. See sections 3.5 Consent to Investigation or Treatment, 3.9 Ethical and Professional Issues, 3.10 Seeking Ethical and Legal Advice, and 3.11 Research Ethics.)

General/Specific Objectives

The competent clinician should be able to demonstrate an understanding that:

- It is mandatory that the patient's consent is obtained for any medical investigation, treatment, or research.

- Consent must be freely given and fully informed.

- Full information must be given, in language that the patient or involved person(s) can understand. This must include information regarding the nature of the proposed treatment or investigation, anticipated effects, material or significant risks, alternatives available, and any information regarding delegation of care, and will be given according to the circumstances of each particular case.

- The obligation of disclosure rests with the clinician who is to carry out the treatment. It may be delegated in appropriate circumstances to another qualified clinician, but responsibility lies with the delegating clinician.

- Consent may be expressed or implied, and given orally or in writing according to the circumstances, noting that by law in some circumstances consent must be written.

- The consenting patient must have the legal capacity to consent; i.e. be of a legal age to consent (different states specify differing ages at which a patient is deemed to be capable of giving consent). The treatment of minors often raises a number of important legal (as well as ethical and practical) issues for clinicians.

- The consenting patient must be competent to consent; i.e. sufficiently capable, e.g. if they are young or mentally incapacitated, they must be able to understand the information required for consent and appreciate the reasonably foreseeable consequences. Competence is to be assessed operationally or functionally; i.e. the patient need only be competent to consent to, or refuse the particular choice in question.

- If the patient is not competent or lacks capacity to consent, then consent may be obtained (according to the law applicable in each state and the specific circumstances) from a court, parent or substitute decision-maker. The law regarding delegation of care is specific to each state and the clinician should be fully aware of local requirements in this regard.

- The patient has the right to refuse consent to treatment and this decision must be respected, even when this may lead to the death of the patient.

- Consent may be withdrawn at any time without penalty or any other impact on the provision of care.

- There are a number of exceptions to the requirement for consent, such as:

  - necessary treatment in a medical emergency;

  - under certain circumstances (including pursuant to mental health legislation) where patients are a danger to the lives or health of others or themselves; and

  - where the law provides for compulsory treatment.

- Treatment is limited to the scope of consent given, including to the identity of the treating clinician.

References

- Australian Medical Association:
  http://www.ama.com.au
  > Policy and Issues > Legal

4.4 Legal Aspects of Confidentiality

Overview

Clinicians are legally (and ethically) bound to hold any and all information obtained from a patient confidential. This duty ensures that the patient's legal rights (including reputation and social status) are protected. Confidentiality is, of course, also recognised as essential for clinician-patient respect and trust. Exceptions arise when the patient waives the right to confidentiality or when provided for in law.

Key Objectives

- The duty of confidentiality: a legal requirement.

- Exceptions to the requirement of confidentiality.

(These issues should be considered in conjunction with corresponding objectives concerning the ethical aspects of medical practice. See sections 3.1 Doctor-Patient Relationship, 3.3 Ethics of Medicine, 3.4 Confidentiality and Privacy, and 3.6 Disclosure.)

General/Specific Objectives

The competent clinician should be able to recognise and apply the following principles in the clinical situation:

- The patient's fundamental right to security of the person, reputation and social status, and various specific provisions in law require that clinicians hold all information concerning a patient confidential.

- A clinician may not disclose patient information (whether about the existence, nature, extent of illness or any other health information) except where expressly authorised by the patient to do so, or when the law permits or requires such disclosure.

- Exceptions to the duty of confidentiality and the requirement of patient consent for its disclosure are provided for in various (state and federal) statutes. These require clinicians to report certain confidential information for the protection of public health and other purposes, and in some cases provide penalties for failure to do so. (See 3.4 Confidentiality and Privacy.)

- In respect of legal processes involving clinicians, clinicians may not disclose confidential information even in the case of service of a subpoena or police investigation, except when ordered to do so by a court or pursuant to a search warrant.

- Consent may reasonably be implied, with caution, where inter-healthcare team communication is essential for the effective provision of care.

- Special care must be exercised not to inadvertently disclose patient confidences, e.g. in unguarded conversation or to patients' friends or relatives.

- Breach of the duty of confidentiality renders the clinician potentially liable for damages to the patient and/or open to disciplinary proceedings before a state medical board.

- A clinician's duty to society may in exceptional circumstances legally justify disclosure of confidential information where, for example it becomes known to a clinician that a patient is about to seriously harm or kill another person. There are limitations in law, however, on the duty to warn.

- Due to the complexity of, and exceptions to, the duty of confidentiality, advice may be sought from state medical boards or legal counsel, when in doubt.

- Special care must be exercised with the use of fax, e-mail or other electronic means for the transmission of patient health information, as these methods of transmission can compromise confidentiality.

References

- Australian Medical Association:
  http://www.ama.com.au

4.5 Clinicians' Legal Liability for Negligence

Overview

Clinicians are legally liable to their patients for causing harm through a failure to meet the standard of duty of care applicable under the circumstances. While there are a number of differing 'causes of action' for such liability including assault and battery, the great majority of civil cases launched by patients against clinicians are based on negligence. A number of elements must be present for a claim against a clinician to succeed.

Issues

- Clinicians' civil liability for their actions and omissions
- Legal foundations for clinicians' civil liability
- The basic elements of clinicians' civil liability to a patient

General/Specific Objectives

Competent clinicians should be able to demonstrate an understanding that:

- Clinicians are legally liable to their patients for causing harm through a failure to meet the standard of duty of care that is applicable under the particular circumstances under consideration.

- This liability arises from the clinician's common law duty of care to his/her patients in the doctor-patient relationship.

- Four basic elements must generally be established by a patient for an action against a clinician to succeed in negligence (or civil liability):

  - a duty of care owed to the patient, and the standard required in such duty;
  - a breach of the duty of care;
  - some harm or injury to the patient; and
  - the harm or injury must have been caused by the breach of the duty of care.

- The duty of care arises out of the doctor-patient relationship. Once such a relationship arises, the clinician is required to attend to the patient attentively, with continuity, and to exercise reasonable care, skill, and judgment (until the relationship is ended through an appropriate process).

- The standard of care expected of a clinician is one that would reasonably be expected under similar circumstances of an ordinary, prudent clinician of the same training, experience, specialisation, and standing.

- In some circumstances, clinicians may be held vicariously liable (i.e. legally liable for the actions of employees or other persons under their control/delegation).

- Actions in negligence (or civil liability) must be launched by patients within a certain prescribed time period, which may differ from state to state.

References

- Australian Medical Association:
  http://www.ama.com.au

- Breen KJ, Pleuckhan VD, Cordner SM. Ethics, law and medical practice. Sydney: Allen & Unwin; 1997.

- Dooley B, Fearnside M, Gorton M. Surgery, ethics and the law. Melbourne: Blackwell Science Asia; 2000.

4.6   Legal Aspects of Clinician Competence and Conduct

Overview

Protection of patients and the public requires that clinicians' competence be assured and maintained; that clinicians' conduct in the context of the clinician/patient relationship be proper; and that mechanisms exist for dealing with incompetent or impaired clinicians, or those who engage in improper behaviour. (See also sections 3.1 Doctor-Patient Relationship and 3.2 Personal and Professional Conduct.)

Issues

- Requirement for clinician licensure

- Legal (and ethical) prohibitions, e.g. those concerning clinicians' sexual conduct with patients

- Clinician's legal (and ethical) obligations of continuity of care, and of competent and accessible care

- Clinicians' obligations to make reports concerning other clinicians' conduct

- Conflict of interest

- Conduct with regard to advertising and soliciting patients

General/Specific Objectives

Competent clinicians should be able to demonstrate an understanding that:

- Clinicians are legally required to be licensed with the appropriate authority.

- Clinicians' competence and conduct is legally (and ethically) regulated in certain respects to protect patients and society in general.

- Clinicians' conduct is of particular concern with respect to:

  - the continuity and accessibility of the care and coverage they provide;

  - in particular, clinicians must ensure that patients have access to continuous on-call coverage and are never abandoned;

  - clinicians' sexual conduct with patients, which irrespective of whether the patient apparently consented, is a serious transgression that could lead to criminal, civil, and disciplinary action against the clinician;

- clinicians' honesty and integrity, including information provided to third parties; e.g. relatives, employers, insurance companies, welfare, and other government departments; and

- conflict of interest, including by virtue of direct financial interest in a pharmaceutical, therapeutic, laboratory or other enterprise, or by virtue of a direct or indirect commission or payment for a service rendered to a patient by another person who is not a formal partner (according to law in some states).

References

- Australian Medical Association:
  http://www.ama.com.au
  > Legal issues

4.7 Statutory Requirements of Clinicians

Overview

It is judged to be in the interest of the public at large and public health that certain information concerning communicable diseases, infirmities, harmful social behaviours, and certain vital statistics be compulsorily reported by clinicians to the appropriate authorities, notwithstanding the clinician's duty of confidentiality.

Key Objectives

- Clinicians' statutory reporting or notification obligations.

- Exceptions to the duty of confidentiality.

(These issues should be considered in conjunction with corresponding objectives concerning organisational and ethical aspects of medical practice. See sections 5. General Organisation and 3.4 Confidentiality and Privacy.)

General/Specific Objectives

Competent clinicians should be able to demonstrate an understanding that:

- Clinicians are legally required under certain provisions of various state and federal laws to report confidential information concerning the health, well-being, morbidity or mortality of a patient to the appropriate authorities.

- Reporting requirements vary from state to state, and often include areas such as:

  - fitness to work in the field of aeronautics;

  - reports to coroners regarding death through violence, misconduct, negligence, malpractice, pregnancy, or unknown cause(s);

  - suspected child abuse or abandonment;

  - fitness to drive a vehicle on public highways;

  - pre-marital health;

- communicable/infectious and certain environmental/occupational diseases;

- details of births and deaths (vital statistics legislation);

- occupational illness and injury;

- the conduct of other clinicians or regulated health professionals;

- conditions in healthcare institutions; and

- neglected persons.

- Failure to make such a statutorily-required report can incur penal sanction (e.g. charges, fines) or civil liability on the part of the clinician concerned.

- These obligations to report constitute legal exceptions to the duty of confidentiality and clinicians making such reports are shielded from any liability for doing so.

References

- Australian Department of Health and Ageing website (with links to various state and territory health websites, and to institutions within those sites): http://www.health.gov.au

- Australian Department of Health and Ageing A–Z guide: http://www.health.gov.au/activities.htm#M

- Australian Commonwealth Government Information website: http://www.fed.gov.au/KSP
  > Health

- Australian Medical Association: http://www.ama.com.au
  > Policy and Issues > Legal

4.8   Legal Aspects of Medical Records

Overview

As a component of adequate care, clinicians are required to maintain adequate (complete, up-to-date, and accurate) medical records concerning each patient. This is essential for adequacy, continuity, and comprehensiveness of care, as well as with respect to malpractice, quality control, and medical/legal reporting. The issues of patient and others' access to records, their ownership and transfer, their use in court proceedings, and the fact that medical/legal reports are regulated by law in most jurisdictions must be recognised.

Key Objectives

- The duty to maintain medical records.

- Access to and disclosure of medical records.

- Ownership and transfer of medical records.

- Use of medical records in court proceedings.

(These issues should be considered in conjunction with corresponding objectives concerning organisational aspects of medical practice. See sections 5.4 Organisation of Medical Practice, and 5.5 Medical Records in Office Practice.)

General/Specific Objectives

Competent clinicians should be able to demonstrate an understanding that:

- Clinicians have a duty to maintain adequate records in respect of each patient they treat.

- The law (and good practice) obliges the clinician to maintain an adequate medical record, which includes:

    - ensuring adequate, continuous, and comprehensive care;

    - quality control;

    - evidence in the context of alleged malpractice; and

    - provision of medical-legal reports.

- The law specifies minimum time-frames for the preservation of medical records (10 years in most jurisdictions, and possibly permanently).

- While patients and their representatives are fully entitled to access to the patient's medical records upon written request, a third party may only have such access with the consent of the patient, by provision of law (e.g. post-mortem insurance company access; post-mortem family access concerning inheritable diseases), or by order of a court.

- Various statutes provide for the compulsory disclosure of part or all of a medical record under certain defined circumstances.

- Under very limited circumstances, a clinician may refuse to permit access to a medical record where the clinician believes that such disclosure would harm the patient or a third party. Such refusal may however be challenged, including in court.

- While the medical record is the property of the clinician or institution, the clinician must provide the patient with full access to the content of the medical record on request.

- A clinician is required to promptly furnish a copy of the medical record to another clinician at the patient's (written) request.

- The clinician may charge the patient a reasonable fee for copying and delivery of the record. The record may not be unreasonably withheld, even where the fee has not been paid (e.g. in the case of financial hardship).

- A clinician must furnish a medical record to a patient's lawyer or insurer on the patient's (written) request.

- Legal confidentiality requirements apply equally to electronic records, in respect of which particular care must be taken with respect to preservation and confidentiality.

- There may be particular legal requirements in some states relating to medical records of which clinicians in certain specialties need to be aware.

References

* *AMA Code of Ethics*
  Australian Medical Association:
  http://www.ama.com.au

Privacy issues:

* *Handbook for the Management of Health Information in Private Medical Practice*
  The Royal Australian College of General Practitioners:
  http://www.racgp.org.au
  > Your practice > Privacy
* Australian Medical Association:
  http://www.ama.com.au
  > Privacy Legislation

4.9   Legal Aspects of Hospitals and the Clinician

Overview

Clinicians' practice in the hospital context raises a number of important legal and institutional concerns.

Key Objectives

* Clinicians' relationship with hospitals.
* Clinicians' legal obligations in the hospital context.

(These objectives should be considered in conjunction with corresponding objectives concerning organisational aspects of medical practice. See 5.2 Hospitals / Medical Care Institutions.)

General/Specific Objectives

Competent clinicians should be able to demonstrate an understanding that:

* While clinicians are mostly not employed by hospitals, clinicians' practice in the hospital context is regulated by common law and a number of statutory provisions.
* Legal provisions concerning medical practice in the hospital context include clinicians' duty to:
  - ensure their own competence;
  - respect hospital by-laws and regulations;
  - practise within the limits of privileges granted; and
  - cooperate with other clinicians and hospital personnel.
* Clinicians are required to maintain adequate hospital records, including ongoing care and discharge treatment.

- The hospital may regulate clinician admission to hospital practice, and clinician conduct and compliance with hospital requirements, through the issue and withdrawal of hospital privileges.

References

- Australian Department of Health and Ageing website (with links to various state and territory health websites, and to institutions within those sites): http://www.health.gov.au

5.1   General Organisation of Medical Care / Healthcare in Australia

Overview

An understanding of the principles and legislative framework of the organisation and the components of the healthcare system in Australia, including the significant Commonwealth, state or territory, and local government laws, is essential for medical practice in Australia.

Issues

- Development of The Australian Healthcare System
- Commonwealth role and authority in healthcare
- Health Insurance Commission (HIC)
- Pharmaceutical Benefits Scheme (PBS)
- States' and territories' roles and authorities in healthcare
- Local government role in healthcare
- Aboriginal and Torres Strait Islander health issues
- Private health insurance

General/Specific Objectives

Competent clinicians will demonstrate appropriate knowledge and principles with respect to:

- The key issues in the development of the The Australian Healthcare System, including Medicare, Veterans' Affairs and private health insurance.
- The structure of government and the enabling legislation and agreements applicable to healthcare in Australia (e.g. *Commonwealth of Australia Constitution Act 1900*, *National Health Act 1953*).
- Commonwealth authority (*Health Insurance Act 1973*, *Health Care (Appropriation) Act 1998*, *Veterans Entitlement Act 1986*).
- The state or territory authority (relevant Acts).
- The public funding and administration of the systems, federal and local, including Medicare, Veterans' Affairs and private health insurance (Commonwealth, state and territory health departments however titled).
- The components of the healthcare system including the referral system.
- Eligibility to use the health system (residents, immigrants, visitors, veterans, pensioners).

References

Commonwealth
- *National Health Act 1953*
- *Health Care (Appropriation) Act 1998*
- *Health Insurance Act 1973*
- *Veterans Entitlements Act 1986*
- *Therapeutic Goods Act 1999*
- *Therapeutic Goods Act Amendment (Medical Devices) Act 2002*
- *Narcotic Drugs Act 1967*

State/Territory

Acts relevant to one state (Queensland) are given as examples:

- Queensland Acts:
  - *Health Act 1937*
  - *Health (Drugs and Poisons) Regulations 1996*
  - *Health Practitioners (Professional Standards) Act 1999*
  - *Medical Practitioners (Professional Standards) Act 1999*
  - *Medical Practitioners Registration Act 2001* and *Medical Practitioners Regulation 2002*
  - *Health Rights Commission Act 1991*
  - *Health Services Act 1991*
  - *Mental Health Act 2000* and *Mental Health Regulation 2002*
  - *Private Health Facilities Act 1999*
  - *Transplantation and Anatomy Act 1979*
  - *Coroners Act 1958*
  - *Local Government Act 1993*

- Similar Acts in the relevant state or territory

- Legislation may be accessed at:
  Australian Law Online:
  http://www.law.gov.au

- Australian Department of Health and Ageing website (with links to various state and territory health websites, and to institutions within those sites):
  http://www.health.gov.au

- Australian Department of Health and Ageing A–Z guide:
  http://www.health.gov.au/activities.htm#M

- Australian Commonwealth Government Information website:
  http://www.fed.gov.au/KSP
  > Health

- Divisions of General Practice Program (DGPP):
  http://www.ruralhealth.gov.au/workers/dgp.htm

- Medicare:
  http://www.hic.gov.au/providers/programs_services/about_medicare.htm

- Pharmaceutical Benefits Scheme (PBS):
  http://www.hic.gov.au/providers/programs_services/about_pbs.htm

- Mental Health and Wellbeing:
  http://www.mentalhealth.gov.au

5.2 Hospitals / Medical Care Institutions

Overview

Clinicians should demonstrate an understanding of hospitals/institutions – their organisation (governance / management / medical staff / other healthcare) and interrelationships. They must be aware that within a hospital or other health institution, they have a contractual arrangement and cannot view themselves as wholly independent operators. Medical students and junior graduates will demonstrate understanding of their role as trainees and as junior hospital medical officers within the various hospital clinical services and departments, and with their immediate medical supervisor / mentor. Medical staff appointees will demonstrate understanding of the duties and obligations of the Chief of Medical Staff, Chief of Department/Service, and individual staff / medical staff members. Appointees should demonstrate an understanding of the accountability as clinicians for medical care rendered and their mandate to review and continuously improve care. They should demonstrate an understanding of the granting of appointment to the staff of a hospital/institution with privileges, and the rights and responsibilities/obligations that accompany a medical staff appointment. They should demonstrate their understanding of the process and sanctions that may be brought to bear for incompetence, incapacity or misconduct as a member of the medical staff. Appropriate and agreed duty and position statements should be made available to each medical staff appointee, including appropriate bylaws and regulations of the institution.

Issues

- Types of service institutions (see 5.3 Support Services in the Community)
- Governance of hospitals/institutions
- Management of hospitals/institutions
- Relationships between teaching hospitals and other institutions, and with universities and clinical schools
- Appropriate integration of clinical service, teaching, research and administrative activities of the institution and of individual staff members
- Medical staff organisation, including general roles of Chief of Staff / department heads / service heads
- Organisation of departments/services
- Appointment/Credentialling/Privileges/Obligations
- Hospital bylaws/regulations
- Occupational health and safety (OH&S)
- Quality assurance / Safety / Management
- Accountability/Discipline
- Legislative authority for hospitals/institutions

General/Specific Objectives

Competent clinicians should demonstrate appropriate knowledge, skills, and attitudes with respect to:

- The statutory authority for public hospitals/institutions and private hospitals/institutions.

- The nature and powers of governance in public hospitals and private hospitals.

- The nature and power of management in public hospitals and private hospitals.

- The nature and power of the medical advisory committee or its equivalent.

- The nature and role of the medical staff association or its equivalent.

- The duties and roles of hospital administrators, including the Chief Executive Officer (CEO) or equivalent, Director of Nursing, Director of Clinical Services.

- The duties of the Director of Medical Services or equivalent.

- The duties of the director or head of department/service/programme/unit.

- The duties of the CEO within the area health service.

- The duties and lines of reporting of the individual medical staff in regard to clinical service, teaching, research and administrative activities.

- The nature of obligations such as on-call and recall arrangement for individual medical staff.

- The nature of by-laws or regulations of institutions/hospitals.

- The requirement for continuous quality of care review.

- The accountability of medical staff members and the process and sanctions for professional misconduct or failure to maintain medical standards.

- The notion of professional self-regulation as it applies to medical staff appointees.

References

- Hospitals services Acts (by state or territory)

- Private health facilities Acts (by state or territory)

- Australian Department of Health and Ageing website (with links to various state and territory health websites, and health services and institutions within those sites):
  http://www.health.gov.au

- Australian Department of Health and Ageing A–Z guide:
  http://www.health.gov.au/activities.htm#M

- Australian Commonwealth Government Information website:
  http://www.fed.gov.au/KSP
  > Health

5.3   Support Services in the Community

Overview

Medical practitioners should demonstrate an understanding of the network and nature of healthcare support services and institutions available in both the community setting and hospital and institutional sites (including specialty hospitals such as mental, paediatric, obstetric and women's, hospice palliative care and rehabilitation). Clinicians will demonstrate that they know how to access and utilise these services for their patients.

Issues

5.3.1   Services in the community

*   Federal support services or institutions (e.g. Australian Radiation Protection and Nuclear Safety Agency (ARPNSA), Therapeutic Goods Administration (TGA))
*   State support services or institutions (state laboratories)
*   Public health system and units
*   District or regional health councils or agencies
*   Australian Department of Health and Ageing
*   Health Insurance Commission (HIC)
*   Pharmaceutical Benefits Scheme (PBS)
*   Australian Red Cross Blood Service
*   Home and Community Care Programme
*   Medical Aids Programme
*   State public health departments and units
*   Regional or district health councils
*   Worker's Compensation boards or equivalent
*   Youth protection agencies (legal and other roles)
*   Consumer associations
*   The Royal Flying Doctor Service
*   Ambulance services
*   Mobile Intensive Care
*   State alcohol and drug information and counselling services

5.3.2   Services provided by institutions

*   Public and private hospitals
*   Nursing homes and chronic care facilities
*   Mental health units and community services

- In-patient services, emergency services, ambulatory and primary care services, specialist consultative services, and other services
- Community health centres

General/Specific Objectives

Competent clinicians should demonstrate knowledge of and how to access services with respect to:

- The nature and role of Commonwealth programmes and services (e.g. Bureau of Drugs and Devices, Medicare, pharmaceutical benefits, therapeutic drugs and devices, and blood transfusion services).
- The nature and role of state programmes and services (public health departments and social service agencies, public hospitals, community health services, mental health services).
- The nature and role of support services for injured workers (Worker's Compensation boards or equivalent).
- The nature and role of support services for road crash and other transport accident victims.
- The nature and role of support services for youth (Children's Aid Society, state human services or families departments, child protection agencies).
- The nature and role of facilities and services for the aged.
- Mechanisms and organisations which provide social services related to health.
- The co-ordination of services (ambulatory, in-patient, chronic care, rehabilitation services).
- Individuals able to assist with access to community services (home care co-ordinator, and home care assessment teams, etc.)

References

- Australian Department of Health and Ageing website (with links to various state and territory health websites, and health services and institutions within those sites):
  http://www.health.gov.au
- Australian Department of Health and Ageing A–Z guide:
  http://www.health.gov.au/activities.htm#M
- Australian Commonwealth Government Information website:
  http://www.fed.gov.au/KSP
  > Health
- Health of indigenous Australians:
  http://www.ama.com.au
  > Policy and Issues > Public Health

5.4 Organisation of Medical Practice

Overview

Clinicians should demonstrate an understanding of the various types of practice situations and appreciate their obligations in managing a practice. The clinician should demonstrate an understanding of the medical regulatory requirements for administrative standards of practice, as well as recognising other requirements relating to fulfilment of labour standards in staffing and other legal obligations under municipal or state regulations.

Issues

- Institutional practice (salaried, visiting medical officer (VMO), independent contractor, fee-for-service private practice)
- Private office practice (solo, group, clinics – including diagnostic and day procedure units)
- Clinician as employer and as office manager (labour law, industrial law, commercial law, industrial relations)
- Medical regulatory requirement in practice (advertising, maintenance of medical records, infection control, medication handling, preservation of records, disposal of human tissue/products, and quality assurance)
- Remuneration models and billing for uninsured services (Medicare, private health insurance, billing arrangements including bulk billing and charges for uninsured services)
- Liabilities: office risk management and coverage
- Relationship to unions in medical practice
- Geographical distribution and workforce issues
- Payment for uninsured services
- Medical indemnity
- Licensing of private health facilities
- Accreditation of healthcare services
- Drugs and poisons regulations
- Occupational health and safety requirements

General/Specific Objectives

Competent clinicians should demonstrate knowledge with respect to:

- The advantages/disadvantages of different practice situations.
- The responsibilities and obligations in the general administration and management of an office.
- The responsibility and obligation to meet the medical regulatory requirements for a medical office practice (medical records, advertising, narcotic and drug control, quality assurance, infection control).

- The requirement for advertising of services not to be false or misleading and to be in good taste, not to create unjustified expectations, and not to impugn the reputation of other medical practitioners or services.

- The different remuneration models available in fee-for-service, salary practice, and capitation (including managed care).

- Principles underlining the policies on billing for services under Medicare and in accordance with Australian Medical Association (AMA) recommendations.

- The requirements of a prior disclosure of fees to patients, opportunities to discuss fees, options for payment of fees and determination of fees in accordance with the nature of service.

- Principles underlying the policies on billing for uninsured services recommended by the state registration authority and/or state medical association/federation (nature of service, patient's ability to pay, notification of fee prior to treatment).

- The special requirements for billing for uninsured services, including prior disclosure of fees to patients, opportunities to discuss fees, option of prior payment of fees, and fees to be determined by the nature of service.

References

- State and territory legislation on drugs and poisons, workplace health and safety

- *Health Insurance Act 1973*

- Australian Department of Health and Ageing website (with links to various state and territory health websites, and health services and institutions within those sites):
  http://www.health.gov.au

- Australian Department of Health and Ageing A–Z guide:
  http://www.health.gov.au/activities.htm#M

- Australian Commonwealth Government Information website:
  http://www.fed.gov.au/KSP
  > Health

- Divisions of General Practice Program (DGPP):
  http://www.ruralhealth.gov.au/workers/dgp.htm

5.5 Medical Records in Office Practice

Overview

Medical records document the nature and continuity of care for each patient and must meet a statutory requirement for their development, maintenance, and security. Patient's right of access has recently been clarified and extended by the courts under Commonwealth legislation. Clinicians must demonstrate an understanding of privacy issues and under what circumstances access can be provided to other persons.

Issues

- Medical practitioner's duty to maintain medical records
- Medical practitioner's ownership of the medical records
- Patient's right of access to and transmission of the medical information to others
- Medical practitioner's duty to transfer patient information upon request and authorisation
- Ownership of patient's medical records and related information

General/Specific Objectives

The competent medical practitioner will be able to demonstrate an understanding that:

- Medical practitioners have a duty to maintain adequate records on each patient.
- Certain basic elements must be included in that record.
- The records must be secure and they are the property of the medical practitioner.
- The records must be maintained for a defined period.
- Patients have a right of access to their records at reasonable times.
- Authorised representatives have right of access to the records or their copies.
- The patient may request transfer of the medical information to another medical practitioner.
- A fee may be charged for this transfer of information or copying of records.
- The medical practitioner may only deny access to a medical record when he or she believes on reasonable grounds that such disclosure may lead to harm to the patient or violate a confidence.

References

- *Privacy Act 1988*
- *Privacy Amendment (Private Sector) Act 2000*
- *Guidelines on Privacy in the Private Health Sector*, Office of the Federal Privacy Commissioner (November 2001):
  http://www.privacy.gov.au/publications/hg_01.html
- State and territory health services legislation and confidentiality requirements
- *AMA Code of Ethics*
  Australian Medical Association:
  http://www.ama.com.au

Privacy issues:

- *Handbook for the Management of Health Information in Private Medical Practice*
  The Royal Australian College of General Practitioners:
  http://www.racgp.org.au
  > Your practice > Privacy

- Australian Medical Association:
  http://www.ama.com.au
  > Policy and Issues > Legal > Privacy Legislation

5.6   Self-Regulation of the Profession

Overview

Clinicians should demonstrate an understanding of the nature of self-regulation under the authority of the medical registration authorities and the responsibilities of the individual practitioner in self-regulation. Clinicians should demonstrate an understanding that, as practising medical doctors, they are registered with the state or territory licensing board with duties and obligations in the common purpose of regulating and governing the practices of medicine. Competent clinicians should demonstrate an understanding that medical self-regulation is a privilege and not a right and that it must be exercised in the public interest.

Issues

Medical self-regulation implies that society grants certain privileges and obligations to the profession and in return requires the profession to act in the public interest through the:

- Role and authority of state and territory registration (state and territory medical boards)

- Medical registration authorities: maintaining standards for registration, definition of restrictive acts, continuing competence, and clinical practice

- Medical registration authorities: maintaining standards or code of ethics

- Medical registration authorities: dealing with complaints, allegations of incompetence, incapacity, or misconduct

- Medical registration authorities: dealing with impaired medical practitioners

- Role of the clinical colleges in certifying competence

- Role of certifying bodies

- Role of the Australian Medical Association (AMA), specialist colleges and specialty societies

- Healthcare institutions: maintaining quality of medical care and handling of complaints; accreditation, credentialling and privileges, complaints management

General/Specific Objectives

Competent clinicians should demonstrate knowledge and attitudes with respect to:

- The role and authority of the medical boards to regulate and govern all members of the profession in the public interest by setting and maintaining standards.

- Their role and obligations as members of the licensing authority (the medical board).

- The requirements for co-operation with the medical board (e.g. access to records, the office).

- The standards for entry to practise (registration requirements).

- The requirements for continuing competence (continuing professional education and recency of practice legislation, quality assurance (QA) and continuing medical education (CME) programmes, peer assessment).

- The requirements for ethical and mandatory reporting to the medical board (code of ethics, public hospitals act, state-specific healthcare legislation, state medical practitioners registration legislation).

- Assistance with processing complaints/allegations about medical practitioner performance/conduct.

- The role of the state or territory health rights commission, health ombudsman or relevant similar authority.

- The distinction between the registering authority (the medical board) and the certifying bodies (university medical schools, professional colleges, the Australian Medical Council (AMC)).

- The distinction between the licensing authority and the AMA and specialty medical groups.

References

- State and territory medical registration Acts

- *AMA Code of Ethics*
  Australian Medical Association:
  http://www.ama.com.au

- Medical boards (various states and territories) – see Appendix 1

- Speciality colleges (various specialities) – see Appendix 2

- Complaints tribunals and ombudsman (by state)

- Australian federal, state, territory & local governments website (with links to various state and territory health websites and services and institutions within those sites):
  http://www.gov.au

5.7   Non-Governmental Organisations (NGOs)

Overview

The clinician should demonstrate an understanding of the large informal network of volunteer groups that exist to assist or advocate in the community on behalf of institutions, specific disease states, or patient groups. The clinician should recognise the major contribution that non-governmental organisations (NGOs) make to fundraising and direct patient or institution support.

Issues

5.7.1   Volunteer support and non-profit groups

- Home care (e.g. AIDS organisations, home and community care services, Meals on Wheels)
- Disease-specific support groups (e.g. Australian Kidney Foundation, Heart Foundation, The Cancer Council Australia, Arthritis Society)
- Community groups offering services or products (e.g. St. John's Ambulance, Red Cross, Community Nursing Services)
- Religious groups (e.g. Salvation Army, church-based food banks or shelters, nursing services and home care)

5.7.2   Advocacy groups

- Patient advocacy (e.g. patient rights associations; Consumers Association of Australia, Consumers Health Forum of Australia, psychiatric patient survivor's groups)
- Disease advocacy (e.g. AIDS groups, The Cancer Council Australia, mental health consumers groups)

5.7.3   Hospital/Institution support groups

- Fundraising foundations
- Hospital-family liaison committees
- Volunteers associations (e.g. fundraising, patient support)
- Consumer committees
- Aboriginal and Torres Strait Islander liaison officers

General/Specific Objectives

Competent clinicians should demonstrate knowledge with respect to:

- The major role volunteer support groups play in fundraising and in providing direct support for patients in or out of institutions.

- The role some advocacy groups play in promoting the interest of sufferers of specific disease states through public awareness, fundraising activities, and direct patient care.

- The role and benefit of non-profit organisations in providing healthcare out of hospital.

- The role of some advocacy groups in challenging current healthcare and care by medical practitioners.

- The role of NGOs in fundraising for health services, programme support, and research.

References

- Medical boards (various states and territories) – see Appendix 1
- Speciality colleges (various specialities) – see Appendix 2

5.8 Professional Associations

Overview

Clinicians should demonstrate an understanding of the nature and roles of major professional medical associations and their distinctive roles as opposed to the role of the state or territory medical boards with which they have a statutory and mandatory relationship.

Issues

5.8.1 Voluntary professional associations

- Australian Medical Association (AMA) and its state or territory divisions
- Resident/Student associations and their state associations
- Hospital medical staff associations / student associations
- Industrial relations association (e.g. Australian Salaried Medical Officers Federation)
- National specialty associations (e.g. Cardiac Society, Gastroenterology Society)
- Medical defence associations
- Non-medical health professions associations (e.g. medico-legal societies, health informatics groups)

5.8.2 Mandatory professional bodies

- Medical boards of states and territories
- Australian Medical Council (AMC) – certification of university and specialty college undergraduate and postgraduate training programmes and overseas qualifications

5.8.3 Certifying/Educational bodies

- AMC
- Universities and medical schools
- The professional colleges

General/Specific Objectives

Competent clinicians should demonstrate knowledge with respect to:

- The role and voluntary nature of the AMA and other professional associations, advocating for and representing the interests of the medical profession in healthcare and health education.
- The role and function of the certifying/evaluating bodies (e.g. the speciality professional colleges, the AMC) in evaluating clinicians and professional courses, and the advocacy role of the specialty colleges, in dealing with the areas of educational standards.
- The role of specialty and other professional associations in providing educational and professional developments, as well as being advocates for their disciplines.
- The role of student and medical staff associations in promoting and protecting their members' interests.
- The role of the medical defence associations in representing the interests of individual medical practitioners.
- The unique role and authority of the medical boards in the self-regulation and governance of the medical profession.
- The roles played by other associations and special interest groups in delineating healthcare, educational, and research policies in Australia.
- The roles played by the other health professional associations in developing health policy.

References

- Breen K, Frank I, Walters T. Medicine in the 21st century: Australian Medical Council: a view from the inside. *Internal Medicine Journal* 2001;31: 243–248.
- State and territory Acts for medical boards
- Charters for colleges and voluntary associations
- Voluntary professional associations
- Australian Medical Association: http://www.ama.com.au
- Doctors Reform Society
- Medical defence organisations

For current issues in medical indemnity:

- Australian Medical Association:
  http://www.ama.com.au

- Professional Medical Indemnity

Also, further information can be obtained at:

- Health Access and Finance, Australian Department of Health and Ageing:
  http://www.health.gov.au/haf/mi/index.htm

- Mandatory professional bodies

- Medical boards (various states and territories) – see Appendix 1

Certifying bodies:

- Australian Medical Council (AMC)

- Speciality colleges (various specialities) – see Appendix 2

5.9 Inter-Professional Issues

Overview

The clinician should demonstrate an understanding of the need for proper professional relations with other healthcare professionals and workers based on respect for others working in a team environment, including an understanding of roles, competencies, and lines of responsibility of each.

Issues

- Regulatory status of other healthcare professions

- Scope of practice of other healthcare professions

- Defining lines of authority, concept and process of delegation of medical responsibilities to other healthcare professionals

- The doctor-nurse (or other healthcare workers) professional working relationship

- Professional communications and interaction with other healthcare workers (e.g. nurses)

- Concepts of team management and shared care

- Multidisciplinary healthcare

General/Specific Objectives

The competent clinician should demonstrate knowledge, skills, and attitudes regarding:

- The role and skills of practice for other healthcare workers who are self-regulated.

- The proper inter-professional relationship based on respect and clear communication.

- The delegation of responsibilities between medical practitioners and other healthcare workers.

- The ability to work in a collegial way within a team structure involving other medical practitioners and healthcare workers.

- Maintenance of respect for the role of the other health professions at all times.

References

- State and territory legislation for health professional registration boards

- *AMA Code of Ethics*
  Australian Medical Association:
  http://www.ama.com.au

- Breen KJ, Pleuckhan VD, Cordner SM. Ethics, Law and medical practice. Sydney: Allen & Unwin; 1997.

5.10 Impact of Particular Laws on Practice

Overview

The clinician should demonstrate an understanding of the wide range of laws that place specific duties, obligations and/or reporting requirements (to various agencies) which fall upon the practitioner under certain circumstances. The clinician will be able to apply these laws from the point of practice viewpoint rather than as a regulator. The knowledge expected at this level is general, but state/territory-specific laws and regulations could be evaluated at that level.

General/Specific Objectives

The competent clinician should demonstrate knowledge, skills, and attitudes concerning:

- The duty to report to specified government agencies under certain circumstances (e.g. child abuse, neglect, fitness to drive, fitness to fly, communicable diseases).

- The duty to comply with statutory/judicial standards for obtaining consent.

- The need to respect advanced health directives or guardianship arrangements for individuals without competence to provide consent.

- The penalties for failing to comply with the act requiring reporting to specific agencies.

- The duty to notify births and deaths, completion of death certificates and cremation certificates.

- The duty to report to the Coroner's Office under specified circumstances.

- The duties with respect to youth and childhood protection.

- Responsibilities under the laws and regulations which control biomedical waste.

References

- Relevant state and territory legislation including:
  - Coroner's Acts
  - Registration of births, deaths and marriages
  - Guardianship Act or equivalent

Communicable diseases:

- Australian Department of Health and Ageing:
  http://www.health.gov.au/pubhlth/cdi/cdna/index.htm

Immunisation:

- Health Insurance Commission (HIC):
  http://www.hic.gov.au/providers/programs_services/about_acir.htm
- Australian Department of Health and Ageing:
  http://www.health.gov.au/pubhlth/immunise/index.htm

5.11 Interstate Issues: Patient Benefits, Clinician Mobility, and Medical Drugs and Devices

Overview

Clinicians should demonstrate an understanding of the various principles and legislative policies which influence interstate movement of patients' benefits and health professionals and regulate the drugs and medical devices. They will understand requirements to practise medicine remotely by electronic or other means while meeting standards or requirements in both their resident jurisdiction and that of their cross-border patient.

Issues

- Nationally recognised qualifications
- Mutual recognition of qualifications between state or territory medical boards
- State or territory specificity of registration
- General and special purpose registration conditions
- Portability of educational degrees
- Portability of other qualifications
- State specificity of licensure
- Portability of certification
- Transferability of Medicare benefits

- Commonwealth and state roles in monitoring narcotics, mechanical devices, chemical devices and radiation, and pharmaceuticals
- Telemedicine/Telehealth as a cross-border practice

General/Specific Objectives

Competent clinicians should demonstrate knowledge with respect to:

- The portability of the medical degree.
- The limited portability of other qualifications (certification for registration status via individual state or territory medical boards).
- The non-transferability of state or territory registration but mutual recognition of qualifications between state medical boards.
- Limitations imposed by special purpose registration and conditions on registration (including internship conditions).
- The portability of patients' benefits between states under the *National Health Act 1953* and the *Health Insurance Act 1973*.
- The role of the Commonwealth Government in monitoring the health system across state borders, certain drugs, devices, and hazards.
- The need to meet medical board standards and registration requirements for the practice of telemedicine/telehealth.

References

- Relevant Commonwealth, state or territory Acts
- Australian Medical Association:
  http://www.ama.com.au

Healthcare cards:

- Centrelink:
  http://www.centrelink.gov.au/internet/internet.nsf/payments/conc_cards.htm

5.12 Unorthodox/Unconventional Medicine

Overview

Orthodox, conventional or scientific medicine refers to medical practices based on scientific principles and subject to scientific evaluation (with various degrees of rigour), ongoing audit and peer review. This system of medical practice, often designated 'Western' medicine, and developed most extensively during the 20th century, is now the dominant healthcare paradigm in the world. 'Scientific' medicine coexists with other less orthodox systems of health practice which may have local cultural origins, which may relate to orthodox medical practice as astrology does to astronomy, and which are in varying degrees less based on scientific or evidence-based principles than mainstream practice.

The use of unorthodox health practices (often, but less appropriately, called 'alternative' or 'complementary' medicine) is widespread in the Australian community. A large proportion of the population currently uses such practices, and some medical practitioners are incorporating them into their practices. About half the Australian population will access 'alternative' medicine at some stage in their lives. About 20% of the population will visit unorthodox practitioners each year.

Acupuncture and chiropractic have had items eligible for Medicare payments since the mid-1980s; and surveys indicate that the expenditure on unconventional medicines and therapies exceeds by several times that spent on prescription medicines, accounting to several hundreds of millions of dollars annually. These figures, and the potential for quackery and quasi-scientific misleading claims, and of misuse and overuse of possible harmful therapies, make it important that medical students and doctors are familiar with educational and management objectives as they relate to unorthodox health practices.

Much of the rhetoric of 'holistic', 'integrative' and 'natural' therapies claimed for unorthodox practices, along with claims to consider the patient as a whole individual within a social context and not just a package of symptoms and signs, are clearly entirely compatible with orthodox medicine. Indeed, an holistic, integrative approach is, and always has been, a prerequisite for best orthodox clinical practice.

The prevalence and diversity of unorthodox health practice is indicated by a United States listing of over 60 unorthodox health practices used in America including complete alternative medical systems or theories, bioelectromagnetic applications, approaches to diet, nutrition, herbal medicine and lifestyle, and variants of manual healing, mind/body control, and pharmaco-biological treatment methods.

Methods of unorthodox health practices in Australia

A listing of unorthodox practices, necessarily incomplete, includes:

- Acupuncture
- Aromatherapy
- Biocellular therapies
- Chiropractic medicine
- Chinese herbal medicine
- Clinical ecology

- Energy therapies (Reiki, Qigong)
- Homoeopathy
- Iridology
- Naturopathy
- Orthomolecular medicine
- Osteopathy
- Reflexology

An Australian Medical Council (AMC) discussion paper (2000)[3] encouraged medical schools to devise teaching and learning strategies addressing the impact of unorthodox health practices on Australian medicine.

Key Objectives

- Familiarity with unorthodox medical practices used in Australia.
- Consideration of potential for benefit and harm from unorthodox medical practices in Australian medicine.

General/Specific Objectives

- Consider role of acupuncture in management of chronic pain syndromes.
- Compare relative roles of chiropractic medicine and osteopathy with that of physiotherapy in management of pain associated with musculoligamentous and skeletal injuries.
- Devise and implement methods of using evidence-based strategies to determine therapeutic effectiveness of unorthodox practices in comparison with mainstream practice.

---

3   Australian Medical Council. Undergraduate medical education and unorthodox medical practice: AMC position statement [discussion paper]. Canberra: AMC; 2000 Jul 21.

Appendix 1.   The medical boards in the various states and territories

The boards can be contacted as follows:

Australian Capital Territory
The Registrar
Medical Board of the Australian
Capital Territory
PO Box 976
CIVIC SQUARE ACT 2608
Ph: (02) 6205 1600
Fax: (02) 6205 1602
http://www.medicalboard.act.gov.au

Medical Practitioners Act 1930

New South Wales
Registrar
New South Wales Medical Board
PO Box 104
GLADESVILLE NSW 1675
Ph: (02) 9879 6799
Fax: (02) 9816 5307
http://www.nswmb.org.au

Medical Practice Act 1992

Northern Territory
Registrar
Medical Board of the Northern Territory
GPO Box 4221
DARWIN NT 0801
Ph: (08) 8999 4157
Fax: (08) 8999 4196
http://www.nt.gov.au
> Health > Licensing, Health Profession

Medical Act 1995

Queensland
Executive Officer
Medical Board of Queensland
GPO Box 2438
BRISBANE QLD 4001
Ph: (07) 3234 0176
Fax: (07) 3225 2527
http://www.medicalboard.qld.gov.au

Medical Practitioners Registration Act 2001

South Australia
Registrar
Medical Board of South Australia
PO Box 359
STEPNEY SA 5069
Ph: (08) 8362 7811
Fax: (08) 8362 7906
http://www.medicalboardsa.asn.au

Medical Practitioners Act 1983

Tasmania
Registrar
Medical Council of Tasmania
PO Box 8
SOUTH HOBART TAS 7004
Ph: (03) 6233 5499
Fax: (03) 6233 7986

Medical Practitioners Registration Act 1996

Victoria
Chief Executive Officer
Medical Practitioners Board of Victoria
GPO Box 773H
MELBOURNE VIC 3001
Ph: (03) 9655 0500
Fax: (03) 9655 0580
http://medicalboardvic.org.au

Medical Practice Act No. 23/1994

Western Australia
Registrar
Medical Board of Western Australia
GPO Box 2754
PERTH WA 6001
Ph: (08) 9481 1011
Fax: (08) 9321 1744
http://www.medicalboard.com.au

Medical Act 1894 (amended 1994)

Appendix 2. The specialty colleges

The specialty colleges are responsible for training and for assessment of local specialist trainees and of overseas-obtained qualifications and experience.

Australian and New Zealand College of Anaesthetists (ANZCA)
'Ulimaroa'
630 St Kilda Road
MELBOURNE VIC 3004
Ph: (03) 9510 6299
Fax: (03) 9510 6786
http://www.anzca.edu.au

Joint Faculty of Intensive Care Medicine (JFICM)
Australian and New Zealand College of Anaesthetists and
The Royal Australasian College of Physicians
'Ulimaroa'
630 St Kilda Road
MELBOURNE VIC 3004
Ph: (03) 9530 2861
Fax: (03) 9530 2862
http://www.jficm.anzca.edu.au

Australasian College for Emergency Medicine (ACEM)
17 Grattan Street
CARLTON VIC 3053
Ph: (03) 9663 3800
Fax: (03) 9663 8013
http://www.acem.org.au

Australasian College of Dermatologists (ACD)
PO Box 2065
BORONIA PARK NSW 2111
Ph: (02) 9879 6177
Fax: (02) 9816 1174
http://www.dermcoll.asn.au

The Royal Australian & New Zealand College of Radiologists (RANZCR)
Level 9
51 Druitt Street
SYDNEY NSW 2000
Ph: (02) 9268 9777
Fax: (02) 9268 9799
http://www.ranzcr.edu.au

Faculty of Radiation Oncology (FRANZCR)
The Royal Australian & New Zealand College of Radiologists
Level 9
51 Druitt Street
SYDNEY NSW 2000
Ph: (02) 9268 9777
Fax: (02) 9268 9799
http://www.ranzcr.edu.au

The Royal Australasian College of Physicians (RACP)
145 Macquarie Street
SYDNEY NSW 2000
Ph: (02) 9256 5444
Fax: (02) 9252 3310
http://www.racp.edu.au

Australasian Faculty of Rehabilitation Medicine (AFRM)
The Royal Australasian College of Physicians
145 Macquarie Street
SYDNEY NSW 2000
Ph: (02) 9256 5402
Fax: (02) 9251 7476
http://www.racp.edu.au/afrm

Australasian Faculty of Occupational Medicine (AFOM)
The Royal Australasian College of Physicians
145 Macquarie Street
SYDNEY NSW 2000
Ph: (02) 9256 5400
Fax: (02) 9247 8082
http://www.racp.edu.au/afom

Australian Faculty of Public Health Medicine (AFPHM)
The Royal Australasian College of Physicians
145 Macquarie Street
SYDNEY NSW 2000
Ph: (02) 9256 5404
Fax: (02) 9252 3526
http://www.racp.edu.au/afphm

Paediatrics & Child Health Division
The Royal Australasian College of Physicians
145 Macquarie Street
SYDNEY NSW 2000
Ph: (02) 9256 5408
Fax: (02) 9256 5465
http://www.racp.edu.au

The Royal Australian and New Zealand College of Ophthalmologists (RANZCO)
94-98 Chalmers Street
SURRY HILLS NSW 2010
Ph: (02) 9690 1001
Fax: (02) 9690 1321
http://www.ranzco.edu

Royal Australian and New Zealand College of Obstetricians and Gynaecologists (RANZCOG)
254-260 Albert Street
EAST MELBOURNE VIC 3002
Ph: (03) 9417 1699
Fax: (03) 9419 0672
http://www.ranzcog.edu.au

Royal College of Pathologists of Australasia (RCPA)
207 Albion Street
SURRY HILLS NSW 2010
Ph: (02) 8356 5858
Fax: (02) 8356 5828
http://www.rcpa.edu.au

Royal Australian and New Zealand College of Psychiatrists (RANZCP)
309 La Trobe Street
MELBOURNE VIC 3000
Ph: (03) 9640 0646
Fax: (03) 9642 5652
http://www.ranzcp.org

Royal Australasian College of Surgeons (RACS)
College of Surgeons' Gardens
Spring Street
MELBOURNE VIC 3000
Ph: (03) 9249 1200
Fax: (03) 9249 1219
http://www.surgeons.org

The Royal Australian College of General Practitioners (RACGP)
1 Palmerston Crescent
SOUTH MELBOURNE VIC 3205
Ph: (03) 9214 1414
Fax: (03) 9214 1400
http://www.racgp.org.au

Royal Australasian College of Medical Administrators (RACMA)
35 Drummond Street
CARLTON VIC 3053
Ph: (03) 9663 5347
Fax: (03) 9663 4117
http://www.racma.org.au

Appendix 3. Australian university medical schools

New South Wales

Faculty of Medicine
University of New South Wales
SYDNEY NSW 2052
Ph: (02) 9385 2454
Fax: (02) 9385 1874
http://www.med.unsw.edu.au/

The School of Medical Practice and
Population Health
Faculty of Health
The University of Newcastle
CALLAGHAN NSW 2308
Ph: (02) 4921 5676
Fax: (02) 4921 5071
http://www.newcastle.edu.au/school/
medprac-pop

Faculty of Medicine
Edward Ford Building (A27)
The University of Sydney
SYDNEY NSW 2006
Ph: (02) 9351 4579
Fax: (02) 9351 6645
http://www.medfac.usyd.edu.au/contact/
dean.html

Queensland

School of Medicine
James Cook University
TOWNSVILLE QLD 4811
Ph: (07) 4781 6232
Fax: (07) 4781 6986
http://www.jcu.edu.au/school/medicine/
index.htm

School of Medicine
Mayne Medical School
Faculty of Health Sciences
The University of Queensland
Herston Road
HERSTON QLD 4006
Ph: (07) 3365 5278
Fax: (07) 3365 5433
http://www.som.uq.edu.au/som/
home.shtml

South Australia

School of Medicine
Faculty of Health Sciences
Flinders University of South Australia
GPO Box 2100
ADELAIDE SA 5001
Ph: (08) 8204 4160
Fax: (08) 8204 5845
http://som.flinders.edu.au

Medical School
Faculty of Health Sciences
University of Adelaide
Ground Floor, Room NG45
Medical School North
Frome Road
ADELAIDE SA 5005
Ph: (08) 8303 5336
Fax: (08) 8303 3788
http://www.health.adelaide.edu.au

Tasmania

School of Medicine
Faculty of Health Sciences
University of Tasmania
GPO Box 252-68
HOBART TAS 7001
Ph: (03) 6226 4860
Fax: (03) 6226 4816
http://www.healthsci.utas.edu.au/
medicine/index.html

Victoria

Faculty of Medicine, Nursing and
Health Sciences
Monash University
PO Box 64
CLAYTON VIC 3168
Ph: (03) 9905 4301
Fax: (03) 9905 4302
http://www.med.monash.edu.au

School of Medicine
Faculty of Medicine, Dentistry and
Health Sciences
University of Melbourne
6th Floor, Medical Building
Grattan Street
PARKVILLE VIC 3052
Ph: (03) 9344 7700
Fax: (03) 9347 7084
http://www.medfac.unimelb.edu.au/med

Western Australia

School of Medicine and
Pharmacology
Department of Medicine
Faculty of Medicine and Dentistry
The University of Western Australia
35 Stirling Highway
CRAWLEY WA 6009
Ph: (08) 9224 0250
Fax: (08) 9224 0246
http://www.meddent.uwa.edu.au/
medicine/index.htm

Appendix 4. The area of need scheme

An **area of need** is where there has been difficulty in obtaining sufficient medical practitioners to provide for the basic healthcare needs of the community. These areas are almost exclusive to rural and remote areas.

Further information can be obtained from:

Western Australian Centre for Rural and Remote Medicine
328 Stirling Highway
CLAREMONT WA 6010
Ph: (08) 9384 2811
Fax: (08) 9385 2938
Email: gregdown@cyllene.uwa.edu.au

Rural Workforce Agency Victoria
Level 4, 458-460 Swanston Street
CARLTON VIC 3053
Ph: (03) 9349 4899
Fax: (03) 9349 4211
Website: http://hna.ffh.vic.gov.au/
vicgovdocs/vacancy.htm

Information Service for Overseas Trained Health Professionals
Locked Mail Bag 961
NORTH SYDNEY NSW 2059
Ph: (02) 9391 9588

Queensland Rural Medical Support Agency
PO Box 167
KELVIN GROVE DC QLD 4059
Ph: (07) 3352 7028
Email: grmsa@gpnetwork.net.au

The National Rural Health Alliance may also be able to provide information on rural positions that are available. The Alliance can be contacted at:

National Rural Health Alliance
PO Box 280
DEAKIN WEST ACT 2600
Ph: (02) 6285 4660
Fax: (02) 6285 4670
email: nrha@ruralhealth.org.au

Additional information may be obtained from:

- Australian Medical Association:
  http://www.ama.com.au

- The Royal Australian College of General Practitioners:
  http://www.racgp.org.au

- Australian College of Rural and Remote Medicine:
  http://www.acrrm.org.au

Appendix 5. Notification of infectious diseases

Procedures in one state (Victoria) are given as an example. This is an excerpt from Schedule 3 of the *Health (Infectious Diseases) Regulations 2001* of the Department of Human Services, Victorian State Government.

Notification in Victoria to Communicable Diseases Section, Department of Human Services.

Pre-printed Reply Paid forms provided.

FORM 1: Group A, B, C Diseases

Group A Diseases: **Immediate notification by phone or fax**
Written notification within five days

Anthrax, arbovirus infection (Australian arboencephalitis, Japanese encephalitis), botulism, cholera, diphtheria, haemolytic uraemic syndrome (HUS), *Haemophilus influenzae* type B (Hib), legionellosis, measles, meningococcal infection, paratyphoid, plague, poliomyelitis, rabies, typhoid, viral haemorrhagic fever, yellow fever.

Group B Diseases: **Written notification within 5 days**

Arbovirus infection (Barmah Forest, Dengue, Kumjin, Ross River virus), brucellosis, campylobacteriosis, cryptosporidiosis, giardiasis, hepatitis virus A, hepatitis virus B, hepatitis virus C, hepatitis virus D, hepatitis virus E, influenza virus, leprosy, leptospirosis, listeriosis, lyssavirus, malaria, mumps, pertussis, invasive pneumococcal infections, psittacosis, Q fever, rubella, salmonellosis, shigellosis, tetanus, tuberculosis (TB), verotoxin-producing *Escherichia coli* (VTEC).

Group C Diseases: **Sexually Transmitted Diseases (STDs)**
Written information within five days

To preclude patient identification, only the first two letters of the family and given name are required.

Chlamydia trachomatis, donovanosis, gonococcal infection, syphilis (congenital, early, late).

FORM 2: Group D Diseases

HIV and AIDS **Written notification within five days**

A separate form is used due to the need to have national uniformity in collection of data.

Appendix 6. Legislation regulating the prescription and use of drugs in Australia

State	Relevant Legislation
New South Wales	*Poisons and Therapeutic Goods Act 1966* *Poisons and Therapeutic Goods Regulation 2002*
Victoria	*Drugs, Poisons and Controlled Substances Act 1981* *Drugs, Poisons and Controlled Substances Regulations 1995* *Therapeutics Goods (Vic) Act 1994*
Queensland	*Health Act 1937* *Health (Drugs and Poisons) Regulation 1996*
South Australia	*Controlled Substances Act 1984* *Controlled Substances (Poisons) Regulations 1996*
Western Australia	*Poisons Act 1964* *Poisons Regulations 1965* (amended 2000)
Tasmania	*Poisons Act 1971* *Poisons Regulations 1975* *Alcohol and Drug Dependency Act 1968* *Therapeutic Goods Act 2001*
Northern Territory	*Poisons and Dangerous Drugs Act 1983* *Poisons and Dangerous Drugs Regulations 1985*
Australia Capital Territory	*Poisons Act 1933* *Poisons and Drugs Act 1978* *Poisons and Drugs Regulations* *Drugs of Dependence Act 1989* *Drugs of Dependence Regulations* *Poisons Regulations 1933* (as updated)

Appendix 7.   Contact details for advice on prescribing drugs of dependence

State	Name and Address	Telephone and Facsimile
New South Wales	Pharmaceutical Services Branch NSW Health Department PO Box 103 GLADESVILLE NSW 1675	Ph: (02) 9879 5239 Fax: (02) 9859 5175
Victoria	Drugs and Poisons Unit PO Box 1670N MELBOURNE VIC 3001	Ph: 1300 364 545 Fax: 1300 360 830
Queensland	Medical Adviser Alcohol, Tobacco and Other Drug Services Queensland Health 147 Charlotte Street BRISBANE QLD 4000	Ph: (07) 3234 0957 Fax: (07) 3234 1699
South Australia	Drugs of Dependence Unit Department of Human Services PO Box 6 Rundle Mall ADELAIDE SA 5000	Ph: (08) 8226 7166 Fax: (08) 8226 7102
Western Australia	Pharmaceutical Services PO Box 8172 Perth Business Centre PERTH WA 6849	Ph: (08) 9388 4980 Fax: (08) 9388 4988
Tasmania	Pharmaceutical Services Branch Department of Health and Human Services GPO Box 125B HOBART TAS 7001	Ph: (03) 6233 2064 Fax: (03) 6233 3904
Northern Territory	Poisons Control Department of Health and Community Services PO Box 40596 CASUARINA NT 0811	Ph: (08) 8922 7341 Fax: (08) 8922 7200
Australian Capital Territory	Chief Pharmacist ACT Department of Health Locked Bag 5 WESTON ACT 2611	Ph: (02) 6207 3974 Fax: (02) 6205 0997

Appendix 8. Legislation requiring the notification of suspected child abuse

State	Authority to be notified	Relevant legislation
New South Wales	Director General of Community Services	*Children and Young Persons (Care and Protection) Act 1998*
Victoria	Victorian Child Protection Service Department of Human Services	*Children and Young Persons Act 1989*
Queensland	Department of Family	*Child Protection Act 1999*
South Australia	Department of Family and Youth Services	*Children's Protections Act 1993*
Western Australia	Department for Community Development	*Child Welfare Act 1947*
Tasmania	Child and Family Services Children and Families Division Department of Health and Human Services	*Children and Young Persons and their Families Act 1997*
Northern Territory	Family and Children's Services Department of Health and Community Services	*Community Welfare Act 1983*
Australian Capital Territory	Department of Family Services	*Children and Young Persons Act 1999* *Community Advocate Act 1991*

Appendix 9. Legislation governing the care of the mentally ill

State	Title
New South Wales	*Mental Health Act 1990*
Victoria	*Mental Health Act 1986* *Mental Health Regulations 1998*
Queensland	*Mental Health Act 2000*
South Australia	*Mental Health Act 1993*
Western Australia	*Mental Health Act 1996*
Tasmania	*Mental Health Act 1996*
Northern Territory	*Mental Health and Related Services Act 1998*
Australian Capital Territory	*Mental Health (Treatment and Care) Act 1994*

Appendix 10. Names and addresses of medical defence organisations operating in Australia

Name	Address	Telephone and Facsimile	Operating in
Medical Defence Association of South Australia	161 Ward Street NORTH ADELAIDE SA 5006	Ph: (08) 8267 5166 Fax: (08) 8267 3411	South Australia
Medical Defence Association of Victoria	Pelham House 165 Bouverie Street CARLTON VIC 3053 PO Box 1059 CARLTON VIC 3053	Ph: (03) 9347 3900 Fax: (03) 9347 3439	Victoria
Medical Defence Association of Western Australia	15 Rheola Street WEST PERTH WA 6005 PO Box 263 WEST PERTH WA 6872	Ph: (08) 9481 0977 Fax: (08) 9481 3686	Western Australia
Medical Defence Society of Queensland	Suites 16 & 17 17 Bowen Bridge Road HERSTON QLD 4029	Ph: (07) 3854 1331 Fax: (07) 3252 3389	Queensland
Medical Defence Union	Level 21 201 Kent Street SYDNEY NSW 2000	Ph: (02) 9247 6011 Fax: (02) 9247 6790	All states
Medical Protection Society	293 Royal Parade PARKVILLE VIC 3052 PO Box 21 PARKVILLE VIC 3052	Ph: (03) 9280 8790 Fax: (03) 9280 8794	All states
Medical Protection Society of New South Wales	Suite 201 22 Belgrave Street KOGARAH NSW 2217	Ph: (02) 9553 8200 Fax: (02) 9553 8133	New South Wales
Medical Protection Society of Tasmania	153A Davey Street HOBART TAS 7000	Ph: (03) 6223 7535 Fax: (03) 6223 2579	Tasmania
United Medical Defence	Level 2 60 Miller Street NORTH SYDNEY NSW 2060 Locked Bag 949 NORTH SYDNEY NSW 2060	Ph: (02) 9922 2022 Fax: (02) 9922 2252	All states

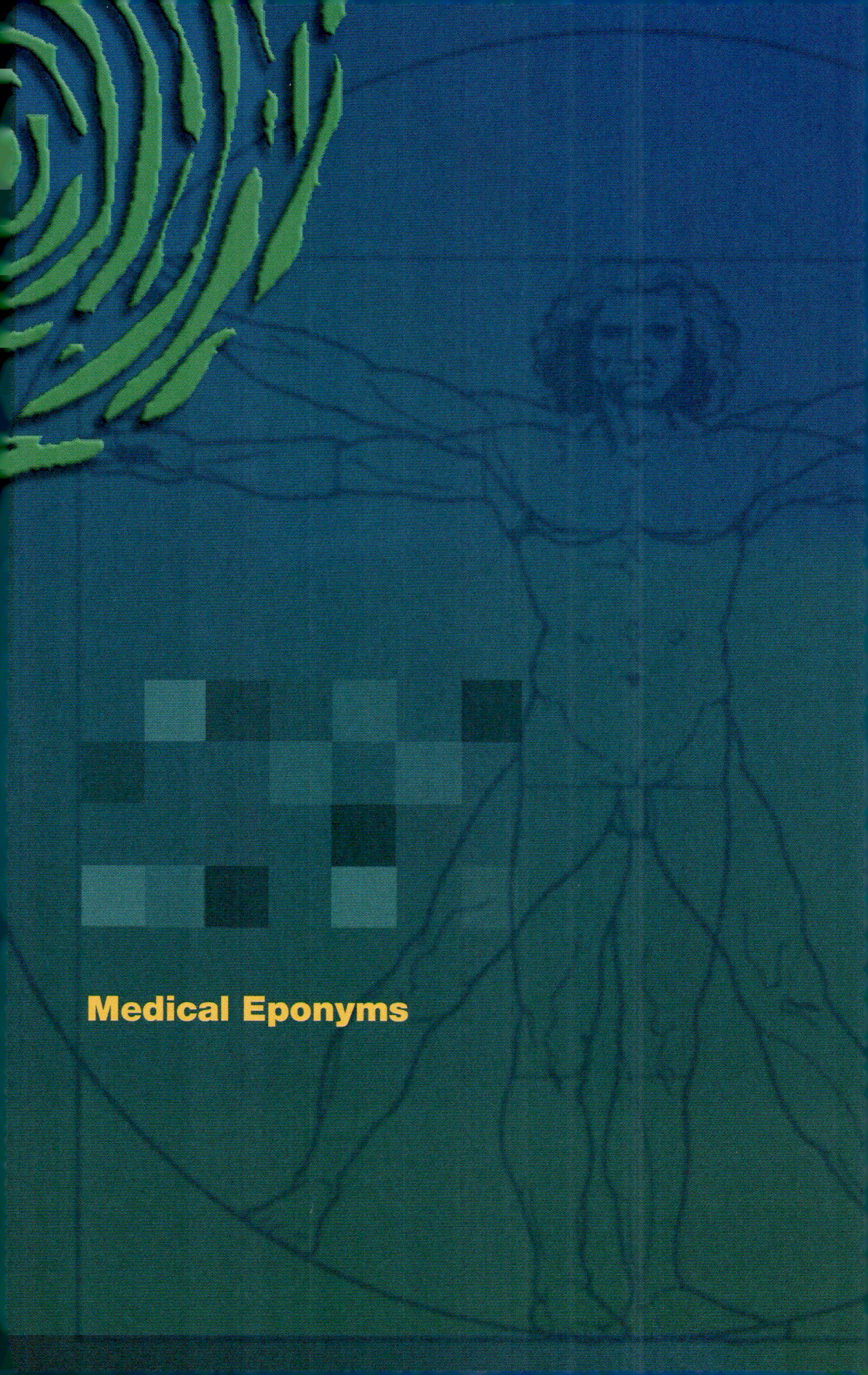

Medical Eponyms

The medical eponyms which follow were all drawn from this *Anthology of Medical Conditions*. A list of the eponyms and their origins is provided not for assessment purposes, but, as in the first Australian Medical Council (AMC) publication (*Annotated Multiple Choice Questions*) for interest and to illustrate – via the diverse origins of the eponymous men, women and other source names – the universality, multiculturality and internationality of Medicine, and its rich history.

Fuller Albright (1900–1969)

Albright syndrome (pseudohypoparathyroidism) Albright-McCune syndrome (polyostotic fibrous dysplasia)
See also D.J. McCune

American physician and clinical investigator who made major contributions to the understanding of calcium metabolism. He described the syndrome of pseudohypoparathyroidism – short stature, bony abnormalities, ectopic ossification without abnormality of parathyroid function.

With McCune, he described the syndrome of polyostotic fibrous dysplasia involving replacement of bone by fibrous tissue at multiple sites, causing deformities and pathological fractures without evidence of hyperparathyroidism (HPT). Accompanying skin pigmentation with melanin and sexual precocity also occur.

Ash leaf

Ash leaf macules

Small de-pigmented leaf-shaped skin macules, commonly on the buttock, associated with tuberous sclerosis – an autosomal dominant condition with the triad of mental retardation, epilepsy and skin lesions.

Joseph Asherman (born 1889)

Asherman syndrome

Israeli clinician, born in Czechoslovakia; described syndrome of secondary amenorrhoea in hormonally normal women with intra-uterine adhesions.

Australia

Australian antigen (hepatitis B)

Hepatitis B antigen was first identified in the serum of an aboriginal Australian by B.S. Blumberg.

Bairnsdale

Bairnsdale ulcer Bairnsdale bacillus

Town in Victoria, Australia. Chronic indolent leg ulcers initially noted in Bairnsdale in rural Victoria; ultimately identified as due to a mycobacterial organism (*Mycobacterium ulcerans*) which had optimal growth characteristics in media at lower temperatures rather than 37°C (Bairnsdale can be quite cold in winter!)

W.M. Baker (1839–1896)   **Baker cyst**

English 19th century surgeon at St. Bartholomew's Hospital in London, and assistant to Sir James Paget. Described a popliteal fossa cyst or bursa; the term is now used to describe cystic herniation of synovial membrane behind the knee joint in association with degenerative osteoarthritis of knee. Spontaneous rupture of the cystic popliteal swelling can occur with pain and oedema mimicking deep venous thrombosis (DVT).

Jack Barnes   *Carukia barnesi*
                                   See also Irukandji syndrome

Contemporary Australian physician and marine biologist.

J.H.S. Beau (1806–1875)   **Beau lines**

French 19th century physician; described the transverse lines and grooves seen on fingernails after serious illness (e.g. a myocardial infarction (MI)).

J.H. Beckwith (born 1933)   **Beckwith syndrome**

Contemporary American paediatric pathologist; his research interests included sudden infant death syndrome (SIDS). He described the congenital syndrome which bears his name and is associated with exophthalmos, macroglossia and gigantism (EMG) and with other skin and endocrine anomalies.

Sir Charles Bell (1774–1842)   **Bell law**
                                                   Bell palsy
                                                   Bell reflex

Kindly early 19th century Scottish physiologist, surgeon, and accomplished artist who held positions in London (where he founded the Middlesex Hospital) and Edinburgh. He recognised that sensory and motor fibres were carried by the spinal nerves and that the anterior roots carried motor fibres and the posterior roots sensory fibres (Bell law). He described reflex turning upwards of the eyes with eyelid closure (Bell reflex). He described the lower motor neuron paralysis of the seventh cranial nerve which bears his name (Bell palsy). He attended the wounded at Waterloo and made sketches of the battle scenes and victims.

A. Biedl (1869–1933)   **Laurence-Moon-Biedl**
                                            syndrome
                                            See T.Z. Laurence

Theodor Maximillian Bilharz (1825–1864)   **Schistosomiasis (bilharziasis)**

German 19th century parasitologist, Professor of Zoology in Cairo. Discovered a previously unknown parasitic trematode in 1851 as the causative organism of schistosomiasis. Originally placed in the genus *Bilharzia,* the three types of worm which cause endemic disease of man in Africa, Asia and South America were subsequently renamed within the genus *Schistosoma* (*S. haematobium*, *S. mansoni* and *S. japonicum*). They all multiply within snail intermediate hosts, and disseminate in fresh water as free swimming cercariae which burrow into the body through the skin ('swimmers itch') and subsequently migrate to visceral venous plexuses of bladder, intestine or liver. Spined eggs are passed in urine and faeces to start a new cycle in the intermediate snail host.

Edward H. Bishop (1913–1995)   Bishop score

American obstetrician; professor at University of Philadelphia. He described in 1964 a pelvic score for elective induction of labour in an attempt to reduce the chance of failed induction. His score evaluates four cervical factors: position (0–2), consistency (0–2), effacement and dilatation (0–2), and station of the presenting part (0–3).

Bornholm   Bornholm disease
                                                   See also Coxsackie virus

Island in the Baltic; site of a painful illness due to Coxsackie virus infection, eponymised by W. Pickles, English epidemiologist.

C.J. Bouchard (1837–1915)   Bouchard nodes

19th century French physician described nodes in osteoarthritis similar to, but less common than Heberden nodes, affecting the proximal interphalangeal joints.

C.E. Brown-Séquard (1817–1894)   Brown-Séquard syndrome

19th century French neurologist and experimental physiologist; described crossed sensory loss after hemisection of spinal cord, causing on the same side loss of touch, position and vibration sense and flaccid motor paralysis; and on the other side loss of pain and temperature sense.

Pedro, Josep and Ramon Brugada   Brugada syndrome

Contemporary brother Spanish cardiologists; they described in 1992 the phenomenon of sudden death in young males (particularly from South-East Asia) due to a tachyarrhythmia of right bundle branch block (RBBB) and ST segment elevation. Although there is no apparent morphological abnormality the condition appears to have genetic predisposition.

Leo Buerger (1879–1943)   Buerger disease
                                                    Buerger test

American surgical pathologist and urologist, described at Mt. Sinai Hospital in New York the disease of thrombo-angiitis obliterans characteristically seen in Jewish smokers; described postural test of arterial insufficiency causing elevational pallor and dependent rubor.

café-au-lait   café-au-lait spots

Light tan skin macules seen in normal individuals and as cutaneous manifestations in von Recklinghausen neurofibromatosis Type 1 (peripheral form), along with axillary freckling, characteristic cutaneous neurofibromas and endocrine tumours (phaeochromocytoma). Neurofibromatosis Type 2 (central form) is associated with acoustic neuromas and other cerebral and spinal neurofibromas without prominent skin manifestations.

Campbell-de-Morgan (1811–1876)   Campbell-de-Morgan spots

English surgeon at Middlesex Hospital, London; described the very characteristic and common non-blanching skin spots (cherry angiomas) which increase in frequency with age and have no known association with disease.

Jerome W. Conn (born 1907)   Conn syndrome

Contemporary American physician from Ann Arbor, Michigan where he directed the Division of Endocrinology and Metabolism. Described primary aldosteronism associated with functioning adrenal adenoma.

Coxsackie   Coxsackie virus

Town in New York state, USA. Home town of patients in whom the virus causing meningitis, pericarditis, pleurodynia, etc. (see Bornholm disease) was isolated.

cri-du-chat   cri-du-chat syndrome

Mewing cry associated with congenital anomaly of microcephaly, mental retardation and deletion of the short arm of Chromosome 5.

J.F. Crigler (born 1919) and   Crigler-Najjar syndrome
V.A. Najjar (born 1914)

Contemporary American paediatricians. VA Najjar, a graduate of Beirut, came from Lebanon to work in America at Johns Hopkins and Vanderbilt. They described the syndrome of inherited jaundice due to inability to conjugate bilirubin with glucuronic acid.

J. Courvoisier (1843–1918)   Courvoisier law and sign

Swiss-born surgeon, with major interests in entomology and botany. Professor of surgery at Basel, and pioneered biliary tract surgery.

His law is usually stated: *if an enlarged gall bladder is palpable in patients presenting with obstructive jaundice, the cause is unlikely to be gallstones (and thus more likely to be due to pancreatic cancer).*

H.A. Danlos

Ehlers-Danlos syndrome
See E. Ehlers

Sister Mary Joseph Dempsey (1856–1939)   **Sister Mary Joseph nodule**

American nursing sister at Mayo Clinic; described via Charles Mayo a metastatic cancer presenting as a firm umbilical nodule. The primary lesion is commonly stomach or ovary, but may be from any intra-abdominal primary.

Charles Donovan (1863–1951)
Leishman-Donovan body
Leishmania donovani
Donovanosis

British surgeon, subsequently Professor of Physiology in Madras, who confirmed in 1903 while on Indian Medical Service on the northwest frontier Leishman's autopsy discoveries by finding the eponymous inclusion bodies in a diagnostic splenic puncture on a living patient with Kala-azar.

I.N. Dubin and F.B. Johnson   **Dubin-Johnson syndrome**

Contemporary Canadian and American pathologists. Described syndrome of jaundice and hepatic melanin pigmentation due to retention of conjugated bilirubin (see also Rotor syndrome).

G.B.A. Duchenne (1807–1875)
Erb-Duchenne palsy
Duchenne disease
See also W.H. Erb

French neurologist who described many neuromuscular syndromes, including progressive bulbar palsy and progressive muscular dystrophy (Duchenne disease) and the upper trunk brachial plexus (Erb-Duchenne) palsy; also used electrical stimulation to analyse mechanisms of facial expression. Superb and painstaking clinician, dubbed by Charcot as 'The Master'.

L.M. Eaton (1905–1958) and   **Eaton-Lambert syndrome**
E.H. Lambert (born 1915)

American neurologists who described a myasthenic syndrome with proximal muscle weakness and sensory paraesthesiae often associated with carcinoma of the lung.

W. Ebstein (1836–1912)   **Ebstein malformation**

German physician who described a congenital malformation of the tricuspid valve.

E. Ehlers (1863–1937) and
Danish dermatologist
H.A. Danlos (1844–1912)
French physician and dermatologist

Ehlers-Danlos syndrome

Described in 1901 an inherited disorder, mostly with autosomal dominant inheritance, characterised by skin laxity and hypermobility of joints due to a defect in collagen synthesis. Skin bruising, ocular fragility, mitral valve prolapse and congenital cardiac defects are associated features. A semi-simulacrum of the condition was the comic-book hero character 'Plastic Man' in the 1930s, who used extensile and adaptable limbs and body tissues to fight crime.

V. Eisenmenger (1864–1932)

Eisenmenger syndrome

German physician who described syndrome of left to right vascular shunting causing pulmonary hypertension with subsequent reversal of the shunt and cyanosis (e.g. in patent ductus arteriosus).

W.H. Erb (1840–1921)

Erb palsy
Erb-Duchenne palsy
See also G.B.A. Duchenne

Eminent German neurologist, first person to use the tendon reflex hammer as a routine in physical examination.

Austin Flint (1812–1886)

Austin Flint murmur

American physician, described late diastolic mitral murmur heard in aortic incompetence.

Hugo Flecker

Chironex fleckeri

Contemporary Australian marine biologist, identified in 1956 the box jellyfish ('sea wasp') responsible for painful and sometimes fatal attacks in Northern Australian coastal waters.

Marshall and Susan Folstein

Folstein Mini–Mental State Examination (MMSE)

Contemporary husband and wife American psychiatrists; described mini–mental state assessment in 1975.

A.H. Freiberg (1868–1940)

Freiberg disease

Professor of orthopaedic surgery at Cincinnati; described aseptic necrosis of metatarsal.

P.C.E. Gaucher (1854–1918)

Gaucher disease

French physician and dermatologist. Described the lipid storage disease bearing his name in 1882.

Augustin Nicholas Gilbert (1858–1927)   Gilbert disease

French physician, Professor of Clinical Medicine at Hôtel-Dieu in Paris, described in 1900 the hereditary jaundice bearing his name. Inherited as autosomal dominant and causes fluctuating benign jaundice secondary to glucuronyl-transferase deficiency with rise in unconjugated bilirubin. The commonest of the hereditary jaundices, often diagnosed by chance investigation, with an incidence of one to two percent in females and around five percent in males.

Glasgow   Glasgow Coma Scale

City in Scotland; the Glasgow Coma Scale, based on eye opening, best verbal and best motor responses to stimuli – ranges from 3 (unresponsive coma) to 15 (oriented, responsive). The scale, introduced by Graham Teasdale and colleagues from the department of neurosurgery since 1974, is now used as a standard for depth of coma.

E.W. Goodpasture (1886–1960)   Goodpasture syndrome

American pathologist, described syndrome of acute glomerulonephritis with haemoptysis and intrapulmonary haemorrhage.

Felix J.S. Guyon (1831–1920)   Guyon canal

French surgeon; described fibrous canal on inner side of carpal ligament transmitting ulnar nerve.

W.M. Heberden (1710–1801)   Heberden nodes

Outstanding 18th century British physician. A posthumous publication in 1802 contained the description of the hard arthritic finger nodules which now bear his name.

Norman Jefferis ('Jeff') Holter (1914–1983)   Holter monitoring

American biophysicist and research scientist who pioneered from the 1970s the development of the ambulatory electrocardiographic (ECG) monitor and data reduction systems.

J. Ramsay Hunt (1874–1937)   Ramsay Hunt syndrome

American neurologist, described geniculate ganglion syndrome in 1907. He also was an early exponent of the importance of carotid artery lesions in people with stroke.

Irukandji Aboriginal Australian tribe   Irukandji disease or syndrome

Disease prevalent around Cairns and northern Australian coastline, named after a local Aboriginal tribe. The minute jellyfish (2.0 cm x 2.5 cm) responsible was discovered in 1961 by Dr Jack Barnes and was later named *Carukia barnesi*. Causing initially only mild local discomfort, the venom produces severe systemic effects of intense abdominal and muscle pains and spasms, marked hypertension and acute pulmonary oedema.

F.B. Johnson

Dubin-Johnson syndrome
See I.N. Dubin

Inspector Johnstone

Crocodylus johnstoni

Collected first museum specimen of the Australian freshwater crocodile from the Herbert River in Queensland. The freshwater crocodile, found in lagoons, rivers and billabongs north of a line from Broome in Western Australia to Johnstone in Queensland, has a narrow snout, is shy and does not attack people. The extremely dangerous estuarine ('saltwater') crocodile (*Crocodylus porosus*) can inhabit both fresh- and saltwater (by shedding salt from the tongue) and devours a wide range of prey up to and including humans. No alligators occur in Australia.

H.F. Klinefelter (born 1912)

Klinefelter syndrome

Contemporary American physician and clinical endocrinologist who described XXY syndrome of feminisation and infertility with small testes and gynaecomastia while working at Harvard with Fuller Albright.

A. Köhler (1874–1947)

Köhler disease

German radiologist; described aseptic necrosis of tarsal navicular bone in 1908.

E.H. Lambert (born 1915)

Eaton-Lambert syndrome
See L.M. Eaton

T.Z. Laurence (1830–1874),
English ophthalmologist
R.C. Moon (1844–1914)
American ophthalmologist, and
A. Biedl (1869–1933)
Czech physician

**Laurence-Moon-Biedl
syndrome**

Laurence and Moon first described in 1866 the syndrome of an inherited disorder affecting mostly males and characterised by retinitis pigmentosa, obesity, polydactyly, mental deficiency and hypogonadism. Biedl, in 1922, elaborated upon the earlier publication.

Sir William Leishman (1865–1926)

Leishmaniasis
Leishmania donovani
Leishman-Donovan body

Scottish pathologist famous for his work on Kala-azar and antityphoid inoculation. His researches into tropical diseases began while he was with the British Army Medical Service in India. In 1900 he detected the parasitic protozoa responsible for Kala-azar ('oriental sore') discovering the nonmotile inclusions of the protozoa in macrophages while performing an autopsy on a soldier serving in India. *Leishmania* are flagellates of the family Trypanosomatidae.

Frederic H. Lewy (Lewey) (1885–1950)   **Lewy body dementia**

German neurologist in the United States; described a type of dementia with cognitive impairment and extrapyramidal features, associated with hyaline material (Lewy bodies) in the cerebral cortex. Similar material occurs in nigral cells in Parkinson disease.

G. Grant Liddle (born 1921)   **Liddle syndrome**

Contemporary American endocrinologist; described familial renal disorder characterised by hypertension, hypokalaemic alkalosis and deficient aldosterone secretion.

Lyme, Connecticut   **Lyme disease**

An acute inflammatory disease with arthralgia, skin lesions and neurological involvement caused by a spirochaete (*Bonelia burgdorferi*) transmitted by a tick vector (*Ixodes dammini*). First reported in patients from Lyme, Connecticut.

D.J. McCune   **McCune-Albright or Albright-McCune syndrome (polyostotic fibrous dysplasia)**

American physician, described syndrome of polyostotic fibrous dysplasia with Fuller Albright.

Albert Hippolyte Malherbe (1845–1915)   **Malherbe benign calcifying epithelioma (pilomatrixoma)**

French surgeon, professor of surgery, histology and anatomy at Nantes and director of the medical school. He described in 1880 an indolent and clinically benign, hard, calcified encapsulated tumour of the dermis with normal overlying skin, arising from sebaceous glands – now usually classified as a hamartoma of the pilosebaceous follicle. He became extensively involved in medical school administration and was a significant force in reform of Continental medical schools, later giving impetus to reform in the United States through the efforts of Flexner and others. He was an admirer of family practice and wrote: 'The various medical fields are like a city with a great port. Family practitioners are the captains of the ship. Specialists are only the pilots who occasionally come aboard to guide the craft through difficult passages.'

G.K. Mallory (born 1900) and   **Mallory-Weiss syndrome**
S.Weiss (1898–1942)

American pathologist and physician, respectively, from Boston. Described syndrome of haematemesis due to a mucosal tear near the oesophagogastric junction following forceful vomiting.

F. Martorell   **Martorell ulcer**

Contemporary Spanish vascular surgeon who described ischaemic leg ulcers in patients with arterial disease secondary to hypertension.

R.A. Mees   **Mees lines**

Dutch physician who described in 1919 transverse white lines in nails of patients with arsenical poisoning. (See also Beau lines.)

H. Meibom (1638–1700)   **Meibomian glands (tarsal glands)**
                                                        Meibomian cyst (chalazion)

German physician who described in 1666 the conjunctival sebaceous glands which produce a fatty secretion lubricating the eyelids. He was appointed Professor of Medicine, History and Poetry at Helmstadt in Germany.

F.L. Meleney (1889–1963)   **Meleney synergistic gangrene**
                                                        Meleney ulcer

American surgeon; in United States army corps in World War I, subsequently worked in Peking and Columbia University in New York. Interested in bacterial infections, introduced use of bacitracin. Described spreading postoperative gangrene with an enlarging chronic ulcer due to synergistic infection with a microaerophilic streptococcus and *Staphylococcus aureus*.

Gregor Mendel (1822–1884)   **Mendel laws**
                                                        Mendelian inheritance
                                                        Mendelian dominant

Austrian monk and botanist, whose work studying the hybridisation of peas in an Augustine monastery uncovered the basic principles of genetics. He described paired elementary units of heredity (genes) which obeyed simple statistical laws.

F.S. Merkel (1845–1919)   **Merkel cells, corpuscles**
                                                        Merkel tumour

German anatomist who described in 1880 tactile nerve ending cells first in the nose of a mole, later found in human skin. He wrote a standard multivolume book of human anatomy and instigated the convention of displaying arteries in red, veins in blue and nerves in yellow. Tumours of Merkel cells comprise malignant skin tumours with features similar to malignant carcinoid.

H. Mondor (1855–1962)   **Mondor disease**

French surgeon; described self-resolving phlebitis of superficial veins / lymphatics producing subcutaneous strings on chest wall, axilla or elbow sometimes mistaken for cancer.

Mongolian   **Mongolian spot**

Mongolian spot (blue naevus); an entirely benign intradermal naevus presenting as a characteristically blue-grey, flat or slightly elevated nodule at base of spine, or on face or limbs. Originally thought more common in infants of Mongoloid racial origin from northern and eastern Asia.

W.F. Montgomery (1797–1859)   **Montgomery follicles/ tubercles/glands**

Irish obstetrician; described enlargement of the apocrine sebaceous glands on the surface of the areola as one of the early signs of pregnancy in 1837, since known as Montgomery tubercles and Montgomery glands.

T.G. Morton (1835–1903)   **Morton metatarsalgia**

American surgeon; described metatarsalgia caused by compression of a digital plantar nerve between metatarsal heads associated with a thickened neuroma, usually between third and fourth toes – said to occur particularly when the second toe is longer than the big toe.

R.C. Moon (1844–1914)   **Laurence-Moon-Biedl syndrome**
                                                                  See T.Z. Laurence

R.S. Muehrcke   **Muehrcke lines**

American physician: described parallel white lines separated by normal nail seen in hypoalbuminaemia.

J. Müller (1801–1858)   **Müllerian (paramesonephric) duct**

German biologist, Professor of Anatomy at Bonn, teacher of Virchow, who made the embryological discovery of the eponymous duct in 1825.

Murray River and Valley   **Murray Valley encephalitis**

River dividing the Australian states of New South Wales and Victoria; popular holiday and recreational area. Location of episodic viral encephalitis associated with mosquito vector.

V.A. Najjar (born 1914)   **Crigler-Najjar syndrome**
                                                                  See J.F. Crigler

Albert Niemann (1880–1921) and   **Niemann-Pick disease**
Ludwig Pick (1868–1944)

German physicians: described an error in lipid metabolism, inherited as an autosomal recessive. Lipid accumulates in early life in macrophages of liver and elsewhere and patients present with hepatosplenomegaly, anaemia, mental retardation and skin pigmentation due to accumulation of sphingomyelin secondary to lack of the enzyme sphingomyelinase. First described by Niemann in 1914, subsequently described in greater detail and differentiated from Gaucher disease by Pick in 1926.

Norwalk, Ohio   **Norwalk agent**

The causative agent of an institutional outbreak of viral gastroenteritis first reported in Norwalk, Ohio.

Sir William Osler (1849–1919)   **Osler nodes**
                                                         Osler hereditary haemorrhagic
                                                         telangiectasia
                                                         Osler polycythaemia rubra
                                                         vera

Canadian-born physician, educator and aphorist. The most outstanding medical personality of his time, his influence was world-wide and persists. He graduated from McGill University, Montreal; and held chairs of medicine successively at four major universities: McGill, Pennsylvania, Johns Hopkins and Oxford. An outstanding diagnostician, he wrote classical papers on hereditary haemorrhagic telangiectasia, polycythaemia vera and the painful embolic finger nodules of subacute bacterial endocarditis. His numerous aphorisms, and his essays (such as 'Aequanimitas' – outlining an optimum approach to the practice of clinical medicine) are as relevant and cogent today as when written.

Ludwig Pick (1868–1944)   **Niemann-Pick disease**
                                                         See Albert Niemann

A. Prader and H. Willi   **Prader-Willi syndrome**

Swiss Paediatricians: described in 1956 a congenital disorder characterised by short stature, obesity, mental retardation, hypotonia and hypogonadism.

Fritz de Quervain (1868–1940)   **de Quervain stenosing**
                                                         tenosynovitis

Swiss physician; described stenosing inflammation of the tendon sheath on thumb side of the wrist containing the tendons of abductor pollicis longus and extensor pollicis brevis, causing pain on thumb movements and local tenderness and/or nodule. Also in 1895 described the acute inflammatory swelling of thyroid now known as de Quervain thyroiditis.

H.C. Reiter (1881–1969)   **Reiter syndrome**

German physician and hygienist. While serving with German forces in World War I, he treated and described a patient with the triad of urethritis, conjunctivitis and arthritis, which he thought initially spirochaetal but subsequently revised this opinion. The syndrome is often associated with a history of venereal contact and diarrhoea; and has a high association with histocompatibility antigen Human Leucocyte Antigen–B27 (HLA-B27).

A. Rett   **Rett disorder/syndrome**

Austrian physician; described autistic behaviour developing in girls aged between one and four years with ataxia, disordered hand movements, and dementia.

Ross River   **Ross River fever**

Northern Australian river; site of infections by arbovirus.

A.B. Rotor   **Rotor syndrome**

Philippine physician; described in the Philippines an inherited disorder with jaundice associated with increased conjugated bilirubin, distinct from Dubin-Johnson syndrome.

Leopold von Sacher-Masoch (1836–1895)   **Sadomasochism**
See Marquis de Sade

Bernard P. Sachs (1858–1944)   **Tay-Sachs syndrome**
See Warren Tay

Marquis de Sade and   **Sadomasochism**
Leopold von Sacher-Masoch

Marquis de Sade (1740–1814)   **Sadism**

French soldier and writer; as a young nobleman consorted with prostitutes and developed a taste for sexual perversions and licentiousness, subsequently described sexual fantasies in his erotic novels. His compulsion for physically, mentally and sexually abusing others originated the term **sadism** – pleasure from the infliction of pain on others. He died in an insane asylum.

Leopold von Sacher-Masoch (1836–1895)   **Masochism**

Austrian erotic novelist, stressed sexual pleasures derived from personal pain; these reflected his own life in which he acted out the sexual fantasies and fetishes described in books such as 'Venus in Furs'. **Masochism**, denoting pleasure in being subjected to pain or humiliation, was an established medical term by the 1890s; along with **sadomasochism**, the derivation of pleasure from infliction of physical or mental pain on others or on oneself.

T.A.H. Schwann (1810–1882)

Schwannoma
Schwann cells
Schwann sheath

German anatomist, founder of modern neurohistology. Described the myelin sheath (neurilemma) of nerve axons and the cells surrounding the myelinated axons between two nodes of Ranvier forming the sheath. Schwannomas (neurilemmomas) are tumours arising from the Schwann cells.

J.W. Sever (born 1878)

Sever disease

American orthopaedic surgeon, described calcaneal apophysitis.

H.L. Sheehan (born 1900)

Sheehan syndrome

British pathologist; described pituitary necrosis with hypopituitism resulting from postpartum haemorrhage.

Adrian van den Spieghel / Spigelius
(1578–1625)

Spigelian hernia

Professor of Anatomy at Padua, also a renowned botanist; described hernia of linea semilunaris.

P.H.M. Sudeck (1866–1945)

Sudeck atrophy

German surgeon; Professor of Surgery in Hamburg, described aseptic bone demineralisation after injury and immobilisation.

J.M. Tanner

Tanner stages

Defined stages of normal pubertal development in females (1969) and males (1970).

Warren Tay (1843–1927) and

Tay-Sachs disease

British surgeon specialising in ophthalmology and paediatrics. Described in 1881 degeneration of the choroid associated with amaurotic idiocy.

Bernard P. Sachs (1858–1944)

American neurologist, published independently in 1887 a comprehensive description of a fatal hereditary error of metabolism characterised by accumulation of sphingolipids in nervous tissue due to an enzyme deficiency (compare Gaucher disease, Niemann-Pick disease) associated with progressive paralysis, dementia and blindness with a cherry-red spot in the retina, inherited as an autosomal recessive, and subsequently shown due to deficiency of hexosamidase A.

Thalassa – Greek – The sea

Thalassaemia major, minor
Mediterranean anaemia

Inherited anaemia common in Greece and other Mediterranean areas. The heterozygous inheritance of the gene causes thallassaemia minor and carriage of the trait. Homozygous inheritance causes the severe disease of thallassaemia major.

A. Tietze (1864–1927)

Tietze syndrome

German surgeon, described costo-chondritis giving chest pain at costo-chondral junctions; more common in females, and often left-sided. Usually self-resolving, but causes diagnostic confusion with pain from other conditions (cardiac pain, mastalgia).

R.B. Todd (1809–1860)

Todd palsy

Irish anatomist and physician, professor of physiology at King's College, London. Described transient localised paralysis with monoparesis or hemiparesis that may follow a focal epileptic seizure.

G. Gilles de la Tourette (1857–1904)

Tourette disease or syndrome

French neurologist, student of Charcot at Saltpêtrière. He described in 1884 the tic disorder bearing his name, characterised by violent facial and limb muscular jerks with spasmodic grunting and involuntary verbalisation, echolalia and coprolalia. The first patient he described died aged 85 years, and the Paris papers published some of her more colourful phrases in her obituary. He pioneered clinical studies in hysteria and hypnotism. He was once shot by one of his previously hypnotised patients. His later career was characterised by increasing eccentricities culminating in his dismissal from office.

G. Grey Turner (1877–1951)

Grey Turner sign

English surgeon; graduate of University of Durham, subsequently Professor of Surgery at the Postgraduate Medical School, London; described sign of loin discolouration due to extraperitoneal extravasation of blood seen in one or both flanks after acute pancreatitis.

S. Weiss

Mallory-Weiss syndrome
See G.K. Mallory

F. Wegener (born 1967)

Wegener granulomatosis

German pathologist, described syndrome of necrotising respiratory granuloma with angiitis and glomerulonephritis.

E.A. von Willebrand (1870–1939)

von Willebrand disease
von Willebrand factor

Finnish physician; described in 1926 the family tree of a bleeding disorder distinguishable from haemophilia (pseudohaemophilia); characterised by a prolonged bleeding time, and an inheritance which is usually autosomal dominant – due to absence of a plasma protein clotting factor (von Willebrand factor).

H. Willi

Prader-Willi syndrome
See A. Prader

A.E.J. Yersin (1863–1943)

Yersinia pestis
Plague bacillus

Swiss bacteriologist who discovered the cause of plague in 1894 in Hong Kong after serving with the Medical Corps of the French Army in Indonesia. The organism *Bacillus pestis*, later *Pasteurella pestis*, was named *Yersinia pestis* in 1944. He also introduced the rubber tree into Indo-China.

Other medical eponyms from A–Z mentioned in the current text are listed below. Their eponymous origins have been described previously in the linked AMC publication of *Annotated Multiple Choice Questions*[4].

Addison disease
Alzheimer disease
Apgar score
Bowen disease
Brucellosis
Celsius
Cock peculiar tumour
Coombs test
Charcot-Marie-Tooth disease
Creutzfeldt-Jakob disease
Crohn disease
Cushing syndrome
Down syndrome
Dupuytren disease or contracture
Epstein-Barr virus (EBV)
Escherichia coli
Fallot tetralogy
Fanconi syndrome
Felty syndrome
Fournier gangrene
Giardiasis
Gram stain
Graves disease
Guillain-Barré syndrome
Henoch-Schönlein purpura
Hirschsprung disease
Hodgkin lymphoma
Horner syndrome
Huntington chorea

Hutchinson melanotic freckle
Kaposi sarcoma
Klumpke paralysis
Legg-Calvé-Perthes disease
Marfan syndrome
Marjolin ulcer
Meckel diverticulum
Ménière disease
Münchausen syndrome
Osgood-Schlatter disease
Paget diseases
Pancoast tumour
Papanicolaou (Pap) test
Parkinson disease
Perthes disease and test
Peutz-Jeghers syndrome
Q fever
Raynaud disease/syndrome
Salmonella
Shigella
Sjögren syndrome
Still disease
Turner syndrome
Volkmann contracture
Whipple disease
Wilson disease
Wolff-Parkinson-White syndrome (WPW)
Zollinger-Ellison syndrome

The eponym list thus *in toto* comprises origins of disease description from every continent and from a spread of countries matching the 70 countries of origin of the numerous immigrant overseas-trained doctors who have since the 1960s passed the AMC assessments to practise medicine in Australia.

---

4   Australian Medical Council Inc.   ?d multiple choice questions.
    Carlton, Vic: Blackwell Scier

Glossary

Glossary

'ABCDE':	*A*irway; *B*reathing; *C*irculation; *D*isability; *E*xposure
ACE:	angiotensin-converting enzyme
ACTH:	adrenocorticotrophic hormone
ADH:	antidiuretic hormone
ADHD:	attention deficit hyperactivity (hyperkinetic) disorder
AGUS:	atypical glandular cells of uncertain significance
AIDS:	acquired immune deficiency syndrome
ALTE:	acute life-threatening event
ARF:	acute renal failure
ASA:	American Society of Anaesthiologists
ASCUS:	atypical squamous cells of uncertain significance
ASD:	atrial septal defect
ATN:	acute tubular necrosis
AVM:	arteriovenous malformation
AVN:	avascular necrosis
BCC:	basal cell carcinoma
BMI:	body-mass index
BP:	blood pressure
BSA:	body surface area
'CAGE':	*C*utting down on your drinking?; *A*nnoyed by criticism of drinking?; *G*uilty about your drinking?; *E*ye opener needed in the morning?
CABG:	coronary artery bypass graft
CAD:	coronary artery disease
CBD:	'common' bile duct
CCF:	congestive cardiac failure
CDH:	congenital dysplasia of hip (now archaic, see DDH)
CEO:	Chief Executive Officer
CIN:	cervical intra-epithelial neoplasia
CK:	creatine kinase
CMV:	cytomegalovirus
CNS:	central nervous system

COPD:	chronic obstructive pulmonary disease
CPR:	cardiopulmonary resuscitation
CSF:	cerebrospinal fluid
CT:	computed tomography
DCIS:	ductal carcinoma-*in-situ*
DDAVP:	1-desamino-8D-arginine vasopressin
DDH, CDH:	developmental dysplasia of hip
DIC:	disseminated intravascular coagulation
DSM-IV-TR:	*The Diagnostic and Statistical Manual 4 – Text Revision*
DVT:	deep venous thrombosis
EBV:	Epstein-Barr virus
ECG:	electrocardiogram, electrocardiography
EDTA:	ethylene diamine tetra-acetic acid
EMG:	electromyelogram, electromyelography
EMG syndrome:	exophthalmos, macroglossla and gigantism
EMST:	emergency management of severe trauma
ENT:	ear, nose and throat
ERCP:	endoscopic retrograde cholangio-pancreatography
ESR:	erythrocyte sedimentation rate
FBE:	full blood examination
FEV$_1$:	forced expiratory volume in one second
FNAC:	fine needle aspiration cytology
FSGS:	focal segmental glomerulosclerosis
GFR:	glomerular filtration rate
GH:	growth hormone
GnRH:	gonadotropin-releasing hormone
hCG:	human chorionic gonadotropin
HDL:	high-density lipoprotein
'HELLP' syndrome:	*H*aemolysis, *E*levated *L*iver enzymes, *L*ow *P*latelets
Hib:	*Haemophilus influenza* type B
HIV:	human immunodeficiency virus
HLA-B27:	Human Leucocyte Antigen–B27
HMG-CoA:	3-hydroxy-3-methylglutaryl coenzyme A
HPT:	hyperparathyroidism
HPV:	human papilloma virus

HRT:	hormone replacement therapy
HS1:	heart sound 1
HS2:	heart sound 2
HUS:	haemolytic uraemic syndrome
IBD:	inflammatory bowel disease
ICD:	implantable cardiac defibrillator
ICSI:	intra-cytopasmic sperm injection
IgA, G:	immunoglobulin A, G
IM:	intramuscular
IQ:	intelligence quotient
IUGR:	intra-uterine growth retardation
IV:	intravenous
IVF:	*in-vitro*-fertilisation
LBBB:	left bundle branch block
LCIS:	lobular carcinoma-*in-situ*
LDL:	low-density lipoprotein
LVH:	left ventricular hypertrophy
MCU:	micturating cysto-urethrogram
MI:	myocardial infarction
MMSE:	(Folstein) Mini–Mental State Examination
MRCP:	magnetic resonance cholangio-pancreatography
MRI:	magnetic resonance imaging
MSDS:	Material Safety Data Sheets
NMS:	neuroleptic malignant syndrome
NSAID:	nonsteroidal anti-inflammatory drug
OCP:	oral contraceptive pill
P_a:	partial arterial pressure
P_A:	partial alveolar pressure
Pap smear:	Papanicolaou smear
PEM:	protein-energy malnutrition
PR:	per rectum
PTH:	parathyroid hormone
PUO:	fever/pyrexia of unknown origin
RA:	rheumatoid arthritis
RBC:	red blood cell

RBBB:	right bundle branch block
SARS:	severe acute respiratory syndrome
SCC:	squamous cell carcinoma
SIADH:	syndrome of inappropriate ADH secretion
SLE:	systemic lupus erythematosus
STD:	sexually transmitted disease
TB:	tuberculosis
TENS:	transcutaneous electric nerve stimulation
TMJ:	temporomandibular joint
'TORCH' infection/s:	*T*oxoplasmosis, *O*ther, *R*ubella, *C*ytomegalovirus, *H*erpes simplex virus
TSH:	thyroid-stimulating hormone
URTI:	upper respiratory tract infection
UTI:	urinary tract infection
UV:	ultraviolet
VIPoma:	vasoactive intestinal peptide tumor
VSD:	ventricular septal defect
WCC:	white cell count
WPW:	Wolff-Parkinson-White syndrome

Index

Index

Page numbers in **bold** indicate major discussions of clinical presentations. Page numbers in *italics* refer to illustrations. Eponymous diseases are indicated by the numeric code of the presenting sign/symptom, e.g. Addison disease *see* [038] indicates Addison disease might present as [038] Fatigue.

ADH (antidiuretic hormone) 77
ADHD (attention deficit hyperactivity
    (hyperkinetic) disorder) 92, 93, 94
adrenal hyperplasia, congenital *228*
Adrenal Mass [002H] **43–44**, *43*
Adult Constipation [027E] **140–141**, *140,
    141*
advertising, of professional services 518,
    535, 548
advice, seeking 527
advocacy groups 552–553
aged persons *see* elderly patients
aggression, defined 464 *see also* Violence/
    Aggression and Mental Illness [119]
agoraphobia 298
AIDS (acquired immune deficiency
    syndrome), notification requirement 567
air pollutants 322
alcohol, cirrhosis caused by 251
alcohol abuse *see* Substance Abuse/
    Addiction [107]
alkalaemia 64–66, 71
alkalosis
    associated deficiencies 71
    Metabolic alkalosis [005B] **65, 66**
    Respiratory alkalosis (due to increased
        alveolar ventilation from overbreathing)
        [005D] **65, 66**
allergic reactions
    Allergic Reactions [127] **493–495**, *493,
        494*
    to amoxycillin *411*
    Anaphylaxis [098A] **388–389**
    rhinitis 372
    see also urticaria
alopecia 205, *205, 206*, 207
ALTE (acute life-threatening event) 390–391
alternative medicine *see* unorthodox
    medicine
Alzheimer disease *see* [024]; [056]; [064]
amaurosis fugax 222
amblyopia 421
AMC *see* Australian Medical Council (AMC)
Amenorrhoea (also Oligomenorrhoea) [063A]
    262–263
American Medical Association 468
Anaemia and Pallor [012] **90–91**, *90*
anaesthesia 284
anal disorders
    acute perianal haematoma *54*
    anal fissure *54*
    anal fistula *55*
    Anal Pain [003E] **54–55**
    haemorrhoids 54, 55, *98*
    Pruritus Ani [086A] **345**
Anal Pain [003E] **54–55**, *54, 55*
Anaphylaxis [098A] **388–389**

anasarca *see* Oedema [034]
androgen, in gynaecomastia 100
aneurysm *34, 213*
angina *see* Childhood Communicable
    Diseases with or without Skin Rash
    [102B]; Rhinorrhoea/Sore Throat [092]
angina pectoris *see* Chest Discomfort [020]
angio-oedema 411–412
animal bites 496–498, *496, 497, 498*
animal research 528
anisocoria 348
ankle pain 363
ankylosing spondylitis *353*
anorexia nervosa 71, 94, 95, 485–486
anorgasmia 384
anovulval warts *461*
Antepartum Care [081A] **330–331**
anti-venoms 496
antidiuretic hormone (ADH) 77
antisocial behaviour *see* violent behaviour
antisocial personalities *see* Personality
    Disorders [078]
anuria 368–369
anus *see* anal disorders
anxiety
    childhood and adolescence 92
    fibromyalgia associated with 350
    Panic and Anxiety [073] **298–299**
    problem gambling associated with 424
    somatisation associated with 268
    see also mood disorders
aortic aneurysm *34*
aortic regurgitation 277
aortic stenosis 274
aphasia 221–225
apnoea
    Cyanosis/Hypoxia/Apnoea in Children
        [023A] **123–124**
    Insomnia/Sleep and Circadian Rhythm
        Disorders/Sleep-Apnoea Syndrome [056]
        246–247
appendices (1–10) 561–572
arachnidism 496, *497*, 498
area of need scheme 566
areola mammae *see* Breast - Skin Changes
    [017E]
ARF (acute renal failure) 368–369
arrhythmia
    hypomagnesaemia associated with 76
    Palpitations (Abnormal Electrocardiogram
        (ECG)/Arrhythmia) [072] **296–297**, *296*
    syncope associated with 428
arterial disease, risk factors for 67
arterial stenosis, renal *234*
arterial ulcer *see* Chronic Leg Ulcer [101A]
arteriovenous malformation, cerebral *213*
arteritis, temporal *213*, 350

blood vessel problem 96
blue naevus (Mongolian spot) *392*
blunt trauma *see* Trauma/Accidents/
Prevention [113]
body-mass index (BMI) 177
boils 404–406
Bone and Joint Injuries [113B] **437–438**,
437, *438 see also* fractures and
dislocations
bone density, in osteoporosis 365
Bornholm disease *see* [020]
Bouchard node *see* [129B]
Boutonnière deformity *see* [129B]
bowel obstruction
Abdominal Distension/Ileus (Ascites,
Bowel Obstruction) [001] **29–31**
adhesions causing *46*
distended caecum *141*
Bowen disease *396*
box jellyfish (*Chironex fleckeri*) 497
bradyarrhythmia 113
bradycardia, fetal 184
brain death 211–212
branchial cyst *282*
breast abscess 107
breast cancer 101, 102, 103, *104*, 108, *109*
Breast Disorders [017] **100–109**
Breast Pain (Mastalgia) [017D] **107**, *107*
Breast - Skin Changes [017E] **108–109**,
108, 109
Female (Breast Lump/Prevention of
Cancer/Screening) [017B] **102–103**, *104*
Male (Gynaecomastia) [017A] **100–101**,
101
Nipple Discharge/Galactorrhoea [017C]
105–106
breast infections 102
Breast Pain (Mastalgia) [017D] **107**, *107*
Breast - Skin Changes [017E] **108–109**,
108, 109
breathing problems
Newborn in Poor Condition/Depressed
Breathing [025] **128–129**
Wheezing/Respiratory Difficulty/Stridor
[126] **489–492**, *489*
see also respiratory disorders
Brown-Séquard syndrome *see* [050A]
Brugada syndromes *see* [109]
bruising 96–97
bruit 432–433
bulimia 94, 95 *see also* weight disorders
bunion 400
Burns [018] **110–112**, *111, 112*, 439, 441
bursa *see* Focal Subcutaneous Lumps
[100C]
bursitis *400*

CAD (coronary artery disease) 67, 115
caecum 90, *141*
café-au-lait spot *see* [077A]
'CAGE' questions 423
calcinosis *359*
calcium/phosphate serum levels
Hypercalcaemia [004A] **58–59**
Hypocalcaemia [004B] **60–61**, 71
Hypophosphataemia/Fanconi Syndrome
[004C] **62–63**
calculus *46, 50, 219, 273*
Campbell de Morgan spot *see* [100A]
camptodactyly 502, *502*
cancer
basal cell carcinoma 395, *395*
of breast 101, 102, 103, *104*, 108, *109*
of caecum 90
Cancer Pain [089K] **366–367**, *366*
of colon 98, 99, 140
common types of 366
hepatocellular *36*
laryngeal *415*
of lip *271*
of lung *158, 366*
lymphangitic *153*
melanoma *see* Focal Skin Lesions -
'Suspicious' Lesions [100B]
metastasis *70, 260, 366, 457*
occult gastrointestinal bleeding associated
with 98
of oesophagus 148, *148*
ovarian *302*
pain relief 367
pharyngeal *260*
prostatic 457, *457*, 458
of rectum *98*, 99
renal *366*
screen-detected excision *104*
squamous cell carcinoma *271*, 396, *396*
of stomach 98
Cancer Pain [089K] **366–367**, *366*
cancer prevention *see* Bleeding with
Defaecation/Acute Lower Gastrointestinal
Bleeding/Melaena/Occult Blood in Stool/
Prevention of Cancer [016]; Dyspnoea
and/or Cough/Prevention of Cancers and
Chronic Respiratory Diseases [032];
Female (Breast Lump/Prevention of
Cancer/Screening) [017B]
capacity of patients
assessment of 521–522
defined 514
legal aspects 531–532
car crash injuries *see* vehicle crash injuries
carbon dioxide poisoning 112
carbon monoxide poisoning 323
carbuncle 404–406

distension, abdominal *see* Abdominal
Distension/Ileus (Ascites, Bowel
Obstruction) [001]
distributive justice, defined 514
diverticular disease *40, 47*, 98
diverticulitis, perforated colonic *47*
Dizziness/Vertigo [029] **144–145**
doctor—patient relationship xxix–xxxi, 516–
517, 519, 534 *see also* LEO (Legal,
Ethical and Organisational) aspects
doctors' responsibilities *see* LEO (Legal,
Ethical and Organisational) aspects
domestic violence *see* family violence
double vision 142–143, *142*
Down syndrome *see* [043]; [043A]
drowning 496, 508
drug addiction *see* Substance Abuse/
Addiction [107]
drugs
of dependence 569
legislation regulating use of 568
Dubin-Johnson syndrome *see* [007]
Duchenne disease *see* [026]
Duchenne muscular dystrophy *see* [043];
[043A]
ductus arteriosus 124
duplex system *451*
Dupuytren disease *503 see also* [129B]
duty of care 534
DVT (deep venous thrombosis) 170–171,
294
Dying Patient [030] 114, **146–147**
dysaesthesia 284
dyslexia 92
dysmenorrhoea 264–265
dysmorphic features 201–204
dyspepsia 52–53, *53*
Dysphagia [031] **148–149**, *148, 149*
dysphonia 415–416, *415*
dysplasia, of hip *499*
Dyspnoea and/or Cough/Prevention of
Cancers and Chronic Respiratory
Diseases [032] **150–165**
Cough [032F] **162–163**, *163*
differentiation between acute and chronic
160
differentiation of causes 150–151
With Diffuse Chest X-Ray Abnormality
[032A] **152–153**, *152*
Dyspnoea/Respiratory Distress, Paediatric
[032G] **164–165**
With Fever [032C] **156–157**, *156*
With Local Chest X-Ray Abnormality
[032D] **158–159**, *158, 159*
With Normal Chest X-Ray [032] **160–161**
With Pleural Chest X-Ray Abnormality
[032B] **154–155**, *154*

Dyspnoea/Respiratory Distress, Paediatric
[032G] **164–165**
dysuria 451–452, *451*, 462

Ear Pain [033] **166–167**
ears
congenital malformation *201*
Ear Pain [033] **166–167**
Hearing Loss/Deafness [047] **215–216**
Tinnitus/Bruit [111] **432–433**
eating disorders 71, 94, 95, 485–486
Eaton-Lambert syndrome *see* [122]
Ebstein anomaly *see* [067A]
EBV (Epstein-Barr virus) *see* [040]; [062];
[105]
ECG (electrocardiogram)
cardiac arrhythmia associated with
syncope 428
hypokalaemia diagnosis 71
Palpitations (Abnormal Electrocardiogram
(ECG)/Arrhythmia) [072] **296–297**, *296*
economic abuse 466 *see also* abuse
edema *see* oedema
EDTA (ethylene diamine tetra-acetic acid) 60
effusion, pleural 154–155, *154*
Ehlers-Danlos syndrome *see* [020]
Eisenmenger syndrome *see* [023]; [067C];
[080]
ejaculation disorders 384
elbow pain *350*, 358–359
Elder Abuse [119B] **468–469**
elderly patients
Elder Abuse [119B] **468–469**
Failure to Thrive in the Elderly [036B]
176–177
falls by 178, 197
fractures/dislocations 197
health considerations for 319
Hypertension in the Elderly [054C] **240–
241**
mouth problems 272
periodic health examination 306–307
prostate cancer 457, *457*, 458
severity of haematemesis in 217
syncope prevalence 427
Urinary Incontinence, Elderly [115B] **455–
456**
see also all other presentations
electrical burns *see* Burns [018]
electrocardiogram (ECG)
cardiac arrhythmia associated with
syncope 428
hypokalaemia diagnosis 71
Palpitations (Abnormal Electrocardiogram
(ECG)/Arrhythmia) [072] **296–297**, *296*
electrocution 508
electrolytes, serum

hypokalaemia diagnosis 71, 72
hyponatraemia detection 77, 78
paediatric diarrhoea affecting 138
electronic records 533, 538 see also
telemedicine
elevated mood see mood disorders
emergencies
Anaphylaxis [098A] **388–389**
Cardiac Arrest/Respiratory Arrest [019]
113–114
Childhood Communicable Diseases with or
without Skin Rash [102B] **413–414**, *413*,
508
Dyspnoea/Respiratory Distress, Paediatric
[032G] **164–165**
Fever and Chills (Adult and Paediatric)
[040] **185–196**
hypertensive 240
Hypothermia [040D] **193–194**, *193*
Life Support Protocol Flow Chart *xxiii*
Life-Threatening Emergencies [131A]
507–508, *508*
Malignant Hypertension [054D] **242–243**,
243
Paediatric Emergencies [011A] **84–85**
Palpitations (Abnormal Electrocardiogram
(ECG)/Arrhythmia) [072] **296–297**
poisoning/drug overdose 326
Shock/Hypotension [098] **386–389**
testicular torsion *376*, 377
emotional abuse 466 see also abuse
emotional disturbance 92, 94, 95
employers, legal obligations of 317
encopresis, paediatric 58, 136–137, *136*
enteritis, in Crohn disease *135*
enterocele 340
enuresis 454–456
envenomations 496–498, *496*, *497*
Environment [077H] **322–323**
environmental emergencies see Hyperthermia
[040E]; Hypothermia [040D]
environmental health issues see Environment
[077H]; Work-Related Health Issues
[077E]
epidermolysis bullosa *405*
epididymal cyst 374, 375
epidural haematoma *211*
Epigastric Mass [002A] **34**, *34*
epigastric pain see Abdominal Pain [003]
epilepsy 378–379
eponyms 575–591 see also *individual
eponymous diseases/syndromes*
Epstein-Barr virus (EBV) see [040]; [062];
[105]
Erb paralysis see [129B]
erythrocyte sedimentation rate (ESR) 350,
351

erythrocytes
ESR in polymyalgia rheumatica 350, 351
Polycythaemia/Elevated Haemoglobin
[080] **328–329**
erythrocytosis 328
eschar *439*
esophagus see oesophagus
ESR (erythrocyte sedimentation rate) 350,
351
ethical dilemmas 513, 519, 526–527
ethical guidelines, breaches of 513, 535
ethical principles 519
ethics
advice on 527
clinicians and commerce 525
confidentiality of patients 519–521
consent to investigation or treatment
521–522
defined 514
dilemma resolution 513, 519, 526–527
of disclosure 522–523
doctor—patient relationship 516–517
key principles 519
of medicine 519
origin of 513
personal conduct of clinicians 517
privacy of patients 519–521
of professional conduct 517–518
professional issues 526–527
of research 527–528
of resource allocation 524
ethylene diamine tetra-acetic acid (EDTA) 60
euthanasia, defined 515
exomphalos *501*
expectoration of blood 226–227, *227*
extra heart sounds see Murmur/Extra Heart
Sounds [067]
Eye Injuries [113F] **441**
Eye Redness [035] **172–173**, *172*
'eye strain' 213
eyes
Diplopia (Double Vision) [028] **142–143**,
142
Eye Injuries [113F] **441**
Eye Redness [035] **172–173**, *172*
'eye strain' 213
Pupil Abnormalities [088] **348–349**, *348*
retinopathy *231*, *239*, *243*
Strabismus and/or Amblyopia [106] *142*,
421
transient monocular blindness 222
Visual Disturbance/Loss [120] **473–475**,
474, *475*

Freiberg disease *see* [089I]
frostbite *193*
full blood examination (FBE), in anaemia 90, 91
fussing child 86–87

Gait Disturbances - Ataxia [042] **199–200**
galactorrhoea 105–106
gambling, pathological/problem 424
ganglion *400 see also* Focal Subcutaneous Lumps [100C]
gangrene *291, 292*, 401, 402, *402*
'gas gangrene' 401, 402
gastric ulcer *217*
gastro-oesophageal reflux disease 148
gastrointestinal bleeding
    Bleeding with Defaecation/Acute Lower Gastrointestinal Bleeding/Melaena/Occult Blood in Stool/Prevention of Cancer [016] **98–99**
    Haematemesis/Melaena [048] **217–218**, *217*
Gaucher disease *see* [058A]
gender, behaviour disorders and 94
gender identity disorder 384–385, *385*
generalised anxiety disorder 298 *see also* mood disorders
Generalised Oedema [034A] **168–169**
Genetic Concerns, Dysmorphic Features [043] **201–204**
    differentiation of causes **201–202**, *201, 202*
    Genetic Concerns, Screening [043A] **203–204**
    see also Congenital Malformations [129A]
genital mutilation 526
genital tract infections 461, *461, 462*
giant cell arteritis *see* temporal arteritis
Gilbert disease *see* [007]
Gilbert syndrome *see* [058]; [058A]
gingivitis 271
Glasgow Coma Scale 118, 211
globus hystericus 148
glomerular haematuria 219–220, *219, 220*
glomerulonephritis 372
glossary
    LEO terminology 514–515
    medical terminology 595–598
goitre
    Neck or Facial Mass/Goitre/Thyroid Disease [068] **281–283**, *281, 282*
    retrosternal, causing stridor *489*
gonorrhoea *462 see also* sexually transmitted diseases (STDs)
Goodpasture syndrome *see* [032A]; [051]
'granny battering' *468 see also* Elder Abuse [119B]

granuloma, pyogenic *398*
Graves disease *see* [044B]; [068]
groin hernia 41, *41, 42, 47, 57*
growing pains 258
growth abnormalities *see* development disorders; Weight (Low) at Birth/Intra-uterine Growth Aberration [123]
growth and development *see* Periodic Health Examination/Growth and Development [077]
Guillain-Barré syndrome *see* [122]
gunshot wounds 435, 436, 439, 445, 449
Guyon canal *see* [089F]
Gynaecomastia [017A] **100–101**, *101*

Haematemesis/Melaena [048] 98, **217–218**, *217*
haematochezia 98, 99
haematoma
    acute perianal *54*
    epidural *211*
    subdural *212*
    subungual *210*
    in vascular injury 449
Haematuria [049] **219–220**, *219, 220*
haemoglobin, elevated 328–329
Haemoptysis [051] **226–227**, *227*
haemorrhage
    retroperitoneal, following warfarin *97*
    sub-conjunctival *172*
    treatment priority 437
    Vaginal Bleeding, Excessive in Amount or Irregular in Timing [117] **459–460**
    in vascular injury 449
    see also bleeding
haemorrhagic stroke 221
haemorrhoids 54, 55, *98*
Hair and Nail Disorders [044] **205–210**
    Hair Disorders [044A] **205–207**, *205, 206*
    Nail Disorders [044B] **208–210**, *208, 209, 210*
    see also Hirsutism and Virilisation [052]
hallucinations 346
hamstring tear *434*
Hand Deformities [129B] **502–504**, *502, 503, 504*
Hand/Wrist/Elbow Pain [089F] **358–359**, *358, 359*
Hand/Wrist Injuries [113H] *438*, **443**, *443*
hCG (human chorionic gonadotropin) 100
HDL (high-density lipoprotein) 67
Head Injuries/Brain Death/Transplant Donation [045] **211–212**, *211, 212*
Headache [046] **213–214**, *213, 214*, 323
health examination *see* Periodic Health Examination/Growth and Development [077]

melanocytic naevus 393

melanoma *see* Focal Skin Lesions - 'Suspicious' Lesions [100B]

Meleney ulcer *see* [100D]

memory disturbances 125–127

menarche 262

Ménière disease *see* [029]; [047]; [111]

meningioma *213*

meningococcal septicaemia *413*, *508*

Menopause [064] **266–267**

Menstrual Cycle Abnormal [063] **262–265**

    Amenorrhoea (also Oligomenorrhoea) [063A] **262–263**

    Pre-Menstrual Syndrome/Dysmenorrhoea [063B] **264–265**

    see also Vaginal Bleeding, Excessive in Amount or Irregular in Timing [117]

mental disorders *see* mood disorders; Violence/Aggression and Mental Illness [119]

mentally ill, legislation governing care of 571

Merkel cell tumour *see* [100B]

mesenteric ischaemia, metabolic (lactic) acidosis associated with *64*

Metabolic acidosis [005A] **64**, **66**, 73

Metabolic alkalosis [005B] **65**, **66**, 71

metastasis

    bony, in lung cancer *366*

    hepatic *70*

    pharyngeal cancer *260*

    prostate cancer *457*

    spinal, in renal cancer *366*

micturating cysto-urethrogram (MCU) *451*

micturition *see* Urinary Frequency [114]

migraine 213, 323

minors

    ethical and professional issues 526

    legal aspects of consent 531–532

    research ethics 527

    right to confidentiality and privacy 520

misconduct *see* conduct, of clinicians

mitral regurgitation *152*, 274

mitral stenosis 277, 278

Mixed acid-base disorders [005E] **65–66**

mole *see* Skin and Subcutaneous Lesions [100]

molluscum contagiosum *413*

Mondor disease *see* [107E]

Mongolian spot *392 see also* [100A]

monocular diplopia *see* Diplopia (Double Vision) [028]

Montgomery follicle *see* [107E]

mood disorders

    childhood and adolescence 92, 94, 95

    family violence predisposing to 470

    fibromyalgia associated with 350

    hyperparathyroidism associated with 58

Mood Disorders [065] **268–270**

    pain precipitating 286

    Panic and Anxiety [073] **298–299**

    Personality Disorders [078] **324–325**

    problem gambling associated with 424

    Psychosis/Disordered Thought [087] **346–347**

    somatisation 288

    Suicidal Behaviour/Prevention [108] **425–426**

    suicidality, defined 425

    see also Violence/Aggression and Mental Illness [119]

Mood Disorders [065] **268–270**

moral issues 526–527

morals, defined 515

Morton metatarsalgia *see* [089I]

motor vehicle crash injuries *see* vehicle crash injuries

Mouth Problems [066] **271–273**, *271*, *272*, *273 see also* Neck or Facial Mass/Goitre/Thyroid Disease [068]

movement disorders *see* Involuntary Movement Disorders/Tic Disorders [057]; locomotion disorders

MRI (magnetic resonance imaging), ischaemic lesions 221

mucous cyst *209*, *272*, *400*

Muehrcke lines 209

Müllerian duct *see* [096B]

multisystem/organ failure *508 see also* emergencies

Münchausen stridor *see* [098A]

Münchausen syndrome *see* [119A]

Murmur/Extra Heart Sounds [067] **274–280**

    Diastolic Murmur [067B] **277–278**, *277*

    Heart Sounds, Pathological [067C] **279–280**

    Systolic Murmur [067A] **274–276**, *275*

Murray Valley encephalitis *see* [040]; [130]

musculofascial pain, chronic 350–351, *350*

musculoligamentous injuries 560

musculoskeletal pain *see* pain

myalgia 258

mycosis fungoides *398*

myeloid leukaemia, chronic 82

myositis, clostridial 401

naevus *see* Skin and Subcutaneous Lesions [100]

Nail Disorders [044B] **208–210**, *208*, *209*, *210*

National Rural Health Alliance 566

'natural' therapies 559

nausea 476–477

Neck or Facial Mass/Goitre/Thyroid Disease [068] **281–283**, *281*, *282*, *489*

Neck Pain [089C] **354–355**

necrotising arachnidism 496, *497*
necrotising infections 401, 402, *402*
neglect, child abuse presenting as 466
negligence, liability for 534–535
Neonatal Jaundice [058A] **252–253**
neonate
    cyanosis 123, 124
    Diarrhoea, Paediatric [027D] **138–139**
    ductus arteriosus closure 124
    Failure to Thrive [036A] **174–175**
    Fever in the Neonate (in Child Less than Four Weeks) [040C] **191–192**
    health considerations for 319
    Hypertension in Childhood [054A] **236–237**
    hypoxaemia 123, 124
    morbidity/mortality due to prematurity 334
    Neonatal Jaundice [058A] **252–253**
    Newborn Assessment/Nutrition [077A] **308–309**
    Newborn in Poor Condition/Depressed Breathing [025] **128–129**
    premature birth 334
    respiratory rate 165
    Sudden Infant Death Syndrome (SIDS) (Acute Life-Threatening Event (ALTE)) [099] **390–391**
    Weight (Low) at Birth/Intra-uterine Growth Aberration [123] **481–482**
    see also all other presentations
nephroblastoma *see* Wilms tumour
Nerve Injuries [113J] **444**
neurally-medicated reflex syncopal syndromes 427
neuroblastoma, adrenal *43*
neuromuscular signs/symptoms, hypomagnesaemia associated with 75
neuropathy *see* Numbness and Tingling [069]
neutropenia 81, 82
neutrophil count, critical 83 *see also* Abnormalities of White Blood Cells [010]
neutrophilia 82
nevus *see* Skin and Subcutaneous Lesions [100]
Newborn Assessment/Nutrition [077A] **308–309**
Newborn in Poor Condition/Depressed Breathing [025] **128–129**
newborn infant *see* neonate
NGOs (non-governmental organisations) 553–554
nicotine abuse *see* Substance Abuse/Addiction [107]
Niemann-Pick disease *see* [011C]; [024]; [058A]
Nipple Discharge/Galactorrhoea [017C] **105–106**

nipples
    accessory nipple *108*
    Nipple Discharge/Galactorrhoea [017C] **105–106**
    Paget disease of *108*
    skin changes 108–109, *108*
nocturia 58 *see also* urinary system disorders
nodularity, of breast 102, 107
nodule *see* Skin and Subcutaneous Lesions [100]
Non-Acute/Recurrent Abdominal Pain in Infancy and Early Childhood [003B] **48–49**
non-governmental organisations (NGOs) 553–554
Non–hypo-osmolar hyponatraemia 77–78
non-profit groups 552–553
non-reassuring fetal status 183–184
Norwalk agent *see* [027D]
notifiable diseases *see* communicable diseases
Numbness and Tingling [069] **284–285**
nutrients, inorganic 487, *487*
nutrition
    Newborn Assessment/Nutrition [077A] **308–309**
    Nutritional Disorders and Deficiencies [125B] **487–488**, *487*, *488*

obesity *see* weight disorders
obsessive-compulsive disorder 298 *see also* mood disorders
Obstetrical Complications [081D] **334–335**
occult blood 98–99
Oedema [034] 77–78, **168–171**
    allergic periorbital *494*
    Generalised Oedema [034A] **168–169**
    hyponatraemia associated with 77–78
    Unilateral Limb Oedema (Swollen Limb) [034B] **170–171**, *171*
oesophagus
    cancer of 148, *148*
    hiatus hernia *53*, 149
    motility disorder *53*
    para-oesophageal hiatus hernia *148*
    tracheo-oesophageal fistula *500*
oestrogen, in gynaecomastia 100
olecranon bursitis *400*
oligomenorrhoea 262–263
oliguria 368–369
onychogryposis 209, *210*
oppositional behaviour 92
opthalmic herpes zoster *405*
organ donation *see* Head Injuries/Brain Death/Transplant Donation [045]
organ/multisystem failure 508 *see also* emergencies

lung metastasis *158*
pulmonary stenosis 275
right middle lobe collapse *158*
see also pneumonia; respiratory disorders
pulmonary oedema 152
pulmonary stenosis 275
PUO (pyrexia of unknown origin) 187–188
Pupil Abnormalities [088] **348–349**, *348*
pustules 404–406, *404*, *405*
pyloric stenosis *29*, *65*
pyoderma gangrenosum *402*
pyogenic granuloma *398*
pyrexia of unknown origin (PUO) 187–188
pyuria 451–452

Q fever *see* [040A]; [130]
quadriplegia 224
qualifications
assessment of overseas 562–563
transferability of 557, 558

ram-horn nail 209, *210*
Ramsay Hunt syndrome *see* [033]
rape *see* Violence: Domestic/Family [119C]
rash
Pruritus [086] **343–344**, *344*
Skin Rash/Dermatitis [102] **410–414**,
410, *411*, *412*, *413*, *493*, *494*, *508*
of SLE *189*
Raynaud disease/syndrome *see* [023A];
[071A]; [089F]
records *see* medical records
rectocele 340
rectum, carcinoma of *98*, 99
recurrent fever 189–190, *189*
red cell lysis 73
red cells *see* erythrocytes
Red, Hot, Tender, Swollen Skin and
Subcutaneous Layers [100D] **401–403**,
401, *402*
references, for further study xxvi–xxviii
reflex syncopal syndromes 427
reflux, gastro-oesophageal 52–53, *53*
Regional Pain [089] **350–367**
Cancer Pain [089K] **366–367**, *366*
Chronic Musculofascial Pain [089A] **350–
351**, *350*
Facial Pain [089D] **356**, *356*
Foot and Ankle Pain [089I] **363**
Hand/Wrist/Elbow Pain [089F] **358–359**,
358, *359*
Hip Pain [089G] **360–361**, *361*
Knee Pain [089H] **362**
Low Back Pain [089B] **352–353**, *353*
Neck Pain [089C] **354–355**
Shoulder Pain [089E] **357**

Spinal Compression/Osteoporosis [089J]
364–365
registration
cross-border transferability 557, 558
of medical practitioners 513, 550
regurgitation 477
Reiter syndrome *see* [060]; [089B]
remote area healthcare 566
renal artery stenosis *234*
renal calculus *219*
renal cell tumour *219*
renal 'colic' *46*
renal failure
Acute (Anuria/Oliguria/Acute Renal Failure
(ARF)) [090] **368–369**
Chronic [091] **370–371**, *370*
herbal medications causing 321
hyperkalaemia associated with 73
see also urinary system disorders
Renal Failure, Acute (Anuria/Oliguria/Acute
Renal Failure (ARF)) [090] **368–369**
Renal Failure, Chronic [091] **370–371**, *370*
reporting requirements 536–537, 556–557
see also notifiable diseases
research ethics 527–528
resource allocation 515, 524
Respiratory alkalosis (due to increased
alveolar ventilation from overbreathing)
[005D] **65**, **66**
respiratory arrest 113–114
respiratory disorders
'common cold' 372
Cyanosis/Hypoxaemia/Hypoxia [023]
121–124
Cyanosis/Hypoxia/Apnoea in Children
[023A] **123–124**
Dyspnoea/Respiratory Distress, Paediatric
[032G] **164–165**
Lower Respiratory Tract Disorders [126B]
491–492
Newborn in Poor Condition/Depressed
Breathing [025] **128–129**
Respiratory alkalosis [005D] **65**, **66**
Respiratory (gaseous) acidosis [005C] **65**,
66
Upper Respiratory Tract Disorders [126A]
489–490, *489*
URTI (upper respiratory tract infection)
372, 491
see also Dyspnoea and/or Cough/
Prevention of Cancers and Chronic
Respiratory Diseases [032]
Respiratory (gaseous) acidosis (due to
decreased alveolar ventilation, usually
with attendant hypoxia) [005C] **65**, **66**
respiratory rate, neonate/child 165
retinoblastoma *474*
retinopathy *231*, *239*, *243*

Speech and Language Abnormalities/
Dysphonia/Hoarseness [103] **415–416**,
415

spermatocele *374*, 375

spider bites 496, *497*

spider naevus *393*

Spinal Compression/Osteoporosis [089J]
364–365

Spinal Injuries [104] **417–418**, *417*

spinal metastasis *366*

spleen, traumatic laceration of *436*

splenectomy 310

Splenomegaly [105] **419–420**, *420*

spondylitis, ankylosing *353*

spouse abuse 470–472

squamous cell carcinoma (SCC) *271*, 396,
396 see also Focal Skin Lesions -
'Suspicious' Lesions [100B]

squint *see* vision disorders

stammer 416

staphylococcal pneumonia *156*

stature, abnormal 430–431, *430*

statutory requirements, of clinicians 536–537

STDs *see* sexually transmitted diseases
(STDs)

steatorrhoea (fatty stool) 134

stenosis
    aortic 274
    mitral 277, 278
    pulmonary 275
    pyloric *29, 65*
    renal artery *234*

stiffness
    Joint Pain, Mono-Articular (Acute, Chronic)
    [059] **254–255**
    Joint Pain, Poly-Articular (Acute, Chronic)
    [060] **256–257**, *256, 257*
    of knee 362
    in polymyalgia rheumatica 351

Still disease *see* [105]

stings 388, 496–498

stomach cancer 98

stone *see* calculus

stool
    Bleeding with Defaecation/Acute Lower
    Gastrointestinal Bleeding/Melaena/Occult
    Blood in Stool/Prevention of Cancer [016]
    98–99
    Diarrhoea/Constipation [027] **132–141**,
    134, 135, 136, 140, 141
    fatty 134
    Haematemesis/Melaena [048] **217–218**,
    217

Strabismus and/or Amblyopia [106] *142*, **421**

strawberry naevus 392

streptococcal infection
    cellulitis *171*
    streptococcal tonsillopharyngitis 372

stridor 489–492, *489*

stroke
    Gait Disturbances - Ataxia [042] **199–200**
    Hemiplegia/Hemisensory Loss/Stroke with
    or without Aphasia/Prevention of Stroke
    [050] **221–225**

structural cardiac disease 428

Sturge-Weber syndrome *201*

stutter 416

stye *172*

subcutaneous lesions *see* Skin and
Subcutaneous Lesions [100]

subdural haematoma *212*

Substance Abuse/Addiction [107] **422–424**
    family violence cause of 470
    Pathological/Problem Gambling [107B]
    424
    Substance Abuse/Drug Addiction/
    Withdrawal [107A] **422–423**, 470

subungual haematoma *210*

Sudden Infant Death Syndrome (SIDS)
(Acute Life-Threatening Event (ALTE))
[099] **390–391**

Sudeck atrophy *see* [089F]

Suicidal Behaviour/Prevention [108] **425–
426**, 470

suicidal tendency
    family violence cause of 470
    problem gambling associated with 424
    suicidality, defined 425
    see also mood disorders

suicidality, defined 425 *see also* suicidal
tendency

suicide, clinician-assisted 514

support groups 552–553

support services, community 545–546

Suprapubic/Pelvic Mass [002E] **39**, *39*

surgery
    Postoperative Patient Evaluation and
    Care [077D] **314–315**, *314*
    Preoperative Assessment [077C] **312–
    313**

swallowing difficulty *see* Dysphagia [031]

Swan neck deformity *see* [129B]

swelling *see* Oedema [034]

swollen limb 170–171, *171*

swollen skin 401–403, *401, 402*

syncopal syndromes 427

Syncope/Pre-Syncope/Loss of
Consciousness [109] **427–429**

syndrome of inappropriate ADH secretion
(SIADH) 77

synovitis 350

systemic lupus erythematosus (SLE) *189*,
412

Systolic Murmur [067A] **274–276**, *275*

tachyarrhythmia 113, 296, 297
tachycardia
    fetal 184
    palpitations due to 297
Tall Stature/Short Stature/Abnormal Stature [110] **430–431**, *430*
Tanner stages *see* [096A]
Tay-Sachs disease *see* [011C]
teeth 271, *272*, 273
telemedicine 557, 558 *see also* electronic records
temporal arteritis *213*, 350
tender skin 401–403, *401*, *402*
tendon rupture *290*
tenesmus 55
terminally ill patient 114, 146–147
termination, of pregnancy 336–337
testicular torsion 376, *376*, 377
testis
    Abdominal Hernia [002G] **41–42**, *41*, *42*, *57*, 499
    Fournier gangrene of scrotum *402*
    Scrotal Mass [093] **374–375**, *374*
    Scrotal Pain (Acute) [094] **376–377**, *376*
testosterone, in gynaecomastia 100
tetany, hypocalcaemia associated with 60
tetralogy of Fallot *see* [023]; [023A]
tetraplegia 224
textbooks, recommended xxvi–xxvii
thiazide diuretics 77
thirst
    excessive 453
    hypernatraemia indicated by 79
    hyperparathyroidism associated with 58
thought disorder *see* Psychosis/Disordered Thought [087]
thrombophlebitis 294
thrombosis 170–171, 294
thyroglossal cyst *282*
thyroid disease 281–283, *281*, *282*, 489
tic disorders
    behaviour disorders associated with 92, 94, 95
    Involuntary Movement Disorders/Tic Disorders [057] **248–249**
'tidy' wounds 445
Tietze syndrome *see* [017D]; [020]
tiger snake *496*
tinea capitis *206*
tingling sensation 284–285
Tinnitus/Bruit [111] **432–433**
toddler *see* child; infant
tongue *see* Mouth Problems [066]
tonsillopharyngitis 372
'TORCH' infections 215, 334, 338, 481
torticollis *see* Involuntary Movement Disorders/Tic Disorders [057]

Tourette syndrome *see* [014]; [057]
trace element deficiencies 487–488, *487*
tracheo-oesophageal fistula *500*
training colleges 562–563
transient ischaemia, defined 221 *see also* Hemiplegia/Hemisensory Loss/Stroke with or without Aphasia/Prevention of Stroke [050]
transplant donation 211–212
Trauma/Accidents/Prevention [113] **434–450**
    'ABCDE' response 435
    Abdominal Injuries [113A] **436**, *436*
    Bone and Joint Injuries [113B] **437–438**, *437*, *438* see also fractures and dislocations
    categories of **434–435**
    Chest Injuries [113D] **439–440**
    Eye Injuries [113F] **441**
    Facial Injuries [113G] **442**
    Hand/Wrist Injuries [113H] *438*, **443**, *443*
    initial assessment/resuscitative measures 435
    Nerve Injuries [113J] **444**
    prevalence of 434
    Skin Injuries [113K] **445–446**
    Urinary Tract Injuries [113M] **447–448**, *447*
    Vascular Injuries [113N] **449–450**
    see also Burns [018]; Head Injuries/Brain Death/Transplant Donation [045]; Hypothermia [040D]; Spinal Injuries [104]
trauma, dementia/memory disturbances associated with 125
Travel Medicine and Tropical Infections [130] **505–506**
traveller's diarrhoea 133, 505
treatment, patients' consent to 521–522
tremor *see* Involuntary Movement Disorders/Tic Disorders [057]
tricuspid regurgitation 275
trigger finger *358*
Troisier sign *260 see also* [062]
tropical infections 505–506
tropical ulcer *408*
tuberculosis *227*
tumour
    of bone, in childhood 362
    of breast 100, 102
    Pancoast *291*
    renal cell *219*
    of testis 374, 375
    Wilms *37*
Turner syndrome *see* [043]; [110]
twins, conjoined *202*

Notes

Notes

Notes